T0229324

The Gastrocnemius

Editors

MARK S. MYERSON
PIERRE BAROUK

FOOT AND ANKLE CLINICS

www.foot.theclinics.com

Consulting Editor
MARK S. MYERSON

December 2014 • Volume 19 • Number 4

ELSEVIER

1600 John F. Kennedy Boulevard • Suite 1800 • Philadelphia, Pennsylvania, 19103-2899

http://www.theclinics.com

FOOT AND ANKLE CLINICS Volume 19, Number 4
December 2014 ISSN 1083-7515, ISBN-13: 978-0-323-32648-3

Editor: Jennifer Flynn-Briggs
Developmental Editor: Meredith Clinton

© **2014 Elsevier Inc. All rights reserved.**

This periodical and the individual contributions contained in it are protected under copyright by Elsevier, and the following terms and conditions apply to their use:

Photocopying
Single photocopies of single articles may be made for personal use as allowed by national copyright laws. Permission of the Publisher and payment of a fee is required for all other photocopying, including multiple or systematic copying, copying for advertising or promotional purposes, resale, and all forms of document delivery. Special rates are available for educational institutions that wish to make photocopies for non-profit educational classroom use. For information on how to seek permission visit www.elsevier.com/permissions or call: (+44) 1865 843830 (UK)/(+1) 215 239 3804 (USA).

Derivative Works
Subscribers may reproduce tables of contents or prepare lists of articles including abstracts for internal circulation within their institutions. Permission of the Publisher is required for resale or distribution outside the institution. Permission of the Publisher is required for all other derivative works, including compilations and translations (please consult www.elsevier.com/permissions).

Electronic Storage or Usage
Permission of the Publisher is required to store or use electronically any material contained in this periodical, including any article or part of an article (please consult www.elsevier.com/permissions). Except as outlined above, no part of this publication may be reproduced, stored in a retrieval system or transmitted in any form or by any means, electronic, mechanical, photocopying, recording or otherwise, without prior written permission of the Publisher.

Notice
No responsibility is assumed by the Publisher for any injury and/or damage to persons or property as a matter of products liability, negligence or otherwise, or from any use or operation of any methods, products, instructions or ideas contained in the material herein. Because of rapid advances in the medical sciences, in particular, independent verification of diagnoses and drug dosages should be made.

Although all advertising material is expected to conform to ethical (medical) standards, inclusion in this publication does not constitute a guarantee or endorsement of the quality or value of such product or of the claims made of it by its manufacturer.

Foot and Ankle Clinics (ISSN 1083-7515) is published quarterly by Elsevier, Inc., 360 Park Avenue South, New York, NY 10010-1710. Months of issue are March, June, September, and December. Periodicals postage paid at New York, NY, and additional mailing offices. Subscription price per year is $315.00 (US individuals), $421.00 (US institutions), $155.00 (US students), $360.00 (Canadian individuals), $506.00 (Canadian institutions), $215.00 (Canadian students), $460.00 (international individuals), $506.00 (international institutions), and $215.00 (international students). To receive student/resident rate, orders must be accompanied by name of affiliated institution, date of term, and the *signature* of program/residency coordinator on institution letterhead. Orders will be billed at individual rate until proof of status is received. Foreign air speed delivery is included in all *Clinics* subscription prices. All prices are subject to change without notice. **POSTMASTER:** Send address changes to *Foot and Ankle Clinics*, Elsevier Health Sciences Division, Subscription Customer Service, 3251 Riverport Lane, Maryland Heights, MO 63043. **Customer Service: 1-800-654-2452 (US and Canada). From outside of the United States and Canada, call 314-447-8871. Fax: 314-447-8029. E-mail: JournalsCustomerService-usa@ elsevier.com (for print support); JournalsOnlineSupport-usa@elsevier.com (for online support).**

Reprints. For copies of 100 or more, of articles in this publication, please contact the Commercial Reprints Department, Elsevier Inc., 360 Park Avenue South, New York, NY 10010-1710. Tel.: 212-633-3874; Fax: 212-633-3820; E-mail: reprints@elsevier.com.

Contributors

CONSULTING EDITOR

MARK S. MYERSON, MD
Director, The Institute for Foot and Ankle Reconstruction, Mercy Medical Center, Mercy Hospital, Baltimore, Maryland

EDITORS

MARK S. MYERSON, MD
Director, The Institute for Foot and Ankle Reconstruction, Mercy Medical Center, Mercy Hospital, Baltimore, Maryland

PIERRE BAROUK, MD
Foot Surgery Center of the Sport Clinic, Bordeaux-Merignac, France

AUTHORS

ANNUNZIATO AMENDOLA, MD
Professor, Department of Orthopaedic Surgery and Rehabilitation, University of Iowa Hospitals and Clinics, Iowa City, Iowa

JAMES AMIS, MD
Lone Star Orthopaedics, Cincinnati, Ohio

JOHN G. ANDERSON, MD
Assistant Program Director; GRMEP Orthopaedic Residency; Associate Director, Grand Rapids Orthopaedic Foot and Ankle Fellowship; Chairman, Spectrum Health Department of Orthopaedics; Orthopaedic Associates of Michigan, PC, Grand Rapids, Michigan

LOUIS SAMUEL BAROUK, MD
Orthopedic Surgeon, Yvrac, France

PIERRE BAROUK, MD
Foot Surgery Center of the Sport Clinic, Bordeaux-Merignac, France

DONALD R. BOHAY, MD, FACS
Director, Grand Rapids Orthopaedic Foot and Ankle Fellowship; Orthopaedic Associates of Michigan, PC, Grand Rapids, Michigan

ANGEL CALVO, MD, PhD
Arthrosport, Institute of Sports Medicine and Advanced Arthroscopy, Centro Milenium Zaragoza, Valencia, Spain

ANDREW CARNE, FRCR
Royal Surrey County Hospital, Guildford, United Kingdom

DANIEL CASANOVA-MARTÍNEZ Jr
Anatomy Unit, Biomedical Department, University of Antofagasta, Antofagasta, Chile

CYRILLE CAZEAU, MD
Foot and Ankle Department, Clinique Geoffroy Saint Hilaire, Paris, France

MIQUEL DALMAU-PASTOR, PodD, PT
Podologist, Physiotherapist, Laboratory of Arthroscopic and Surgical Anatomy, Human Anatomy Unit, Department of Pathology and Experimental Therapeutics, School of Medicine, University of Barcelona, Barcelona, Spain

MARK S. DAVIES, FRCS (Tr&Orth)
London Foot and Ankle Centre, London, United Kingdom

CHRISTOPHER W. DIGIOVANNI, MD
Visiting Professor; Chief, Foot and Ankle Service and Fellowship Program, Department of Orthopaedic Surgery, Harvard Medical School, Massachusetts General Hospital, Boston, Massachusetts

ERIK B. ELLER, MD
The CORE Institute, Novi, Michigan

BETLEM FARGUES-POLO Jr
Podology Student, Laboratory of Arthroscopic and Surgical Anatomy, Human Anatomy Unit, Department of Pathology and Experimental Therapeutics, School of Medicine, University of Barcelona, Barcelona, Spain

†PAU GOLANÓ, MD
Laboratory of Arthroscopic and Surgical Anatomy, Human Anatomy Unit, Department of Pathology and Experimental Therapeutics, School of Medicine, University of Barcelona, Barcelona, Spain; Department of Orthopaedic Surgery, School of Medicine, University of Pittsburgh, Pittsburgh, Pennsylvania

RAYMOND Y. HSU, MD
Orthopaedic Resident, Department of Orthopaedic Surgery, Rhode Island Hospital, The Warren Alpert Medical School of Brown University, Providence, Rhode Island

JAVIER PASCUAL HUERTA, PhD
Podiatrist, Private Practice, Clínica del Pie Embajadores, Madrid, Spain

ERNESTO MACEIRA, MD
Co-Director, Foot and Ankle Unit, Department of Orthopaedic Surgery, Hospital Universitario Quirón Madrid, Madrid, Spain

MANUEL MONTEAGUDO, MD
Co-Director, Foot and Ankle Unit, Department of Orthopaedic Surgery, Hospital Universitario Quirón Madrid, Madrid, Spain

†Deceased

MARK S. MYERSON, MD
Director, The Institute for Foot and Ankle Reconstruction, Mercy Medical Center, Mercy Hospital, Baltimore, Maryland

PHINIT PHISITKUL, MD
Associate Professor, Department of Orthopaedic Surgery and Rehabilitation, University of Iowa Hospitals and Clinics, Iowa City, Iowa

NICHOLAS R. SEIBERT, MD
Orthopedic Physician Associates, Swedish Orthopedic Institute, Seattle, Washington

MATTHEW C. SOLAN, FRCS (Tr&Orth)
Consultant; Orthopaedic Foot & Ankle Surgeon, Royal Surrey County Hospital; University of Surrey; Surrey Foot and Ankle Clinic, Guildford, United Kingdom; London Foot and Ankle Centre, London, United Kingdom

YVES STIGLITZ, MD
Foot and Ankle Department, Clinique Geoffroy Saint Hilaire, Paris, France

ALTUG TANRIOVER, MD
Orthopaedic Surgeon, Department of Orthopaedic Surgery, Cankaya Hospital, Kavaklıdere, Ankara, Turkey

JOSHUA N. TENNANT, MD, MPH
Assistant Professor, Department of Orthopaedics, University of North Carolina School of Medicine, Chapel Hill, North Carolina

EUGENE P. TOOMEY, MD
Orthopedic Physician Associates, Swedish Orthopedic Institute, Seattle, Washington

C. NIEK VAN DIJK, MD, PhD
Department of Orthopaedic Surgery, Academic Medical Center, University of Amsterdam, Amsterdam, The Netherlands

SCOTT VANVALKENBURG, MD
Orthopaedic Foot & Ankle Fellow, Department of Orthopaedic Surgery, Harvard Medical School, Massachusetts General Hospital, Boston, Massachusetts

JORDI VEGA, MD
Unit of Foot and Ankle Surgery, Hospital Quirón, Barcelona, Spain

BRYAN L. WITT, DO
Suncoast Orthopedics, Largo, Florida

STEFANO ZAFFAGNINI, MD
Laboratorio Di Biomeccanica Ed Innovazione Tecnologica, Sports Traumatology Department, II Orthopaedic Clinic, Instituto Ortopedico Rizzoli, Bologna, Italy

Contents

> Gastrocnemius contracture has recently gained relevance owing to its
> suggested relationship with foot disorders such as metatarsalgia, plantar
> fasciopathy, hallux valgus, and others. Consequently this has induced a
> renewed interest in surgical lengthening techniques, including proximal
> gastrocnemius release, to resolve gastrocnemius contracture in patients
> with foot disorders. This article describes and discusses the general anat-
> omy of the triceps surae and the surgical anatomy of the gastrocnemius.

> A silent gastrocnemius contracture can gradually do much harm when left
> undetected and unattended. The calf is a common source of a majority of
> acquired, nontraumatic adult foot and ankle problems. When it comes to
> surgical lengthening procedures, whether at the Achilles, at the musculo-
> tendinous junction, or more proximal, the search must find the safest, most
> accurate, and quickest recovery method possible. Addressing the calf
> contracture as definitive treatment and, better yet, as prevention will no
> doubt become a mainstay of the treatment of many foot and ankle
> problems.

> The gastrocnemius is the main muscle of the posterior compartment of the
> leg. As a biarticular muscle it has specific biomechanical properties. This

article discusses these properties combining the major biomechanical topics of anatomy, dynamics, kinetics, and electromyography. This muscle is remarkable in that it has very low energy consumption and very high mechanical efficacy. In addition to the biomechanical features, the consequences of its tightness are discussed. The dysfunction also appears in all the biomechanical topics and clarifies the reasons for the location of symptoms in the midfoot and on the plantar aspect of the forefoot.

The diagnosis of gastrocnemius tightness is primarily clinical using the Silfverskiold test, which shows an equinus deformity at the ankle with the knee extended but that disappears with the knee flexed. The manner in which the Silfverskiold test is performed must be consistent with respect to the applied strength of the maneuver, correction of a flexible hindfoot valgus deformity while performing the test, and reproducibility. Although this is a diagnosis based on the clinical examination, this article presents additional clinical signs that can help to make the diagnosis when the retraction is not clinically evident. These include knee recurvatum, hip flexion, lumbar hyperlordosis, and forefoot overload.

Functional hallux rigidus is a clinical condition in which the mobility of the first metatarsophalangeal joint is normal under non-weight-bearing conditions, but its dorsiflexion is blocked when the first metatarsal is made to support weight. In mechanical terms, functional hallux rigidus implies a pattern of interfacial contact through rolling, whereas in a normal joint contact by gliding is established. Patients with functional hallux rigidus should only be operated on if the pain or disability makes it necessary. Gastrocnemius release is a beneficial procedure in most patients.

Although anatomic and functional relationship has been established between the gastrocnemius muscle, via the Achilles tendon, and the plantar fascia, the exact role of gastrocnemius tightness in foot and plantar fascia problems is not completely understood. This article summarizes past and current literature linking these 2 structures and gives a mechanical explanation based on functional models of the relationship between gastrocnemius tightness and plantar fascia. The effect of gastrocnemius tightness on the sagittal behavior of the foot is also discussed.

Pain and reduced function caused by disorders of either the plantar fascia or the Achilles tendon are common. Although heel pain is not a major public health problem it affects millions of people each year. For most patients, time and first-line treatments allow symptoms to resolve. A proportion of patients have resistant symptoms. Managing these recalcitrant cases is a challenge. Gastrocnemius contracture produces increased strain in both the Achilles tendon and the plantar fascia. This biomechanical feature must be properly assessed otherwise treatment is compromised.

Gastrocnemius proximal lengthening was first performed to correct spasticity in children, and was adapted for the patient with no neuromuscular condition in the late 1990s. Since then, the proximal gastrocnemius release has become less invasive and has evolved to include only the fascia overlying the medial head of the gastrocnemius muscle. The indications for performing this procedure are a clinically demonstrable gastrocnemius contracture that influences a variety of clinical conditions in the forefoot, hindfoot, and ankle. It is a safe and easy procedure that can be performed bilaterally simultaneously, and does not require immobilization of the ankle after surgery.

Hallux valgus is the most common foot disorder associated with gastrocnemius tightness, and there is a particularly strong association with juvenile hallux valgus. This article describes an oblique windlass mechanism that can be a causative or a contributory factor in the pathogenesis of juvenile hallux valgus. This article presents a study of 108 patients who underwent a proximal gastrocnemius release and hallux valgus correction using a scarf osteotomy. We believe that assessment of gastrocnemius tightness in juvenile hallux valgus is important and that gastrocnemius lengthening should be routinely considered as part of the operative strategy.

FOOT AND ANKLE CLINICS

**DOWNLOAD
Free App!**

Review Articles
THE CLINICS

NOW AVAILABLE FOR YOUR iPhone and iPad

Foreword

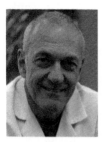

Mark S. Myerson, MD
Consulting Editor

It is remarkable how our thinking has changed over the past few decades regarding the influence of the gastrocnemius on foot and ankle pathology. While the debate still continues and skepticism remains, it is quite clear to many surgeons that contracture of the gastrocnemius has a role in the development of clinical pathology of the foot. I too was a "nonbeliever" up until recently. Gastrocnemius recession? You have to be kidding me. This was my attitude two decades ago. My understanding of the role of the gastrocnemius in the pathogenesis of various foot problems was so limited, albeit naïve. While I recognized the need to perform a gastrocnemius release using a modification of the Strayer procedure for many flatfoot conditions, this was the only indication that I had for this procedure, and I used it sparingly. Now I recognize that gastrocnemius recession has a role in the treatment of forefoot pathology, including metatarsalgia as well as the more proximal conditions such as Achilles tendinopathy.

As well noted by Ernesto Maceira and other contributors to this issue, there is a significant range of joint movements of the lower limb predominantly in the sagittal plane. If one limits the movement of any of these joints in the sagittal plane, some compensatory mechanism must occur to allow the foot to move forward through foot flat and toe off. Although these compensatory changes generally have to occur in the sagittal plane, it will inevitably cause changes by way of abnormal movement or development of deformity in multiple planes. For example, a lack of dorsiflexion in the ankle may be compensated for by dorsiflexion of the foot, but this can only occur if the foot pronates. We see this so commonly in a patient with a flatfoot deformity where dorsiflexion of the foot no longer occurs through the ankle but in an oblique plane through the subtalar joint. If you lock the hindfoot in a neutral position, then you are able to demonstrate the severity of the gastrocnemius contracture on the flatfoot deformity. Of course, the contracture may be secondary to a rupture of the posterior tibial tendon, such that the foot gets flat and there is a secondary effect on the Achilles as the heel moves into valgus. However, we have to assume that regardless of what comes first, a gastrocnemius contracture accompanies a flatfoot deformity.

While stretching should be the initial focus of treatment for all patients with this contracture, as we age, the effect of stretching becomes less effective and, under these circumstances, surgical treatment of the gastrocnemius becomes necessary.

Foot Ankle Clin N Am 19 (2014) xiii–xiv
http://dx.doi.org/10.1016/j.fcl.2014.09.003
1083-7515/14/$ – see front matter © 2014 Published by Elsevier Inc.

For most surgeons, this is performed in the mid-calf at the musculotendinous junction. However, as we are all aware, there is the risk of causing permanent weakness through lengthening of both the gastrocnemius and the soleus fascia; in other words, a lengthening of the tendon is performed. The article by Eugene P. Toomey and Nicholas R. Seibert in this issue highlights the need to identify and accurately locate the gastrocnemius fascia such that inadvertent lengthening of the soleus is not performed. However, in practice, even if the correct location for the release is identified, the gastrocnemius and soleus fascia are adherent and difficult to separate. Much work has been done by Dr Pierre Barouk and Dr Louis Samuel Barouk to clarify and popularize the concept of a more proximal release of the gastrocnemius. This is a relatively novel concept, and one that has minimal morbidity and is not likely to cause any weakness in the leg, making the more proximal release a procedure of choice for certain patients.

I would like to acknowledge the remarkable contribution by Pau Golanó and his colleagues to this issue. Pau will be remembered. He was unique as an anatomist, an artist, and an extraordinary educator.

Mark S. Myerson, MD
The Institute for Foot and Ankle Reconstruction
Mercy Medical Center
Mercy Hospital
Baltimore, MD 21202, USA

E-mail address:
mark4feet@aol.com

Preface

Introduction to Gastrocnemius Tightness

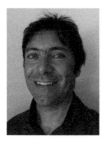

Pierre Barouk, MD
Editor

Looking for a retraction of the gastrocnemius should be an essential part of the foot and ankle examination for practitioners, not just surgeons. Even though the equinus has been recognized for 50 years as having an influence on the foot, only a few practitioners routinely search for it. The proportion of gastrocnemius tightness is high in the normal population, but it is significantly higher in populations that have foot and ankle problems. Why do we have short gastrocs? The evolution of the human race, especially walking at a certain pace and extending the knee, is probably one of the explanations. In addition to this, there is also the problem of sitting for long periods of time and the frequent use of high-heeled shoes. With this issue of *Foot and Ankle Clinics of North America*, you will gain a better understanding of how to recognize gastrocnemius tightness (the clinical Silfverskiold test is essential), how to treat it, and understand why it has an influence on many of the current pathologies that we see every day. Attaching some symptoms (calf cramps, lower limb instability, difficulty in walking without a heel, lumbar pain) to gastrocnemius tightness is essential to treating patients in a global manner. I hope you will be convinced of the importance of this, and no longer do without!

Pierre Barouk, MD
Foot Surgery Center
Clinique du Sport
2 Rue Georges Nègrevergne
33700 Bordeaux-Mérignac, France

E-mail address:
pierre.barouk@wanadoo.fr

Dedication

In Memory of Pau Golanó
1964-2014

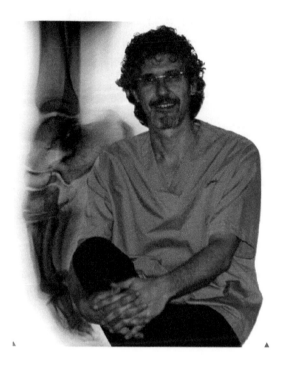

Pau Golanó was an anatomist by profession and a gifted artist in his chosen field. He was an amazing individual whose work will be a resource for surgeons for decades to come. His work was always done to perfection and is exemplified in this issue with his profound insight into the gastrocnemius complex. I have asked his coauthors to write a dedication in Spanish, which I have not translated so as to maintain the sentiment expressed by his friends and coworkers. An additional dedication has been provided by Professor C. Niek van Dijk.

Foot Ankle Clin N Am 19 (2014) xvii–xviii
http://dx.doi.org/10.1016/j.fcl.2014.09.004
1083-7515/14/$ – see front matter © 2014 Published by Elsevier Inc.

foot.theclinics.com

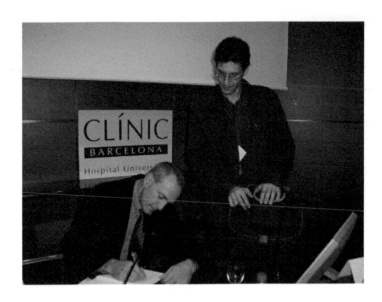

I first met Pau Golanó in 2004 at a meeting in Barcelona in 2001 held at the University Hospital in Barcelona. His English at the time was rudimentary, and my Spanish language skills not much better, but we rapidly developed a friendship based on our mutual interests. I have admired him ever since. He will remain an icon in this field.

Mark S. Myerson, MD
The Institute for Foot and Ankle Reconstruction
Mercy Medical Center
Mercy Hospital
Baltimore, MD 21202, USA

E-mail address:
mark4feet@aol.com

Dedication

In memoriam Pau Golanó (1965–2014)—Anatomist, Scientist, Artist, Teacher, and Friend

It was a Saturday in April 2004. At 4.00 AM, at the Luz de Gas discotheque, we were celebrating our successful 2-day dissection course for my residents. We talked about life. "I will not get old," he said. And he looked serious, "another 10 years." Then, we laughed and took another beer.

Pau Golanó died on Wednesday July 23, 2014 from a massive stroke. Out of the blue, at the top of his career. So many plans, NS so many horizons to cross. Pau Golanó was 49 years old.

Pau was Professor of Pathology and Experimental Therapeutics at the University of Barcelona. His exceptional anatomic dissection skills and passion for education were quickly recognized by the orthopedic surgeons around him. Nor did it take long for his skills to be recognized worldwide, and he became the last decade's leading expert on orthopedic anatomy.

He devoted his career and life to the education of orthopedic surgeons, making them better doctors by teaching anatomy right down to the smallest detail. The door of his department in Barcelona was always open.

Over the years, he wrote many inspiring papers on orthopedic surgical anatomy in the *KSSTA Journal* and his lectures at ESSKA courses and congresses were always extremely well attended. His contributions involved a wide spectrum such as the shoulder, hip, knee, and ankle. He was a teacher for all the orthopedic surgeons involved in ESSKA and a highly respected member of the orthopedic ESSKA community. Together with the love of his life, Celine, he enjoyed traveling the world, meeting friends, and sharing his knowledge.

He was a scientist who devoted his energy to orthopedics in general and ESSKA in particular. Pau Golanó enabled us to be better doctors for our patients. In 2012, he won the Knee Surgery, Sports Traumatology, Arthroscopy (KSSTA) Best Paper Award for *Anatomy of the Ankle Ligaments: A Pictorial Essay.*[1] In May 2014, at the ESSKA Congress in Amsterdam, he was honored with the prestigious ESSKA award for the Most Dedicated Individual ESSKA Member. This award gave him the international recognition he deserved. This recognition was very important to him.

Pau Golanó was a nonconformist. His unique strength was his artistic vision. He was not quickly satisfied with his achievements and set an extremely high standard for

---

From van Dijk CN, Calvo A, Zaffagnini S. In memoriam Pau Golanó (1965-2014)—anatomist, scientist, artist, teacher and friend. Knee Surg Sports Traumatol Arthrosc 2014;22:1961-3; with kind permission from Springer Science+Business Media.

http://dx.doi.org/10.1016/j.fcl.2014.09.005
foot.theclinics.com
1083-7515/14/$ – see front matter © 2014 Elsevier Inc. All rights reserved.

himself. No concessions! As a result, he sometimes collided with the people around him, who were not always able to understand or follow him. However, he was an artist who always had a smile on his face. With his charm, he was liked by everyone. He worked best under pressure. Deadlines were never met. And the projects and deadlines kept piling up. He was at the top of his career. Projects in Qatar, Pittsburgh, Amsterdam, and the ESSKA Academy lay ahead. Recently, he also started a career as a contemporary artist. The first successful Pau Golanó Art Exhibition in Bologna and the second one planned in October in Beirut demonstrated his capacity for being at the top in everything in which he was involved: where anatomy becomes art!

Although he was a team player, he liked to work on his own, spending hours in the laboratory, listening to music while making the best anatomical preparation, no rush, only the perfection of the anatomy and pictures was his goal.

An anatomist among orthopods. Alone among many friends. Friends who characterize him as extremely generous, creative, and a genius. At the same time, he was also eccentric, meticulous, and temperamental.

His work became better and better. He was always in search of new techniques and better ways to expose our inner world. He collaborated with surgeons worldwide. The interaction was always fruitful, and many ideas were born in his laboratory, showing new insights into different joints (hip, knee, and shoulder). His favorite joint was the ankle. The recent publication of almost 100 pieces of his artwork represented the culmination of his skills.[2] Each picture is an example of his unsurpassed eye for detail and his skill in disclosing the beauty of the human body. One of his contributions to world literature is the rediscovery of the forgotten Rouvière-Canela ligament. Together with Peter de Leeuw, he started working on this publication in 2006. It is ready to be submitted.

His legacy will live on. The "Golanos" will pop up now and then in future presentations all over the world. And you will recognize a Golanó when you see one.

The man who made anatomy an art! An anatomist among orthopods. He was one of us!

We will miss him.

Niek van Dijk, Angel Calvo, Stefano Zaffagnini

C. Niek van Dijk, MD, PhD
Department of Orthopaedic Surgery
Academic Medical Center
University of Amsterdam
P.O Box 226600, 1100 DD Amsterdam
The Netherlands

Angel Calvo, MD, PhD
Institute of Sports Medicine and Advanced Arthroscopy
Centro Milenium Zaragoza, Cirilo Amoros 25
Valencia 46004, Spain

Stefano Zaffagnini, MD
Laboratorio Di Biomeccanica Ed Innovazione Tecnologica
Sports Traumatology Department
II Orthopaedic Clinic
Instituto Ortopedico Rizzoli, via di Barbiano 1/10
Bologna 40136, Italy

E-mail addresses:
c.n.vandijk@amc.uva.nl (C. N. van Dijk)
angelcalvo@me.com (A. Calvo)
stefano.zaffagnini@unibo.it (S. Zaffagnini)

REFERENCES

1. Golano P, Vega J, De Leeuw PA, et al. Anatomy of the ankle ligaments: a pictorial essay. Knee Surg Sports Traumatol Arthrosc 2010;18(5):557–69.
2. van Dijk CN, Golano P. Ankle arthroscopy: techniques developed by the Amsterdam Foot and Ankle School. Berlin: Springer; 2014.

Dedication

Recientemente, nuestro amigo y maestro Pau Golanó se nos fué para siempre y sin avisar.

Pau fue anatomista, maestro, sabio, artista, y por encima de todo un amigo. Tenía una personalidad rebelde, seductora e inigualable. Fue un apasionado de su trabajo, innovador, perfeccionista, y sobretodo genial.

Durante sus estudios en la Facultad de Medicina de Barcelona mostró un gran interés por la anatomía y la cirugía ortopédica, de las que fue estudiante-interno casi desde el principio. Tras acabar la carrera de medicina, intentó ser cirujano ortopeda, pero el miedo a cometer un error con consecuencias sobre el paciente le hicieron rectificar y volcarse en su otra pasión, la anatomía. Sin embargo, ese periodo inicial le marcó enormemente su trayectoria profesional. Fue capaz de darse cuenta de que la anatomía, tal y como se describía en los libros clásicos o se enseñaba en las universidades, no era suficiente para alertar a los cirujanos de cuales eran los riesgos quirúrgicos. Además, los tiempos habían cambiado y una cirugía ortopédica moderna, con técnicas que evolucionaban rápidamente como la artroscopia, no podía basarse en el estudio de libros de anatomía clásicos. Pau lo entendió y dedicó el resto de su vida a cambiar el modo de ver la anatomía, y la adaptó a los tiempos modernos. Sin quererlo, también nos cambio a todos.

Supo mostrarnos una anatomía amable y hermosa, alejada de la imagen convencional. Nos enseñó una anatomía perfecta, tan perfecta que la convirtió en arte.

Pero no sólo nos enseño anatomía, sino a vivir la vida, a disfrutarla y a luchar por lo que creemos y por lo que nos gusta, a pesar de todo y de todos.

Su amor por la vida, el trabajo, los suyos, y por todo lo que hacía, era tan grande que se dedicó con pasión y lo dio todo. Lo que hacía te enamoraba, como lo explicaba te seducía, y como lo vivía te fascinaba.

Pau no ha pasado desapercibido. Su amistad, sus consejos, y todos aquellos momentos compartidos quedarán en nuestra memoria. Y su trabajo, por el que tanto luchó, perdurará para siempre.

Gracias por todas las horas que te robamos, por tus enseñanzas, por tu amistad, y por todo aquello que no puede expresarse con palabras.

Tus amigos y colaboradores.

Jordi Vega, MD
Hospital Quirón Barcelona
Plaça d'Alfonso Comín 5
Barcelona 08023, Spain

E-mail address:
jordivega@hotmail.com

Foot Ankle Clin N Am 19 (2014) xxiii
http://dx.doi.org/10.1016/j.fcl.2014.09.006
foot.theclinics.com
1083-7515/14/$ – see front matter © 2014 Elsevier Inc. All rights reserved.

Anatomy of the Triceps Surae: A Pictorial Essay

Miquel Dalmau-Pastor, PodD, PT[a], Betlem Fargues-Polo Jr[a],
Daniel Casanova-Martínez Jr[b], Jordi Vega, MD[c],*,
Pau Golanó, MD[a,d,†]

KEYWORDS

- Anatomy • Surgical anatomy • Gastrocnemius • Gastrocnemius-soleus complex
- Soleus • Calcaneal tendon • Plantaris muscle

KEY POINTS

- The triceps surae is a muscular group formed by the gastrocnemius, the soleus, and the plantaris muscles. The gastrocnemius and soleus muscles join to form the calcaneal tendon while the plantaris muscle inserts independently.
- Gastrocnemius and/or triceps surae lengthening is helpful in resolving foot disorders.
- There exist 5 different anatomic levels at which surgical lengthening of the triceps surae can be achieved. Mastering the anatomy of every level is the basis of these surgical procedures.

INTRODUCTION

Since the beginning of the twentieth century, several techniques have been reported for the treatment of triceps surae contracture in patients with cerebral palsy.[1–6] The objective of these techniques was to lengthen this muscle group. However, it was not until the publications by Kowalski and colleagues[7] in early 1999 and DiGiovanni and colleagues[8] in 2002 that interest in the anatomy of the triceps surae gained relevance, owing to the suggestion by these investigators that gastrocnemius contracture

Disclosure: The authors declare no conflicts of interest.
[a] Laboratory of Arthroscopic and Surgical Anatomy, Human Anatomy Unit, Department of Pathology and Experimental Therapeutics, School of Medicine, University of Barcelona, C/Feixa Llarga, s/n, 08907, Hospitalet de Llobregat, Barcelona, Spain; [b] Anatomy Unit, Biomedical Department, University of Antofagasta, Av. Universidad de Antofagasta s/n (Campus Coloso), Antofagasta 1240000, Chile; [c] Unit of Foot and Ankle Surgery, Hospital Quirón, Plaça d'Alfonso Comín 5, Barcelona 08023, Spain; [d] Department of Orthopaedic Surgery, School of Medicine, University of Pittsburgh, 4200 Fifth Avenue, Pittsburgh, PA 15213, USA
[†] Deceased
* Corresponding author.
E-mail address: jordivega@hotmail.com

Foot Ankle Clin N Am 19 (2014) 603–635
http://dx.doi.org/10.1016/j.fcl.2014.08.002
1083-7515/14/$ – see front matter © 2014 Elsevier Inc. All rights reserved.

foot.theclinics.com

in the healthy individual is associated with conditions affecting the midfoot and fore-foot, such as calcaneal tendon injury, metatarsalgia, plantar fasciopathy, diabetic ulcer, hallux valgus, flat foot, and digital deformity.[8-10]

Therefore, an article on the anatomy of the triceps surae is a key contribution to this special issue on contracture of the gastrocnemius muscle. This article is divided into two parts: one discussing the general anatomy of the triceps surae and one address-ing the surgical anatomy of the gastrocnemius, a key area of knowledge for surgeons applying lengthening techniques.

TRICEPS SURAE

The triceps surae is the muscular group that occupies the superficial posterior compartment of the leg and comprises the gastrocnemius, soleus, and plantaris. The junction of the gastrocnemius and soleus forms the longest and most powerful tendon in the human body,[11,12] the calcaneal tendon. The plantaris, which is present in more than 90% of the population,[13-16] can merge with this muscle group to form the calcaneal tendon.

In recent years, the term gastrocnemius-soleus complex has been used to refer to the triceps surae.[17-20] Although the authors agree that gastrocnemius-soleus complex is a more clinical term and that, from a functional perspective, the gastrocnemius and soleus act as a single unit, the International Anatomical Terminology[21] has established the term triceps surae to refer to the group formed by the gastrocnemius and soleus. Therefore, triceps surae is the term used in this article.

Similarly, the calcaneal tendon is usually referred to as the Achilles tendon. How-ever, as this term is not included in the International Anatomical Terminology,[21] calca-neal tendon is the preferred term here.

Gastrocnemius

The gastrocnemius comprises 2 heads, medial and lateral, at its origin. These heads insert proximally in the posterosuperior region of the corresponding femoral condyle (**Fig. 1**). However, the origin of the muscle varies depending on whether one is referring to the medial or lateral head.

Medial head
The medial head of the gastrocnemius originates in a triangular area on the popliteal aspect of the distal epiphysis of the femur. A medial and a lateral origin can be consid-ered. The medial origin comprises a flattened, thick, and resistant tendon that extends over the medial condyle immediately below the insertion of the tendon of the adductor magnus muscle and along the medial supracondylar ridge. The lateral origin, less important, inserts by means of short tendinous and muscle fibers on the popliteal aspect of the medial femoral condyle, at the site of a small eminence known as the medial supracondyloid tubercle[22] (also called the medial supracondylar tubercle), and on the capsule of the knee joint (see **Fig. 1**; **Fig. 2**).

Lateral head
The lateral head of the gastrocnemius muscle originates from a tendon in a fossa situated posterior to the lateral epicondyle and proximal to the insertion of the popliteal muscle tendon in the lateral supracondylar ridge (see **Figs. 1** and **2**). Short tendinous fibers and muscle fibers situated medial to this tendon originate on the capsule of the knee joint and on the popliteal aspect, where a small bony eminence known as the lateral supracondyloid tubercle[22] (also called the lateral supracondylar tubercle) can be observed, albeit less often than on the medial side (**Fig. 3**).

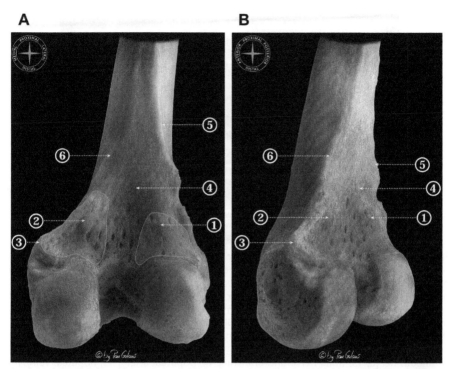

Fig. 1. Posterior (*A*) and posteromedial (*B*) views of the femoral distal epiphysis showing the bony prominences and insertional areas of gastrocnemius muscle (insertional areas of the medial and lateral head of gastrocnemius muscle have been marked in *green*). 1, lateral supracondyloid tubercle; 2, medial supracondyloid tubercle; 3, adductor tubercle; 4, popliteal surface of the femur; 5, lateral supracondylar line; 6, medial supracondylar line. (Figure Copyright © Pau Golanó 2014.)

An accessory ossicle, the fabella, which is found in 10% to 30% of the population, can be found embedded within the tendon of the lateral head (**Fig. 4**).[18] This small sesamoid bone is generally round or oval, with its major axis (5–20 mm) running parallel to the tendinous fibers of the lateral head of the gastrocnemius.[23] It is a casual finding in imaging studies and is usually bilateral.[24] Although the fabella does not generally cause symptoms, it can lead to posterolateral knee pain,[25] and can be fractured[26] or dislocated.[27]

The anterior aspect of the fabella is covered in hyaline cartilage and articulates with the lateral femoral condyle.[25] Its posterior aspect, which is generally convex, is embedded in the tendon and serves as an anchor point for various capsular-ligamentous structures in the posterolateral region of the knee (oblique popliteal ligament, fabellofibular ligament, and arcuate popliteal ligament) (**Fig. 5**).[28] Occasionally an accessory sesamoid bone can be observed on the tendon of the medial head.[12,29]

The medial head is wider and thicker than the lateral head (see **Fig. 2**).

The muscle fibers that originate in these divergent proximal fibers form 2 muscle bellies. As these course distally they converge on themselves, thus delimiting the lower triangle of the popliteal fossa, which is rhomboid in shape. Both muscle bellies are in contact with the posterior capsule of the knee and its reinforcements. The medial head slides across a serous bursa that is generally in direct contact with the joint. This bursa is responsible for the formation of a popliteal cyst (Baker cyst) in cases of

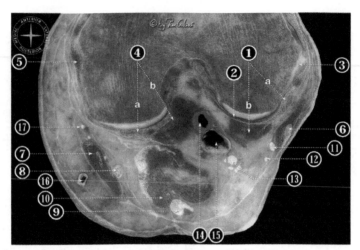

Fig. 2. Transversal section at the level of femoral condyles revealing the proximal insertion of the medial and lateral heads of gastrocnemius muscle (neurovascular structures have been painted with Adobe Photoshop). 1, proximal insertion of the lateral head of gastrocnemius muscle: a. tendinous insertion, b. muscular insertion; 2, knee capsule joint; 3, lateral collateral ligament of the knee joint; 4, proximal insertion of the medial head of gastrocnemius muscle: a. tendinous insertion, b. muscular insertion; 5, medial collateral ligament of the knee joint; 6, biceps femoris muscle; 7, sartorius muscle; 8, gracilis tendon; 9, semitendinosus tendon; 10, semimembranosus muscle; 11, common peroneal nerve; 12, lateral sural cutaneous nerve; 13, tibial nerve and branches; 14, popliteal artery; 15, popliteal vein; 16, great saphenous vein; 17, saphenous nerve. (Figure Copyright © Pau Golanó 2014.)

knee disorder.[28] In addition, the bursa can come into contact with the semimembranosus muscle bursa, thus favoring movement between the bulky tendon and the medial head of the gastrocnemius. The latter is referred to herein as the gastrocnemius-semimembranosus bursa, which may also be associated with the formation of a popliteal cyst (**Fig. 6**).

A corresponding inconstant serous bursa can also be found at the lateral head.

The muscle bellies finish on the posterior aspect of a wide tendinous lamina, or aponeurosis, which almost completely covers the anterior aspect of the corresponding muscle belly. This lamina, which is in contact with each head proximally, finishes as a single lamina with no muscle fibers at its distal end.[11] At the mid-calf, this aponeurosis joins the tendinous lamina of the soleus distally to form the calcaneal tendon (**Fig. 7**). The site and mechanism of union between the tendinous laminas play a key anatomic role in gastrocnemius recession.[30,31]

Plantaris

The plantaris, which is absent in 6% to 8% of the population, is found in the superficial posterior compartment of the leg.[13–16] It arises proximally just superior to the lateral condyle, on the lateral supracondylar ridge, proximal and medial to the lateral head of the gastrocnemius, with which it is in close contact (**Fig. 8**). A small belly measuring 5 to 12 cm emerges from this point[32] and runs distally from lateral to medial crossing the posterior aspect of the knee. At the origin of the soleus, the belly finishes in a long, flat, thin, and almost filiform tendon (approximately 25–35 cm long[32–34]) that varies between 1.5 and 5 mm in width depending on the report (**Fig. 9**).[16,33,34] This tendon runs down the leg between the bellies of the gastrocnemius and soleus until it reaches

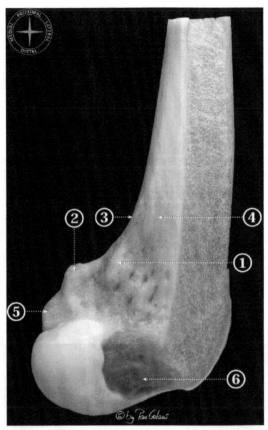

Fig. 3. Posterolateral view of the medial half of the femur distal epiphysis, showing in detail the medial supracondyloid tubercle of the femur. 1, medial supracondyloid tubercle; 2, adductor tubercle; 3, medial supracondylar line; 4, popliteal surface of the femur; 5, medial epicondyle; 6, intercondylar notch (footprint of the posterior cruciate ligament). (Figure Copyright © Pau Golanó 2014.)

the medial border of the calcaneal tendon. Although it has been reported to join the calcaneal tendon, thus contributing to its formation,[32] anatomic studies show that this is not the case[13,34] or that it only joins the calcaneal tendon in very rare cases.[14] The location of the insertion point of the plantaris tendon varies widely. It is most often located in the medial area of the superior calcaneal tuberosity (47%),[13,14,34] anterior and medial to the calcaneal tendon, and thus independent of it (**Fig. 10**). Consequently, it often remains intact in cases of calcaneal tendon rupture. The variable nature of this distal insertion could be due to the loss of the plantar insertion of this muscle, a vestige from when man began to adopt an upright position.[14]

The plantaris can be injured at the level of the musculotendinous junction, either in isolation[35] or simultaneously with a partial rupture of the medial head of the gastrocnemius or soleus.[36]

Soleus

The soleus is the third component of the triceps surae, together with the medial head and the lateral head of the gastrocnemius and the plantaris, when present. The soleus

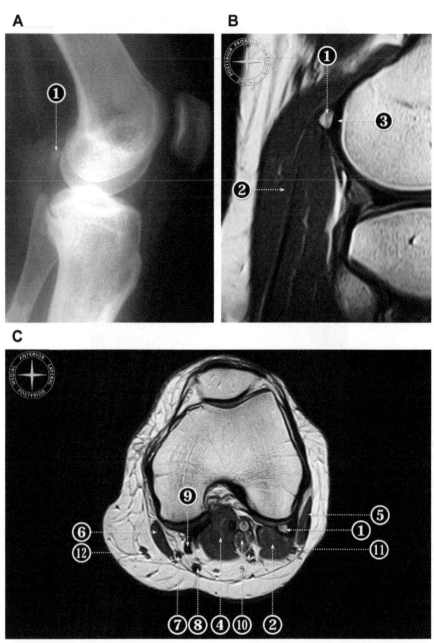

Fig. 4. Os fabella. (*A*) Lateral radiographic view of a right knee with an os fabella. (*B*) Sagittal T1-weighted magnetic resonance (MR) image of the knee showing an os fabella. (*C*) Transversal T1-weighted MR image of the knee showing an os fabella and its relation with surrounding structures. 1, os fabella; 2, lateral head of gastrocnemius muscle; 3, knee joint capsule; 4, medial head of gastrocnemius muscle; 5, biceps femoris muscle; 6, sartorius muscle; 7, gracilis tendon; 8, semitendinosus tendon; 9, semimembranosus tendon; 10, popliteal neurovascular bundle (tibial nerve and popliteal artery and vein); 11, common peroneal nerve; 12, saphenous nerve and great saphenous vein. (Figure Copyright © Pau Golanó 2014.)

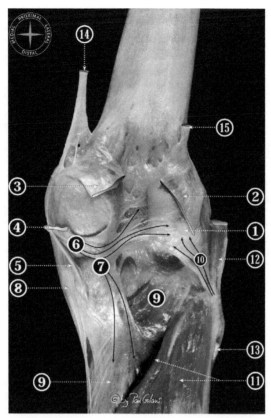

Fig. 5. Dissection of the popliteal region showing the posterior knee joint capsule and an os fabella. Neurovascular structures have been resected. 1, os fabella; 2, lateral head of gastrocnemius muscle (cut); 3, medial head of gastrocnemius muscle (cut); 4, semimembranosus tendon (cut); 5, expansion of the semimembranosus tendon (anterior arm); 6, expansion of the semimembranosus tendon (oblique popliteal ligament, *black arrows*); 7, expansion of the semimembranosus tendon (inferior arm, *black arrows*); 8, medial collateral ligament of the knee joint; 9, popliteus muscle; 10, arcuate popliteal ligament (and *black arrows*); 11, soleus muscle and its tendinous arch; 12, biceps femoris tendon (cut); 13, common peroneal nerve (cut); 14, adductor magnus tendon (cut); 15, lateral intermuscular septum (cut). (Figure Copyright © Pau Golanó 2014.)

is a broad and bulky muscle that lies deep to the gastrocnemius and plantaris and superficial to the muscles of the deep posterior compartment (tibialis posterior, flexor digitorum longus, and flexor hallucis longus muscles), which it covers for most of its course.

The soleus has both a fibular and tibial origin. The fibular origin is on the posterior aspect of the head and upper fourth of the diaphysis. The tibial origin is at the inferior border of the soleal line, a bony ridge running obliquely lateral-proximal to medial-distal that is situated on the upper third of the posterior aspect of the tibia, and the posteromedial border of the tibia (middle third) (**Fig. 11**).

Both origins, which are made of tendinous fibers, merge distally to form a fibrous arch known as the tendinous arch of the soleus, which enables the passage of the tibial nerve and posterior tibial artery and accompanying veins from a superficial position toward the deep posterior compartment (**Fig. 12**).

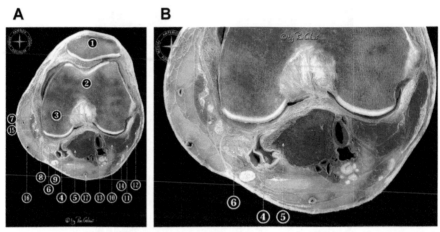

Fig. 6. Popliteal cyst. (*A*) Transversal section at the level of the knee joint showing a popliteal cyst (Baker cyst) at the gastrocnemius-semimembranosus bursa. (*B*) Photomacrography. 1, patella; 2, femur; 3, intercondylar notch; 4, popliteal cyst; 5, medial head of gastrocnemius muscle; 6, semimembranosus tendon; 7, sartorius muscle; 8, gracilis tendon; 9, semitendinosus tendon; 10, lateral head of gastrocnemius muscle; 11, plantaris muscle; 12, biceps femoris muscle; 13, neurovascular bundle (tibial nerve and popliteal artery and vein); 14, common peroneal nerve; 15, saphenous nerve; 16, great saphenous vein; 17, lesser saphenous vein. (Figure Copyright © Pau Golanó 2014.)

The tendinous lamina resulting from the union of these origins gives rise to muscle fibers on both aspects (anterior and posterior). Although most muscle fibers arise from the posterior aspect, some muscle fibers detach from the anterior aspect. Thus, the tendinous lamina is part of the muscle mass and forms the so-called intramuscular aponeurosis of the soleus (**Fig. 13**). Although the tibial nerve innervates the soleus muscle as a whole, each aspect of the muscle (anterior and posterior) has independent branches.[11,32,37,38]

The muscle fibers that originate on the posterior aspect converge downward to finish on the anterior aspect and on the borders of a new tendinous lamina, known as the insertion lamina. This lamina extends proximally along the posterior aspect of the muscle belly (see **Fig. 13**). Wide in its proximal part, it gradually narrows until it joins the tendinous lamina from the gastrocnemius to form the calcaneal tendon. The site and mechanics of the union of both tendinous laminas are an important anatomic detail that should be taken into account in the surgical techniques described later.

Lastly, the bipennate fibers arising on the anterior aspect of the tendinous lamina, or intramuscular aponeurosis, finish in another tendinous formation, known as the median septum.[39,40] This thin component, which takes the form of a short septum, originates on the anterior aspect of the aponeurosis (**Fig. 14**).

The complexity of the muscle fibers, aponeurosis, and innervation of the soleus muscle has motivated studies about its muscular architecture and intramuscular innervation.[37–42]

Calcaneal Tendon

The calcaneal tendon is formed by the union of the soleus and gastrocnemius muscles. It may also include the plantaris (see earlier discussion) (**Fig. 15**).

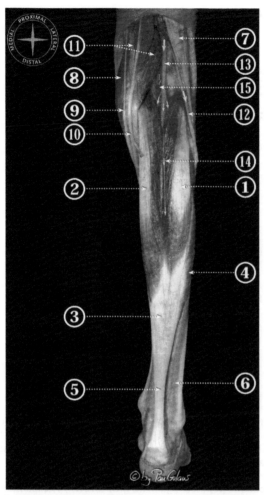

Fig. 7. Superficial dissection of the leg and popliteal area showing a posterior view of the triceps surae and its components and surrounding structures. 1, lateral head of gastrocnemius muscle; 2, medial head of gastrocnemius muscle; 3, gastrocnemius aponeurosis; 4, soleus muscle; 5, calcaneal tendon; 6, posterior deep fascia of the leg; 7, biceps femoris muscle; 8, sartorius muscle; 9, gracilis tendon; 10, semitendinosus tendon; 11, semimembranosus muscle; 12, common peroneal nerve; 13, tibial nerve and branches; 14, sural nerve; 15, popliteal artery and vein. (Figure Copyright © Pau Golanó 2014.)

The calcaneal tendon is the longest and strongest tendon in the human body.[11,12] On average, it can measure up to 2.5 cm in diameter[13] and approximately 15 cm in length.[12] It is also the most frequently injured tendon in the leg (20% of all tendon lesions).[43,44]

The union of the gastrocnemius tendinous lamina to the soleus at mid-calf gives rise to the calcaneal tendon. The contribution of the different muscles to the formation of the calcaneal tendon varies between individuals. Cummins and colleagues[13] observed that the soleus accounts for two-thirds of the tendon in 52% of subjects, both the soleus and the gastrocnemius account for half of the tendon in 35%, and the gastrocnemius accounts for two-thirds of the tendon in the remaining 13%.

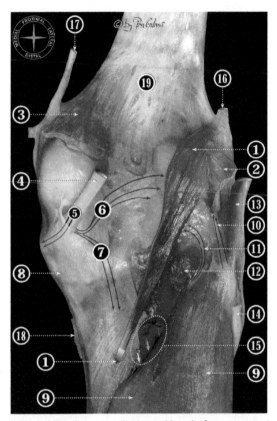

Fig. 8. Dissection of the popliteal region. The lateral head of gastrocnemius muscle has been cut and rejected to show the entire muscle belly of the plantaris muscle. 1, plantaris muscle (*large gray arrow* shows direction of the tendon); 2, lateral head of gastrocnemius muscle (cut); 3, medial head of gastrocnemius muscle (cut); 4, semimembranosus tendon (cut); 5, expansion of the semimembranosus tendon (anterior arm); 6, expansion of the semimembranosus tendon (oblique popliteal ligament, *gray arrows*); 7, expansion of the semimembranosus tendon (inferior arm, *gray arrows*); 8, medial collateral ligament of the knee joint; 9, soleus muscle; 10, fabellofibular ligament (and *gray arrows*); 11, arcuate popliteal ligament (and *gray arrows*); 12, popliteus muscle; 13, biceps femoris tendon (cut); 14, common peroneal nerve (cut); 15, neurovascular bundle passing through the tendinous arch of the soleus; 16, lateral intermuscular septum (cut); 17, adductor magnus tendon (cut); 18, pes anserinus distal insertion (cut); 19, popliteal surface of the femur. (Figure Copyright © Pau Golanó 2014.)

The calcaneal tendon is wide at its origin, although it narrows slightly as it descends, reaching its minimum width at the level of the ankle joint, before widening again and inserting on the calcaneus.[32] The narrowest point results from rotation of the fibers (**Fig. 16**).[13] Consequently, the medial fibers rotate posteriorly and the posterior fibers rotate laterally. The anterior aspect is composed of fibers from the lateral gastrocnemius, and the anteromedial part of the tendon is composed of fibers from the soleus.[45] Torsion of the fibers of the tendon gives it greater mechanical resistance.[46] However, this torsion also creates a poorly vascularized area of stress 2 to 5 cm proximal to its insertion in the calcaneus.[13]

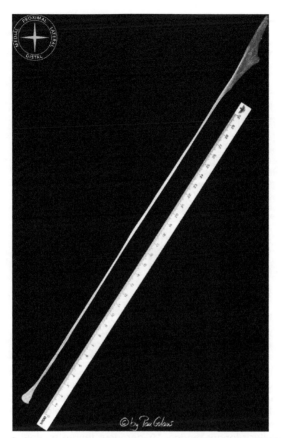

Fig. 9. Overview of plantaris muscle. (Figure Copyright © Pau Golanó 2014.)

Vascularization of the calcaneal tendon has been widely studied.[47–50] It receives its blood supply from the myotendinous junction, the osteotendinous junction, and the paratenon. Vascular supply is via 2 arteries: the posterior tibial artery and the fibular artery. The posterior tibial artery irrigates the proximal and distal sections of the tendon, whereas the fibular artery irrigates the mid-section.[50] The supply from the posterior tibial artery is rich, whereas the mid-section of the tendon, irrigated by the fibular artery, has fewer vessels and therefore a poorer supply.[47]

Sections of the tendons with poor irrigation are more likely to rupture. Therefore, it is no surprise that most ruptures of the calcaneal tendon are in the mid-section.[50]

The bursa of the calcaneal tendon, or retrocalcaneal bursa, is found at the insertion point of the tendon on the posterior aspect of the calcaneus.[51] This bursa, which lies between the calcaneal tendon and the calcaneus, enables proper sliding of the tendon (**Fig. 17**). A second bursa, the subcutaneous calcaneal bursa, is constant and lies between the tendon and the skin (**Fig. 18**).

Knowledge of vascularization of the skin and subcutaneous tissue surrounding the calcaneal tendon is essential in avoiding complications during scarring after surgery. The skin covering the medial and lateral borders of the tendon is better vascularized than that of the posterior aspect. Therefore, it is advisable to avoid incisions on the posterior aspect, because they could lead to complications during scarring.[52]

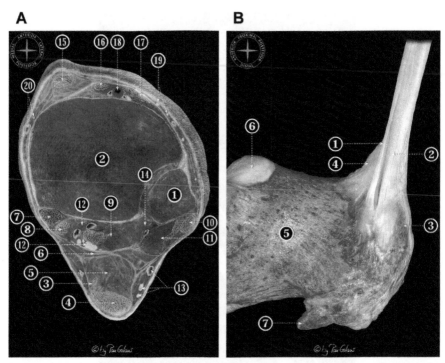

Fig. 10. Plantaris muscle distal insertion. Both preparations show the independent insertion of the plantaris tendon from the calcaneal tendon. (*A*) Transversal section at the level of tibio-fibular syndesmosis (neurovascular structures have been painted with Adobe Photoshop). 1, fibula; 2, tibia; 3, plantaris tendon; 4, calcaneal tendon; 5, precalcaneal fat tissue (Kager fat pad); 6, posterior deep fascia of the leg; 7, tibialis posterior tendon; 8, flexor digitorum longus tendon; 9, flexor hallucis longus tendon; 10, peroneus longus tendon; 11, peroneus brevis tendon; 12, posterior neurovascular bundle (tibial nerve, posterior tibial artery and veins); 13, sural nerve and lesser saphenous vein; 14, peroneal artery; 15, tibialis anterior tendon; 16, extensor hallucis longus tendon; 17, extensor digitorum longus and peroneus tertius tendons; 18, anterior neurovascular bundle (deep peroneal nerve, anterior tibial artery and veins); 19, branches of the superficial peroneal nerve; 20, Saphenous nerve and greater saphenous vein. (*B*) Dissection showing the insertion of the calcaneal and plantaris tendons on the calcaneus. 1, plantaris tendon; 2, calcaneal tendon; 3, posterior calcaneal spur; 4, calcaneal tendon bursa; 5, medial surface of the calcaneus; 6, posterior articular surface for the talus (posterior subtalar joint); 7, calcaneal spur. (Figure Copyright © Pau Golanó 2014.)

Incisions made on the lateral aspect of the tendon carry the risk of injury to the sural nerve and lesser saphenous vein; therefore, incisions made on the medial side seem to be the most appropriate.

Innervation

The triceps surae is innervated by branches from the tibial nerve, which provide motor innervation to the popliteal area.

Function of the Triceps Surae

The gastrocnemius and soleus share an insertion tendon in the calcaneus; therefore, they exercise the same function on the foot. Contraction of the triceps surae produces plantar flexion with adduction and medial rotation of the foot.[11] Despite this similarity

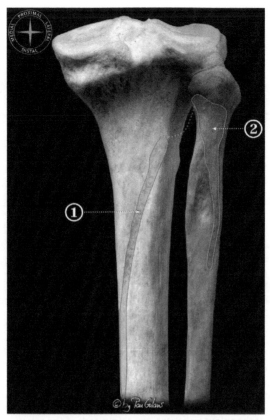

Fig. 11. Posterior view of the proximal half of tibia and fibula bones. Fibular and tibial proximal insertions of the soleus muscle are shown in green. Dotted line indicates the tendinous arch of the soleus muscle. 1, tibial proximal insertion of the soleus muscle on the soleal line; 2, fibular proximal insertion of the soleus muscle. (Figure Copyright © Pau Golanó 2014.)

in function, the power of each muscle differs considerably. In their study on muscle balance, Silver and colleagues[53] found the soleus to be the main plantar-flexor muscle of the foot and the most powerful muscle of those crossing the ankle. The soleus provides more than double the plantar-flexor force of the gastrocnemius, whose medial head provides 71% of its force, with the lateral head contributing only a small part to the plantar-flexor force.

The gastrocnemius also crosses the knee joint, and its contraction leads to flexion of the knee. The flexion force of the gastrocnemius is greater when the knee joint is fully extended.[54] It was traditionally believed that the gastrocnemius and the soleus helped to push the body forward during walking[55]; however, recent studies show that this may not be the case. It seems that the function of the triceps surae during walking has more to do with control of balance and indirect modulation of walking speed.[56] In addition, the soleus acts as a peripheral vascular pump.[57]

Given their function in the foot, it seems logical to consider that the soleus and gastrocnemius enable maximal plantar flexion of the foot and the tiptoe position. However, some investigators state that the plantar aponeurosis plays a fundamental role in this movement, mainly owing to a system that integrates the calcaneal tendon with

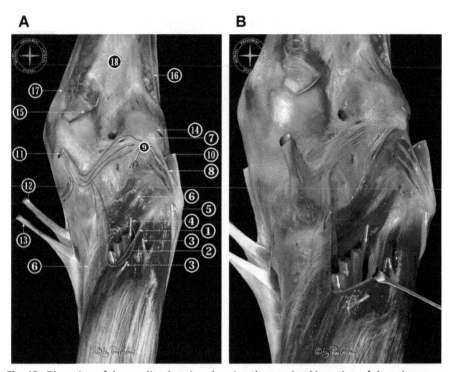

Fig. 12. Dissection of the popliteal region showing the proximal insertion of the soleus muscle and the passage of the neurovascular bundle trough the tendinous arch of the soleus (gastrocnemius muscle has been resected). (*A*) posterior view of the popliteal region. (*B*) posteromedial view (photomacrography) of the popliteal region (surgical instrument is retracting the tendinous arch of the soleus muscle); 1, tendinous arch of the soleus muscle; 2, neurovascular bundle (posterior tibial vein, posterior tibial artery, tibial nerve); 3, motor branches of the tibial nerve entering the soleus muscle (cut) (posterior part of the soleus has usually 2 or 3 motor branches[37]); 4, motor branch for the anterior aspect of soleus and flexor hallucis longus muscles (cut); 5, common peroneal nerve (cut); 6, popliteus muscle; 7, os fabella; 8, fabellofibular ligament; 9, arcuate popliteal ligament; 10, biceps femoris tendon (cut); 11, semimembranosus tendon (cut) and its expansions (*gray arrows*); 12, gracilis tendon (cut); 13, semitendinosus tendon (cut); 14, lateral head of gastrocnemius muscle (cut); 15, medial head of gastrocnemius muscle (cut); 16, lateral intermuscular septum; 17, adductor magnus tendon; 18, popliteal surface of the femur. (Figure Copyright © Pau Golanó 2014.)

structures on the sole (plantar fascia and plantar intrinsic foot muscles) with transmission of forces through the calcaneus. This system was first described by Arandes and Viladot in 1953, and is known as the Achilles-calcaneal-plantar system.[58]

Achilles-Calcaneal-Plantar System

The Achilles-calcaneal-plantar system comprises the calcaneal tendon, the posteroinferior portion of the calcaneus and its trabecular system, the plantar aponeurosis, and the plantar intrinsic foot muscles (**Fig. 19**).

Several investigators have demonstrated continuity between the fibers of the calcaneal tendon and the plantar aponeurosis[51,59]; however, this continuity was only obvious in the fetus and gradually diminished with age until adulthood, when it disappeared, leaving only periosteum between the tendon insertion and the plantar

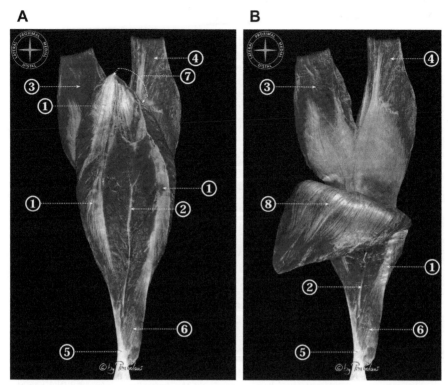

Fig. 13. Overview of the triceps surae components. Muscles have been disinserted. (*A*) Anterior view. (*B*) Anterior view with soleus muscle retracted. 1, intramuscular aponeurosis of the soleus muscle; 2, median septum; 3, lateral head of gastrocnemius muscle; 4, medial head of gastrocnemius muscle; 5, calcaneal tendon; 6, accessory soleus muscle; 7, tendinous arch of soleus muscle; 8, soleus posterior aponeurosis. (Figure Copyright © Pau Golanó 2014.)

aponeurosis.[59] A recent study ruled out a connection between the calcaneal tendon and the plantar aponeurosis, and showed that the only connection is between the paratenon and the plantar aponeurosis.[60]

Some studies associate an excess of tension in the posterior muscles of the thigh and leg with plantar fasciopathy.[61] Furthermore, it seems that proximal release of the medial head of the gastrocnemius is an effective approach to chronic plantar fasciopathy.[62] However, the investigators suggest that reduced dorsiflexion of the ankle is at least partly responsible for plantar fasciopathy, and not the existence of the Achilles-calcaneal-plantar system.

Therefore, despite an apparent functional connection between the structures, the authors believe that the lack of anatomic evidence and reports in the literature makes it possible to rule out the existence of the Achilles-calcaneal-plantar system.

Plantar Aponeurosis

The plantar aponeurosis (plantar fascia) is the fascial covering of the sole.[63] It lies deep to the skin and is separated therefrom by a thick layer of fatty tissue,[11] the plantar fat pad (**Fig. 20**). This fascia is organized into longitudinal, transversal, and vertical bands and tracts. Together with the encapsulated fat lying between the tracts, the fascia connects the skin to the skeleton and enables passage for vessels, nerves, and tendons,

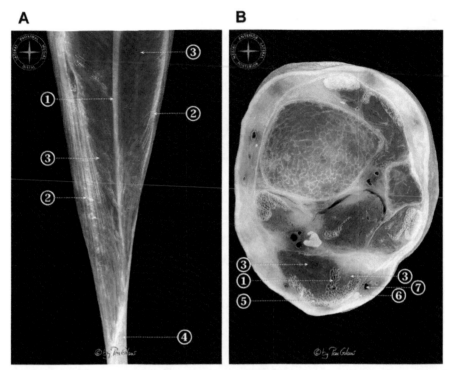

Fig. 14. The median septum of soleus muscle. (*A*) Photomacrography of an anterior view of the soleus muscle showing the median septum and the insertion lamina, finishing in the calcaneal tendon. (*B*) Transversal section at the distal third of the leg showing the sagittal orientation of the median septum. 1, median septum of soleus muscle; 2, intramuscular aponeurosis of the soleus; 3, muscle fibers of the bipennate anterior aspect of soleus muscle; 4, calcaneal tendon; 5, gastrocnemius aponeurosis; 6, sural nerve; 7, lesser saphenous vein. (Figure Copyright © Pau Golanó 2014.)

which it protects from the load of the metatarsal heads.[64] The plantar aponeurosis is also the main support structure of the medial longitudinal arch of the foot.[63]

The plantar aponeurosis is divided into 3 components; medial, central, and lateral. It is triangular in shape, with the apex posterior (calcaneal) and the base anterior (toes). It originates in both apophyses (medial and lateral) of the calcaneal tuberosity. Anteriorly, the fascia finishes at the metatarsophalangeal joints of the first to fifth toes, with some fibers reaching the skin and others contributing to the plantar plate and natatory ligament. The lateral and medial components adhere to the corresponding edge of the foot, in continuity with the dorsal fascia of the foot.[11]

Medial component
The medial component is the smallest of the 3 and forms the fascia of the abductor muscle of the great toe. It originates in the medial tuberosity of the calcaneus and continues medially with the dorsal fascia of the foot.[65]

Lateral component
The lateral component originates on the lateral calcaneal tuberosity[11] or on the lateral side of the medial tuberosity.[63] It then continues anteriorly before bifurcating medially and laterally at the cuboid. The medial component inserts on the base of the fifth metatarsal and the lateral tract on the fascia of the abductor of the fifth toe.[63]

A   **B**

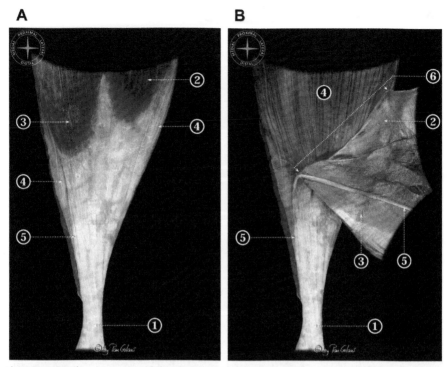

Fig. 15. Muscular dissection of the distal part of the triceps surae showing the aponeurosis of gastrocnemius and soleus muscles and its fusion to form the calcaneal tendon. There is a degenerative lesion (tendinosis) on the medial part of the calcaneal tendon (*yellow area*). (*A*) Posterior view. (*B*) Posterior view with gastrocnemius muscle retracted, showing the fusion of gastrocnemius aponeurosis with soleus posterior aponeurosis. 1, Calcaneal tendon; 2, lateral head of gastrocnemius muscle; 3, medial head of gastrocnemius muscle; 4, soleus posterior aponeurosis; 5, plantaris tendon; 6, area of insertion of gastrocnemius aponeurosis into soleus posterior aponeurosis. (Figure Copyright © Pau Golanó 2014.)

Central component

The central component is the largest of the 3 and is triangular, with the apex posterior and the base anterior. It originates on the medial apophysis of the calcaneal tuberosity.[63]

The fibers of the central component of the plantar aponeurosis become longitudinal in orientation and expand anteriorly. Proximally, at the head of the metatarsals, they divide into 5 divergent superficial bands,[64] each of which in turn divides into 3 parts, 1 superficial and 2 deep. The superficial fibers insert into the dermis distal to the metatarsophalangeal joints, thus contributing to the formation of the superficial transverse intermetatarsal ligament,[21] also known as the natatory ligament.[66,67]

The 2 deep components (sagittal septa), which arise from the longitudinal bands, are arranged as septa situated in the sagittal plane and surrounding the corresponding flexor tendons, thus contributing to the formation of its fibrous sheath.[65] These septa insert into the plantar plate and/or sesamoid bones (great toe) and into the deep transverse metatarsal ligament. Both septa continue with vertical fibers that insert into the skin. Moreover, these sagittal septa divide the plantar fat pad into compartments, thus

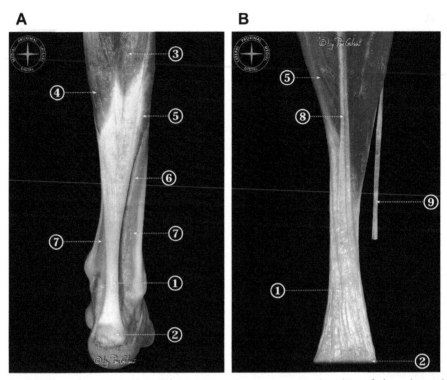

Fig. 16. The calcaneal tendon. (*A*) Dissection showing a posterior view of the calcaneal tendon. (*B*) Anterior view of the calcaneal tendon demonstrating the characteristic rotation of its fibers (specimen is the same in *A* and *B*). 1, calcaneal tendon; 2, insertional area of the calcaneal tendon; 3, lateral head of gastrocnemius muscle; 4, medial head of gastrocnemius muscle; 5, soleus muscle; 6, lateral intermuscular septum; 7, posterior deep fascia of the leg; 8, median septum; 9, plantaris tendon. (Figure Copyright © Pau Golanó 2014.)

creating bodies of adipose tissue between the flexor tendons that protect the neuro-vascular bundle and fibrous tunnels that enable passage of the lumbrical tendons (see **Fig. 20**).

SURGICAL ANATOMY

Several procedures have been described for the treatment of contracture of the gastrocnemius and soleus.[1–6,68–72] Over the years, the original techniques have undergone various modifications with the aim of preventing or reducing complications (especially those affecting the sural nerve), predicting potential anatomic variations, reducing postsurgical convalescence, and improving cosmetic outcome.

The main complications arising from surgical procedures in the area described here include neurologic lesions,[10,73,74] especially those affecting the sural nerve, and poor cosmetic outcome resulting from an excessively wide incision.[75] The intimate relationship between the sural nerve and the triceps surae and its components means that the nerve is at risk of injury during surgery (**Fig. 21**).

Irrespective of the technique applied, knowledge of the local anatomy is a prerequisite if complications, which occur in 0% to 22.2% of cases, are to be reduced or avoided.[10,76–84]

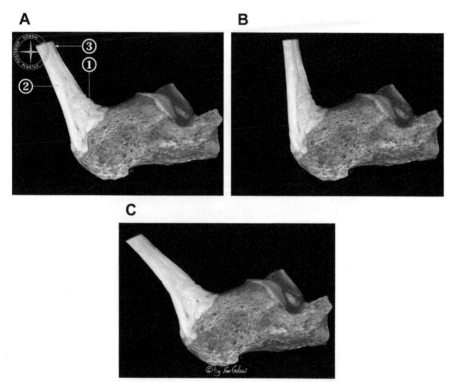

Fig. 17. Dissection of the calcaneal tendon and its insertion on the calcaneus showing the retrocalcaneal bursa through ankle's range of motion (calcaneus has been disarticulated from the foot skeleton). (*A*) Ankle in neutral position. (*B*) Ankle in dorsiflexion. (*C*) Ankle in plantar flexion. 1, retrocalcaneal bursa; 2, calcaneal tendon; 3, plantaris tendon. (Figure Copyright © Pau Golanó 2014.)

The type of technique is also important. The current trend is to propose minimally invasive open procedures in addition to endoscopic procedures. Fewer complications have been reported with these techniques.[10,76–84]

The anatomic site chosen to divide the triceps surae or any of its components is important. The surgeon should be fully acquainted with the various anatomic structures, because the difficulty of the technique and the number of complications will depend on this knowledge. Therefore, and following the schedule proposed by Lamm and colleagues,[85] the authors have divided surgical anatomy into 5 levels, of which level 5 is the most proximal and 1 the most distal (**Fig. 22**).

Level 5 comprises the proximal insertions and tendons of the medial and lateral heads of the gastrocnemius.

Level 4 comprises the medial and lateral bellies of the gastrocnemius.

Level 3 starts where the muscle bellies of the gastrocnemius merge to form the calcaneal tendon and finishes where the aponeuroses of the soleus and gastrocnemius merge.

Level 2 starts in the common aponeurotic tendon of the soleus and gastrocnemius and finishes at the distal end of the soleus muscle.

Level 1 consists of the calcaneal tendon.

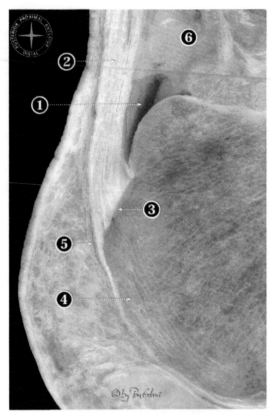

Fig. 18. Sagittal section showing the insertion of the calcaneal tendon and the adjacent bursae. 1, bursa of the calcaneal tendon; 2, calcaneal tendon; 3, insertional area of the calcaneal tendon; 4, calcaneal tuberosity; 5, subcutaneous calcaneal bursa; 6, precalcaneal fat tissue (Kager fat pad). (Figure Copyright © Pau Golanó 2014.)

A 3-level classification of the gastrocnemius-soleus complex based on the surgical procedures used at each level has been proposed.[20] However, the authors use the classification proposed by Lamm and colleagues,[85] considering that it is more anatomic.

The division into levels serves a didactic need and not an anatomic one, because levels 3 and 2 are not always easy to define owing to the anatomic variability of the way the aponeurosis of the gastrocnemius joins the soleus.[30] Nevertheless, the division enables the surgeon to identify the neurovascular structures at risk, depending on the level at which the surgical procedure is performed, thus enabling a safer and more complication-free procedure.

Level 5

Proximal gastrocnemius tenotomy can be performed at this level.

The original procedure for proximal release of the gastrocnemius was described by Silfverskiöld.[2] This procedure consisted of transferring the proximal insertions of the gastrocnemius from the femur to the tibia, thus converting the gastrocnemius into a second soleus muscle. The original technique described section of both the medial and lateral head; today, however, only section of the medial head is performed.[68–72]

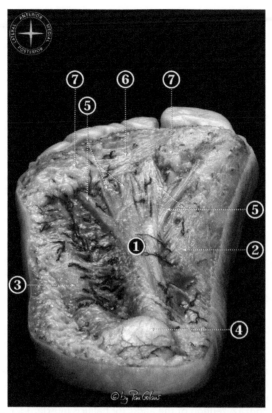

Fig. 19. Posteroplantar view of a dissection of the ball of the foot showing the plantar aponeurosis (arterial network was filled with *black latex*). 1, central component of the plantar aponeurosis; 2, medial component of the plantar aponeurosis; 3, lateral component of the plantar aponeurosis; 4, medial apophysis of the calcaneal tuberosity; 5, superficial bands; 6, transversal bands of the plantar aponeurosis; 7, bodies of adipose tissue. (Figure Copyright © Pau Golanó 2014.)

At this level, certain anatomic details are worthy of mention.

Adequate localization of skin reference points in the medial zone of the popliteal region is essential. In nonobese patients, a small cutaneous fossa can be easily observed in the medial popliteal area; this area results from the proximal-distal course of the semitendinosus and semimembranosus tendons (**Fig. 23**). It is worth remembering that this reference can disappear or be reduced in patients who have undergone anterior cruciate ligament reconstruction using a hamstring graft. The skin incision (3–5 cm) should be made at this level, coinciding with the fold of the flexed knee.[68] Although this medial incision respects neurovascular structures, possible variations in the lesser saphenous vein should be taken into consideration.[86] Of note, an excessively lateral incision could place neurovascular structures at risk (eg, common fibular nerve, lateral and medial sural cutaneous nerve, tibial nerve, and lesser saphenous vein).[86]

In addition to anatomic reasons, there are clinical reasons for isolated tenotomy of the medial head of the gastrocnemius, which plays a much more important role than the lateral head.[68] Cohen[57] found greater tension in the medial head than in the lateral

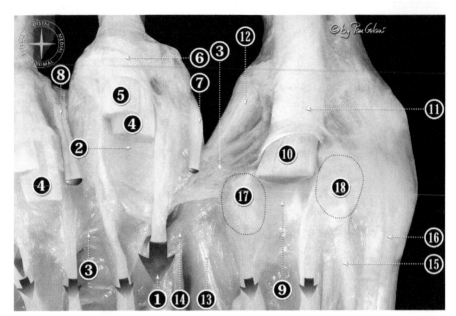

Fig. 20. Dissection of the plantar aspect of the metatarsophalangeal joints of a right foot showing the insertion of the sagittal septa into the plantar plate. 1, sagittal septa (and *black arrows*); 2, plantar surface of the plantar plate of the second toe; 3, deep transverse interme-tatarsal ligament; 4, tendons of flexor digitorum longus muscle; 5, tendons of flexor digitorum brevis muscle; 6, fibrous tendinous sheet for the flexor tendons of the second toe; 7, first lumbrical muscle; 8, second lumbrical muscle; 9, plantar surface of the plantar plate of the great toe; 10, tendon of flexor hallucis longus muscle; 11, fibrous tendinous sheet for the flexor hallucis longus tendon; 12, tendon of the adductor hallucis muscle; 13, oblique head of the adductor hallucis muscle; 14, transverse head of the adductor hallucis muscle; 15, flexor hallu-cis brevis muscle; 16, tendon of the abductor hallucis muscle; 17, lateral sesamoid (*outlined area*); 18, medial sesamoid (*outlined area*). (Figure Copyright © Pau Golanó 2014.)

head. Hamilton and colleagues,[86] on the other hand, found that the aponeurosis of the medial head was 2.4-fold larger than the lateral head (transversal section). Probably for these reasons, Barouk and colleagues[68] and later, Colombier[87] abandoned tenot-omy of both heads in favor of isolated tenotomy of the medial head of the gastrocnemius.

Level 4

The only technique performed at this level is deep gastrocnemius or soleus recession.

The technique is known as the Baumann procedure[6] and involves division of the deep fascia of the gastrocnemius muscle using 1 or 2 parallel transverse incisions.[86,88]

The incision is made on the medial side at mid-calf and runs posteriorly, after blunt dissection, to the interval between the gastrocnemius and soleus muscles. The deep fascia of the gastrocnemius muscle is divided using 1 or more transverse incisions. The posterior aponeurosis of the soleus muscle can also be divided, bearing in mind that the transverse incision must be more distal than the others to avoid overlap.[6]

From an anatomic perspective, the incision endangers the greater saphenous vein and saphenous nerve[6]; therefore, these structures must be identified and retracted during surgery.

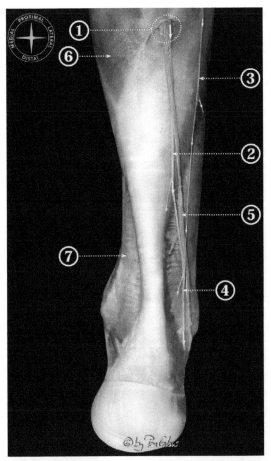

Fig. 21. Posterior view of a superficial dissection of the leg demonstrating the relationship between the sural nerve and the calcaneal tendon. 1, perforation point of the superficial fascia of the leg for the sural nerve (and in this case for the lesser saphenous vein too); 2, medial sural cutaneous nerve (branch of tibial nerve); 3, lateral sural cutaneous nerve (branch of common peroneal nerve); 4, sural nerve; 5, lesser saphenous vein; 6, posterior superficial fascia of the leg; 7, posterior deep fascia of the leg. (Figure Copyright © Pau Golanó 2014.)

Some investigators advise that to avoid injury to these structures, the incision should be made 2 fingerbreadths' distance posterior to the posteromedial aspect of the tibia[88] or 1 fingerbreadth's distance posterior to the palpable area between the bellies of the soleus and gastrocnemius.[6]

Level 3

The procedures that can be performed at level 3 include open gastrocnemius recession (Strayer procedure),[4] endoscopic gastrocnemius recession,[69,70] and gastrocnemius intramuscular aponeurotic recession.[89]

Today, most approaches at this level are endoscopic. In 2002, Trevino and Panchbhavi[69] first described endoscopic gastrocnemius recession. In a cadaver study, Saxena[70] described use of the endoscopic approach in 5 patients.

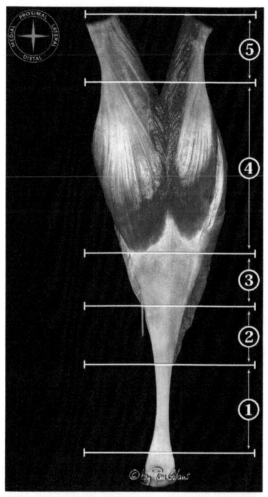

Fig. 22. Surgical anatomy of the triceps surae. The triceps surae is divided into 5 levels for a better understanding of the structures resected during surgery at each level, following the division proposed by Lamm and colleagues.[85] 1, Level 1: calcaneal tendon; 2, Level 2: starts in the common aponeurotic tendon of the soleus and gastrocnemius and finishes at the distal end of the soleus muscle; 3, Level 3: starts where the muscle bellies of the gastrocnemius merge to form the calcaneal tendon and finishes where the aponeuroses of the soleus and gastrocnemius merge; 4, Level 4: comprises the medial and lateral bellies of the gastrocnemius; 5, Level 5: comprises the proximal insertion and tendons of the medial and lateral heads of the gastrocnemius. (Figure Copyright © Pau Golanó 2014.)

The gastrocnemius aponeurosis is defined anatomically as the aponeurotic fascia. This fascia arises below the distal point of the medial head and finishes when it merges with the deep aponeurotic fibers of the soleus to form the calcaneal tendon.[31] This junction, known as the conjoint junction, is the area where the entry points for endoscopic gastrocnemius recession are made (**Fig. 24**). Elson and colleagues[30] and Tashjian and colleagues[90] based their measurements to locate this area on the length of the fibula. The authors believe that this approach is more suitable than that proposed

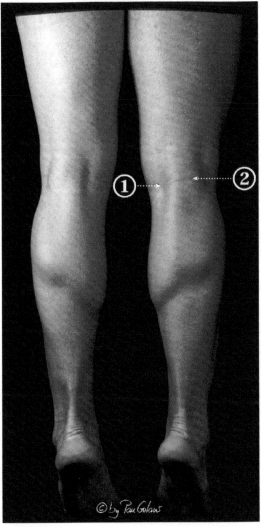

Fig. 23. Cutaneous references at the popliteal region. 1, cutaneous fossa; 2, flexion crease of the knee. (Figure Copyright © Pau Golanó 2014.)

elsewhere,[31] because it provides a value based on the relative length of the leg. However, most surgeons use the distance in centimeters from the calcaneal tuberosity as their reference point. Carl and Barrett[31] suggested that the ideal placement of surgical instruments is a reference point 16.4 cm proximal to the calcaneal tuberosity, because this area is considered safe for endoscopy. Furthermore, this safe area extends 1.79 cm distal and proximal to the reference point.[31] Endoscopy, which can be performed using 1 or 2 entry points, should ensure that the cannula is placed between the sural fascia and the aponeurosis of the insertion of the gastrocnemius to enable recession of the fascia. However, the authors' experience, based on 10 cadaveric dissections to study the anatomy of the triceps surae, is not consistent with the belief that recession at this level (the "safe endoscopic zone" described by Carl and

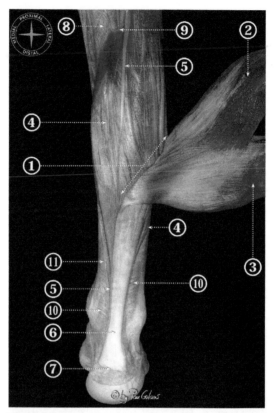

Fig. 24. Muscular dissection of the leg to show the components of the triceps surae (gastrocnemius muscle is rejected to reveal soleus posterior aponeurosis). 1, area of insertion of the gastrocnemius aponeurosis into the soleus posterior aponeurosis (conjoint junction); 2, lateral head of gastrocnemius muscle; 3, medial head of gastrocnemius muscle; 4, soleus posterior aponeurosis; 5, plantaris tendon; 6, calcaneal tendon; 7, insertional area of the calcaneal tendon; 8, popliteus muscle; 9, tendinous arch of the soleus muscle; 10, posterior deep fascia of the leg; 11, medial intermuscular septum. (Figure Copyright © Pau Golanó 2014.)

Barrett[31]) only affects the aponeurosis of the gastrocnemius; it also affects the posterior aponeurosis of the soleus. Therefore, sensu stricto, the term "endoscopic gastrocnemius recession" is not appropriate. In the authors' opinion, a more appropriate term is "endoscopic triceps surae recession."

Endoscopy provides a better cosmetic outcome, although it carries a considerable risk of sural nerve injury. The complication rate can reach 22.2%.[76] The importance of the association between the sural nerve and the endoscopic entry point led to the study by Tashjian and colleagues,[74] who found the distance between the sural nerve and the lateral border of the gastrocnemius and soleus to be 12 mm (range, 7–17 mm). This short distance justifies the use of a medial entry point in this type of endoscopic procedure.

Another procedure performed at this level is the technique originally described by Strayer,[4] which involves recession of the gastrocnemius aponeurosis using open surgery. This approach has the disadvantage of a poor cosmetic outcome, namely, excessively large scars. Consequently, several investigators have improved this

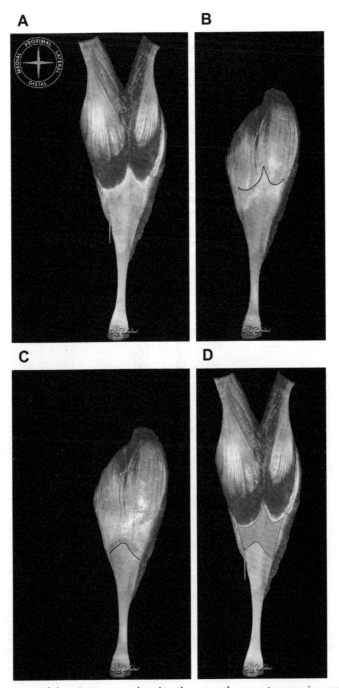

Fig. 25. Dissection of the triceps surae showing the area where gastrocnemius aponeurosis is not fused with soleus posterior aponeurosis. (*A*) Posterior view of the triceps surae. (*B*) Posterior view of the triceps surae (muscular bellies of medial and lateral head of gastrocnemius muscle have been resected). (*C*) Posterior view of the triceps surae (gastrocnemius aponeurosis has been resected until the level of fusion of gastrocnemius and soleus aponeuroses). (*D*) Posterior view of the triceps surae, showing the area where gastrocnemius aponeurosis can be transected in isolation before fusion with soleus posterior aponeurosis (area has been marked using Adobe Photoshop). (Figure Copyright © Pau Golanó 2014.)

technique using minimally invasive entry points. An example of these improvements is gastrocnemius intramuscular aponeurotic recession, as described by Blitz and Rush,[89] who used the minimally invasive technique and also defined the term gastroc run-out to illustrate the zone of gastrocnemius aponeurosis free of both gastrocnemius muscular belly and of soleus aponeurosis. Within this area the gastrocnemius aponeurosis can be transected in isolation (**Fig. 25**). The authors consider this anatomic detail to be of high importance, because a recession of both the soleus and gastrocnemius muscle will produce a more debilitating effect in the leg of the patient, using either the Strayer or the endoscopic gastrocnemius recession procedures.

Based on anatomic studies,[91,92] it has been demonstrated that the aponeurosis of the lateral head of the gastrocnemius is longer than that of the medial head. It has also been observed that the insertion of the aponeurosis of the gastrocnemius into the soleus can be by direct, long, or short insertion (conjoint junction) (**Fig. 26**), thus leading to variations in the difficulty of the surgical procedure. In a long insertion, it is easier to perform an isolated recession of the aponeurosis of the gastrocnemius. On the other hand, in a short or direct insertion, the difficulty in separating the aponeuroses

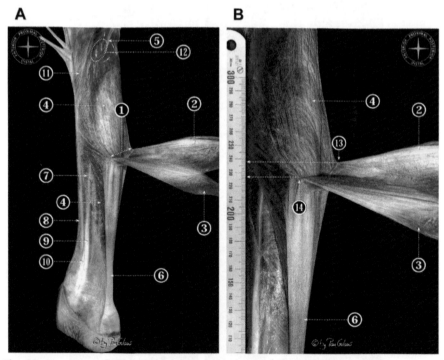

Fig. 26. Dissection of the superficial muscular layer of the leg showing the insertion of gastrocnemius aponeurosis into the soleus (conjoint junction). (*A*) Posteromedial view. (*B*) Photomacrography showing the conjoint junction in detail. 1, conjoint junction; 2, lateral head of gastrocnemius muscle; 3, medial head of gastrocnemius muscle; 4, posterior aponeurosis of soleus muscle; 5, tendinous arch of soleus muscle; 6, calcaneal tendon; 7, posterior deep fascia of the leg; 8, medial surface of the tibia; 9, flexor digitorum longus muscle; 10, tibialis posterior tendon; 11, popliteus muscle; 12, neurovascular bundle passing through the tendinous arch of the soleus muscle (posterior tibial vein, posterior tibial artery, tibial nerve); 13, level of insertion of the lateral head of gastrocnemius muscle; 14, level of insertion of the medial head of gastrocnemius muscle. (Figure Copyright © Pau Golanó 2014.)

of the gastrocnemius and soleus can lead to an iatrogenic recession of the soleus aponeurosis (see earlier discussion).

Levels 2 and 1

Given that this article is about the surgical anatomy of gastrocnemius, the surgical anatomy of more distal levels is not discussed, as they involve recession of the whole triceps surae.[1,3]

SUMMARY

A broad knowledge of the anatomy and biomechanics of the triceps surae is essential for an understanding of the etiology of the shortening or contracture of the gastrocnemius and its treatment.

ACKNOWLEDGMENTS

The authors are grateful to Thomas O'Boyle for editorial assistance. We thank Dr Cristina Manzanares for her institutional support at the University of Barcelona.

REFERENCES

1. Vulpius O, Stoffel A. Orthopädische operationslehre. Stuttgart (Germany): Verlag von Ferdinand Enke; 1913 [in German].
2. Silfverskiöld N. Reduction of the uncrossed two-joint muscles of the leg to one-joint muscles in spastic conditions. Acta Chir Scand 1924;56:315–30.
3. Baker LD. A rational approach to the surgical needs of the cerebral palsy patient. J Bone Joint Surg Am 1956;38:313–20.
4. Strayer LM Jr. Recession of the gastrocnemius: an operation to relieve spastic contracture of the calf muscles. J Bone Joint Surg Am 1950;32:671–6.
5. Barouk LS. Les brièvetés musculaires de l'infime moteur cérébral (IMC). Rev Chir Orthop Reparatrice Appar Mot 1984;70(S2):163–6 [in French].
6. Baumann JU, Koch HG. Lengthening of the anterior aponeurosis of the gastrocnemius muscle. Operat Orthop Traumatol 1989;1(1):254–8 [in German].
7. Kowalski C, Diebold P, Pennecot GF. Le tendon calcanéen court. Encyclopédie medico-chirurgicale. Paris: Elsevier; 1999. p. 27–60. [in French].
8. DiGiovanni CW, Kuo R, Tejwani N, et al. Isolated gastrocnemius tightness. J Bone Joint Surg Am 2002;86(6):962–70.
9. Barouk LS. Gastrocnemius proximal release. In: Barouk LS, editor. Forefoot reconstruction. Paris: Springer; 2003. p. 158–67.
10. Rush SM, Ford LA, Hamilton GA. Morbidity associated with high gastrocnemius recession: retrospective review of 126 cases. J Foot Ankle Surg 2006;45(3): 156–60.
11. Rouviere H, Delmas A. 11th edition. Anatomía humana, vol. 3. Barcelona (Spain): Masson; 2005. p. 421 [in Spanish].
12. Gray H. Gray's anatomy. New York: Barnes and Nobles Inc; 2010. p. 412.
13. Cummins EJ, Anson BJ, Carr BW, et al. The structure of the calcaneal tendon [of Achilles] in relation to orthopaedic surgery: with additional observations on the plantaris muscle. Surg Gynecol Obstet 1946;83:107–16.
14. Daseler EH, Anson BJ. The plantaris muscle: an anatomical study of 750 specimens. J Bone Surg Am 1943;25(4):822–7.
15. Nayak SR, Krishnamurthy A, Ramanathan L, et al. Anatomy of plantaris muscle: a study in adult Indians. Clin Ter 2010;161(3):249–52.

16. Vanderhooft E. The frequency of and relationship between the palmaris longus and plantaris tendons. Am J Orthop 1996;25(1):38–41.
17. Tylkowski CM, Horan M, Oeffinger DJ. Outcomes of gastrocnemius-soleus complex lengthening for isolated equinus contracture in children with cerebral palsy. J Pediatr Orthop 2009;29(7):771–8.
18. El Shewy MT, El Barbary HM, Abdel-Ghani H. Repair of chronic rupture of the Achilles tendon using 2 intratendinous flaps from the proximal gastrocnemius-soleus complex. Am J Sports Med 2009;37(8):1570–7.
19. Shalabi A, Kristoffersen-Wilberg M, Svensson L, et al. Eccentric training of the gastrocnemius-soleus complex in chronic Achilles tendinopathy results in decreased tendon volume and intratendinous signal as evaluated by MRI. Am J Sports Med 2004;32(5):1286–96.
20. Firth GB, McMullan M, Chin T, et al. Lengthening of the gastrocnemius-soleus complex: an anatomical and biomechanical study in human cadavers. J Bone Joint Surg Am 2013;95(16):1489–96.
21. Federative Committee on Anatomical Terminology. International anatomical terminology. Stuttgart (Germany): Thieme; 1998.
22. Stopford JS. The supracondyloid tubercles of the femur and the attachment of the gastrocnemius muscle to the femoral diaphysis. J Anat Physiol 1914;49(Pt 1):80–4.
23. Minowa T, Murakami G, Kura H, et al. Does the fabella contribute to the reinforcement of the posterolateral corner of the knee by inducing the development of associated ligaments? J Orthop Sci 2004;9:59–65.
24. Duncan W, Dahm DL. Clinical anatomy of the fabella. Clin Anat 2003;16(5):448–9.
25. Robertson A, Jones SC, Paes R, et al. The fabella: a forgotten source of knee pain? Knee 2004;11(3):243–5.
26. Heideman GM, Baynes KE, Mautz AP, et al. Fabella fracture with CT imaging: a case report. Emerg Radiol 2011;18(4):357–61.
27. Franceschi F, Longo UG, Ruzzini L, et al. Dislocation of an enlarged fabella as uncommon cause of knee pain: a case report. Knee 2007;14(4):330–2.
28. Fritschy D, Fasel J, Imbert JC, et al. The popliteal cyst. Knee Surg Sports Traumatol Arthrosc 2006;14(7):623–8.
29. Kawashima T, Takeishi H, Yoshitomi S, et al. Anatomical study of the fabella, fabellar complex and its clinical implications. Surg Radiol Anat 2007;29(8):611–6.
30. Elson DW, Whiten S, Hillman SJ, et al. The conjoint junction of the triceps surae: implications for gastrocnemius tendon lengthening. Clin Anat 2007;20(8):924–8.
31. Carl T, Barrett SL. Cadaveric assessment of the gastrocnemius aponeurosis to assist in the preoperative planning for two-portal endoscopic gastrocnemius recession (EGR). Foot 2005;15(3):137–40.
32. Testut L, Latarjet A. 2nd edition. Anatomía humana, vol. 1. Barcelona (Spain): Salvat; 1990. p. 1165 [in Spanish].
33. Jakubiet MG, Jakubietz DF, Gruenert JG, et al. Adequacy of palmaris longus and plantaris tendons for tendon grafting. J Hand Surg Am 2011;36(4):695–8.
34. Dos Santos MA, Bertelli JA, Kechele PR, et al. Anatomical study of the plantaris tendon: reliability as a tendo-osseous graft. Surg Radiol Anat 2009;31(1):59–61.
35. Delgado GJ, Chung CB, Lektrakul N, et al. Tennis leg. Clinical US study of 141 patients and anatomic investigation of four cadavers with MR Imaging and US. Radiology 2002;224(1):112–9.
36. Spina AA. The plantaris muscle: anatomy, injury, imaging and treatment. J Can Chiropr Assoc 2007;51(3):158–65.

37. Parratte B, Tatu L, Vuillier F, et al. Intramuscular distribution of nerves in the human triceps surae muscle: anatomical bases for treatment of spastic drop foot with botulinum toxin. Surg Radiol Anat 2002;24(2):91–6.
38. Loh EY, Agur AM, McKee NH. Intramuscular innervation of the human soleus muscle: A 3D model. Clin Anat 2003;16(5):378–82.
39. Finni T, Hodgson JA, Lai AM, et al. Mapping of movement in the isometrically contracting human soleus muscle reveals details of its structural and functional complexity. J Appl Physiol (1985) 2003;95(5):2128–33.
40. Agur AM, Thow-Hing VN, Ball KA, et al. Documentation and three-dimensional modelling of human soleus muscle architecture. Clin Anat 2003;16(4):285–93.
41. Reid DG. On the structure of the human soleus muscle. J Anat 1918;52(Pt 4): 442–8.
42. Sinha U, Sinha S, Hodgson JA, et al. Human soleus muscle architecture at different ankle joint angles from magnetic resonance diffusion tensor imaging. J Appl Physiol (1985) 2011;110(3):807–19.
43. Edwards DA. The blood supply and lymphatic drainage of tendons. J Anat 1946;80(Pt 3):147–52.
44. Gillies H, Chalmers J. The management of fresh ruptures of the tendon achillis. J Bone Joint Surg Am 1970;52(2):337–43.
45. Szaro P, Witkowski G, Śmigielski R, et al. Fascicles of the adult human Achilles tendon: an anatomical study. Ann Anat 2009;191(6):586–93.
46. Doral MN, Alam M, Bozkurt M, et al. Functional anatomy of the Achilles tendon. Knee Surg Sports Traumatol Arthrosc 2010;18(5):638–43.
47. Lagergren C, Lindholm A. Vascular distribution in the Achilles tendon: an angiographic and microangiographic study. Acta Chir Scand 1959;116(5–6):491–5.
48. Carr AJ, Norris SH. The blood supply of the calcaneal tendon. J Bone Joint Surg Br 1989;71(1):100–1.
49. Schmidt-Rohlfing B, Graf J, Schneider U, et al. The blood supply of Achilles tendon. Int Orthop 1992;16(1):29–31.
50. Chen TM, Rozen WM, Pan WR, et al. The arterial anatomy of the Achilles tendon: anatomical study and clinical implications. Clin Anat 2009;22(3):377–85.
51. Shaw HM, Vázquez OT, Gonagle DM, et al. Development of the human Achilles tendon enthesis organ. J Anat 2008;213(6):718–24.
52. Yepes H, Tang M, Geddes C, et al. Digital vascular mapping of the integument about the Achilles tendon. J Bone Joint Surg Am 2010;92(5):1215–20.
53. Silver RL, Garza J, Rang M. The myth of muscle balance. J Bone Joint Surg Br 1985;67(3):432–7.
54. Li L, Landin D, Grodesky J, et al. The function of gastrocnemius as a knee flexor at selected knee and ankle angles. J Electromyogr Kinesiol 2002; 12(5):385–90.
55. Winter DA. Energy generation and absorption at the ankle and knee during fast, natural, and slow cadences. Clin Orthop Relat Res 1983;(175):147–54.
56. Honeine JL, Schieppati M, Gagey O, et al. The functional role of the triceps surae muscle during human locomotion. PLoS One 2013;8(1):e52943.
57. Cohen JC. Anatomy and biomechanical aspects of the gastrocsoleus complex. Foot Ankle Clin N Am 2009;14(4):617–26.
58. Arandes R, Viladot A. Biomecánica del calcáneo. Med Clín 1953;23:25–34 [in Spanish].
59. Snow SW, Bohne WH, DiCarlo E, et al. Anatomy of the Achilles tendon and plantar fascia in relation to the calcaneus in various age groups. Foot Ankle Int 1995;16(7):418–21.

60. Stecco C, Corradin M, Macchi V, et al. Plantar fascia anatomy and its relationship with Achilles tendon and paratenon. J Anat 2013;223(6):665–76.
61. Bolívar YA, Munuera PV, Padillo JP. Relationship between tightness of the posterior muscles of the lower limb and plantar fasciitis. Foot Ankle Int 2013; 34(1):42–8.
62. Monteagudo M, Maceira E, Garcia-Virto V, et al. Chronic plantar fasciitis: plantar fasciotomy versus gastrocnemius recession. Int Orthop 2013;37(9):1845–50.
63. Hedrick MR. The plantar aponeurosis. Foot Ankle Int 1996;17(10):646–9.
64. Bojsen-Moller F, Flagstad KE. Plantar aponeurosis and internal architecture of the ball of the foot. J Anat 1976;121(Pt 3):599–611.
65. Moraes do Carmo CC, Almeida Melão LI, Lemos Weber MF, et al. Anatomical features of plantar aponeurosis: Cadaveric study using ultrasonography and magnetic resonance imaging. Skeletal Radiol 2008;37(10):929–35.
66. Grapow M. Die Anatomie und physiologische bedeutung der palmar aponeurose. Archiv für Anatomie und Physiologie, Anatomische Abteilung. 1887. p. 143–58. [in German].
67. Henkel A. Die aponeurosis plantaris. Archiv fiur Anatomie und Physiologie, Anatomische Abteilung, Supplemenit-Band. 1913. p. 113–23. [in German].
68. Barouk LS, Barouk P, Toullec E. Brièveté des muscles gastrocnémiens et pathologie de l'avant-pied: La libération proximale chirurgicale. Med Chir Pied 2005; 21:143–52 [in French].
69. Trevino SG, Panchbhavi VK. Technique of endoscopic gastrocnemius recession: a cadaver study. Foot Ankle Surg 2002;8(1):45–7.
70. Saxena A. Endoscopic gastrocnemius tenotomy. J Foot Ankle Surg 2002;41(1): 57–8.
71. Kiewiet NJ, Holthusen SM, Bohay DR, et al. Gastrocnemius recession for chronic noninsertional Achilles tendinopathy. Foot Ankle Int 2013;34(4):481–5.
72. De los Santos-Real R, Morales-Muñoz P, Payo J, et al. Gastrocnemius proximal release with minimal incision: a modified technique. Foot Ankle Int 2012;33(9): 750–4.
73. Apaydin N, Bozkkurt M, Loukas M, et al. Relationships of the sural nerve with the calcaneal tendon: an anatomical study with surgical and clinical implications. Surg Radiol Anat 2009;31(10):775–80.
74. Tashjian RZ, Appel AJ, Benerjee R, et al. Anatomic study of the gastrocnemius-soleus junction and its relationship to the sural nerve. Foot Ankle Int 2003;24(6): 473–6.
75. Donley BG, Pinney SJ, Holmes J. Gastrocnemius recession. Tech Foot Ankle Surg 2003;2(1):35–9.
76. Adelman VR, Szczepanski JA, Adelman RP, et al. Endoscopic gastrocnemius recession ultrasound-guided analysis of length gained. Tech Foot Ankle Surg 2009;8(1):24–9.
77. Trevino S, Gibbs M, Panchbhavi V. Evaluation of results of endoscopic gastrocnemius recession. Foot Ankle Int 2005;26(5):359–64.
78. Roukis TS, Schweinberger MH. Complications associated with uni-portal endoscopic gastrocnemius recession in a diabetic patient population: an observational case series. J Foot Ankle Surg 2010;49(1):68–70.
79. Di Domenico LA, Adams HB, Garchar D. Endoscopic gastrocnemius recession for the treatment of gastrocnemius equinus. J Am Podiatr Med Assoc 2005; 95(4):410–3.
80. Saxena A, Widtfeldt A. Endoscopic gastrocnemius recession: preliminary report on 18 cases. J Foot Ankle Surg 2004;43(5):302–6.

81. Saraph V, Zwick EB, Uitz C, et al. The Baumann procedure for fixed contracture of the gastrosoleus in cerebral palsy: evaluation of function of the ankle after multilevel surgery. J Bone Joint Surg Br 2000;82(4):535–40.
82. Takahashi S, Shrestha A. The Vulpius procedure for correction of equinus deformity in patients with hemiplegia. J Bone Joint Surg Br 2002;84(7):978–80.
83. Kohls-Gatzoulis JA, Solan M. Results of proximal medial release of gastrocnemius. J Bone Joint Surg Br 2009;91(S2):361.
84. Javors JR, Klaaren HE. The Vulpius procedure for correction of equinus deformity in cerebral palsy. J Pediatr Orthop 1987;7(2):191–3.
85. Lamm BM, Paley D, Herzenberg JE. Gastrocnemius soleus recession: a simpler, more limited approach. J Am Podiatr Med Assoc 2005;95(1):18–25.
86. Hamilton PD, Brown M, Ferguson N, et al. Surgical anatomy of the proximal release of the gastrocnemius: a cadaveric study. Foot Ankle Int 2009;30(12):1202–6.
87. Colombier JA. Libération proximale pure dans la prise en charge thérapeutique des gastrocnemiens courts. Med Chir Pied 2006;22:156–7 [in French].
88. Herzenberg JE, Lamm BM, Corwin C, et al. Isolated recession of the gastrocnemius muscle: the Baumann procedure. Foot Ankle Int 2007;28(11):1154–9.
89. Blitz NM, Rush SM. The gastrocnemius intramuscular aponeurotic recession: a simplified method of gastrocnemius recession. Foot Ankle Surg 2007;46(2):133–8.
90. Tashjian RZ, Appel AJ, Benerjee R, et al. Endoscopic gastrocnemius recession: evaluation in a cadaver model. Foot Ankle Int 2003;24(8):607–13.
91. Blitz NM, Eliot DJ. Anatomical aspects of the gastrocnemius aponeurosis and its insertion: a cadaveric study. J Foot Ankle Surg 2007;46(2):101–8.
92. Blitz NM, Eliot DJ. Anatomical aspects of the gastrocnemius aponeurosis and its muscular bound portion: a cadaveric study. Part II. Foot Ankle Surg 2008;47(6):533–40.

The Gastrocnemius
A New Paradigm for the Human Foot and Ankle

 CrossMark

James Amis, MD

KEYWORDS

- Gastrocnemius • Calf contracture • Calf stretching • Surgical lengthening

KEY POINTS

- A silent gastrocnemius contracture can gradually do significant harm to the foot and ankle when left undetected and unattended.
- The calf is a common source of a majority of acquired, nontraumatic adult foot and ankle problems, such as plantar fasciitis, nontraumatic midfoot osteoarthritis, insertional Achilles tendinosis, posterior tibialis tendon dysfunction, and Achilles tendinitis.
- When it comes to surgical lengthening procedures, whether at the Achilles, at the musculotendinous junction, or more proximal, the search must move on to find the safest, most accurate, and quickest recovery method possible.
- Addressing the calf contracture as definitive treatment and, better yet, as prevention, will no doubt become a mainstay of the treatment of many foot and ankle problems.

INTRODUCTION

Until recently, attention to the gastrocnemius as a primary etiology in the foot and ankle has been sparse and not well understood. Understanding in this matter, however, is coming of age. As addressed in this issue of *Foot and Ankle Clinics of North America*, there is more to the gastrocnemius than meets the eye.

In order to move forward, 2 vital questions must be answered: Why would the calves tighten? and, more importantly, How does a tight calf actually cause problems remotely in the foot and ankle? In this overview I proffer a concept that explains why the human calf might tighten in otherwise normal people. Javier Pascual Huerta explains in detail elsewhere in this issue how an isolated gastrocnemius contracture mechanically damages the foot and ankle, with a particular emphasis on plantar fasciitis.

Once it is accepted that the gastrocnemius contracture, which is usually silent, is an integral problem, then 2 final challenges can be considered. The first is to identify all

Disclosures: None.
Lone Star Orthopaedics, 3219 Clifton Avenue, Suite 300, Cincinnati, OH 45220, USA
E-mail address: jamesamis@mac.com

Foot Ankle Clin N Am 19 (2014) 637–647
http://dx.doi.org/10.1016/j.fcl.2014.08.001
1083-7515/14/$ – see front matter Published by Elsevier Inc.

the problems that result, in part or principally, from this seemingly benign process. If the calf can be accurately linked to a particular pathologic entity, such as plantar fasciitis, then treatment in turn becomes more accurate. Then and only then can treating the calf be definitely chosen rather than just treating the result of this contracture (ie, symptomatic treatment of the foot). The second challenge is to refine the treatment of the gastrocnemius contracture itself, whether conservative stretching regimens or surgical lengthening. The ultimate challenge is the realization that if the gastrocnemius contracts with age, then this pathology can be avoided by appropriate preventative treatments.

A LIMITED REVIEW OF LITERATURE

The literature is now replete with evidence to support the association of the gastrocnemius and several foot and ankle conditions, including plantar fasciitis, insertional Achilles tendinosis, posterior tibialis tendon rupture, metatarsalgia, neuropathic ulcers, and others.[1–30] The expense of treating just plantar fasciitis every year in the United States is staggering. Tong and Furia[31] "...projected that in 2007 the cost of treatment to third-party payers ranged from \$192 to \$376 million." They went on to state, "Our estimates do not account for all diagnostic tests and treatments common for PF [plantar fasciitis]. As a result, it is likely that this study understates the true costs of care for the disease."

A consensus on a standard nonoperative treatment protocol has not been established,[2,12,17,19,29,32–45] in part because a majority of these studies have addressed only the apparent problem in the foot and not the cause (ie, the tight calf). The other problem with these protocols is that the treatment options are lumped together in a variety of combinations, including calf stretches, immobilization, rest, orthotics, injections, platelet-rich plasma and cortisone injections, physical therapy, ice, stretching, extracorporeal shock wave therapy, surgery, and so forth. Although each of these treatments alone might help symptoms to some extent, the variety of treatments available only serves to reinforce that the cause of the problem has not been well understood. Although calf stretching has been shown effective,[5,10,11,30,44–46] it has been mostly discounted because of a general feeling of lack of compliance in study groups. Yet, a prospective, randomized, double-blinded study on definitive Achilles stretching by Porter and colleagues[47] was a seminal yet largely overlooked work. Porter and colleagues standardized conservative treatment by examining "one of the more effective nonsurgical modalities for treatment of painful heel syndrome" comparing 2 calf stretching regimens and confirmed that Achilles stretching alone was an effective treatment. Other studies have shown the benefits of calf stretching also. This was subsequently confirmed by DiGiovanni and colleagues,[8] who concluded the "existence of isolated gastrocnemius contracture in the development of forefoot and/or midfoot pathology in otherwise healthy people. These data may have implications for preventative and therapeutic care of patients with chronic foot problems." They stated that it is the gastrocnemius muscle that is contracted, not the Achilles: "such equinus positioning of the foot has frequently been called an Achilles contracture. However, this is a misnomer because the majority of the perceived stiffness or stretch occurs within the muscle bellies themselves, not in the tendon; the tendon can be responsible for only about 3% to 5% of this change in position"; they further noted, "We suspect that this pathologic entity plays a vital role in chronic mechanical breakdown or inflammation of both the foot and ankle."

In many of these works, the measurement method is the Silfverskiöld test.[48] The amount of or lack of dorsiflexion an individual exhibits with this test may be supportive, but a negative Silfverskiöld test does not rule out the calf as the source of the pathology. In other words, a negative Silfverskiöld test does not confirm that there is not a clinically significant calf contracture present. More recently, Barouk and Toulec[49] and Abbassian and colleagues[1] described what I term the *modern method* to surgically lengthen the isolated gastrocnemius contracture, a proximal medial gastrocnemius release. Abbassian and colleagues commented, "Despite this, the exact etiology of the condition is still subject to debate...more recent study, however, reduced ankle dorsiflexion was associated with a much greater risk of developing the condition [plantar fasciitis] than either BMI [body mass index] or activity type." Although it is somewhat a leap of faith to surgically lengthen the gastrocnemius behind the knee to fix plantar fasciitis, this procedure has been demonstrated effective. It is possible in the future that this will be the gastrocnemius lengthening procedure of choice for the isolated gastrocnemius contracture after failed conservative treatment because it directly addresses the contracted gastrocnemius, the degree of release is controlled, and it allows for immediate weight bearing.

None of these concepts is new, as John Joseph Nutt[23] published his book *Diseases and Deformities of the Foot* in 1913, in which he discusses similar principles described by Dr Huerta in this issue. Nutt goes on to state, "Treatment consists in lengthening the gastrocnemius. As a very slight lengthening is all that is necessary, the tendo-Achilles being attached to so short a lever arm, an operation is scarcely demanded." The work of Barouk and Toulec[49] and Abbassian and colleagues,[1] follows this statement; however, I would contend that calf stretching would be equally as effective in a high percentage of cases. Nutt stated, "The chief characteristic of this condition is a shortening of the gastrocnemius and the soleus. This shortening is not enough to produce the deformity of equinous but limits dorsal flexion." What he essentially described in 1913 is the isolated gastrocnemius contracture.[8] The biggest takeaway from Nutt's work is the understanding of the ubiquitous source of calf contractures in otherwise normal humans, and he alludes to the mechanism of injury placed on the foot as a result (**Figs. 1** and **2**).

THE ORIGINS OF THE CALF CONTRACTURE

Where there may be many reasons why this progressive gastrocnemius tightness occurs, there are 4 common categories described in this article: activity changes, physiologic changes in muscles and tendons, genetics, and reverse evolution. Three of these principles generally apply to all muscles, whereas the fourth, reverse evolution, applies particularly to the calf, hamstring, and hip flexors.

The current thoughts on epidemiology of many acquired foot and ankle problems are addressed first. The prevailing thought on the epidemiology of these resulting problems may not be correct.[16,25,41,50] The factors cited—obesity, sedentary life style, medical comorbities, shoe wear, concrete floors, overuse, and so forth—although commonly associated with various foot and ankle problems, all may have a common pathway as the cause of these problems via calf contractures. In other words, although they are indeed present, these factors may not directly cause the resulting foot or ankle problems or pathology. Each of these factors creates an avenue to an increase in the human calf contracture, which in turn causes the foot and ankle pathology. If a tightened gastrocnemius is implicated as the cause of foot and ankle problems, then how and why would this happen in otherwise normal people? My premise is based on the notion that a gastrocnemius contracture is a contracture of the connective tissue surrounding and within the muscle, and less the tendon,[8] and may have little to do with the muscle fibers themselves.

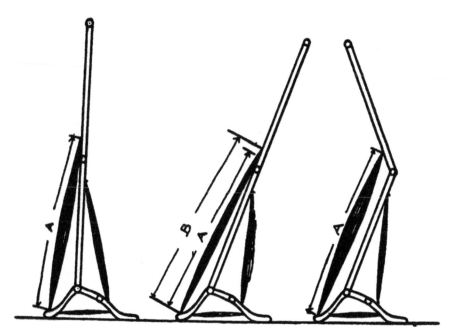

Fig. 1. Nutt depicts the effect gastrocnemius has as the passenger passes over the planted foot. (*From* Nutt J. Diseases and deformities of the foot. New York: E.B.Treat & Co; 1913. Available at: books.google.com/books?id=UWgQAAAAYAAJ.)

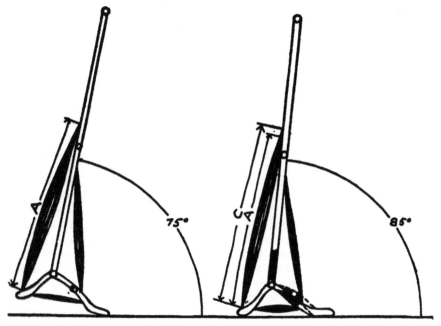

Fig. 2. Nutt depicts the strain of the plantar supportive tissue placed under additional tension and "lowering of the dome" or additional dorsal compressive forces placed on the longitudinal arch. (*From* Nutt J. Diseases and deformities of the foot. New York: E.B.Treat & Co; 1913. Available at: books.google.com/books?id=UWgQAAAAYAAJ.)

ACTIVITY CHANGES: LIFESTYLE INFLUENCES
General Decreased Activities as People Age

As people age, they are simply not as active as they may have been when they were children. Because of this more limited exposure to range of motion, muscle-tendon units fail to reach their ultimate length with regularity. A society of an increasingly sedentary lifestyle does not help matters either. If these stationary habits occur consistently and over a long enough period of time, the muscle-tendon units will shorten. The law of Davis[23] says that over time soft tissue contracts to the shortest position possible, given the opportunity. The isolated gastronemius contracture is a slower process, taking years to develop, but is the most common form of contraction of the lifestyle changes. This concept occurs every day when people experience the start-up stiffness or pain that settles as they get going. When sitting or sleeping, the ankles are in relaxed equinus and the calves tighten, only to stretch out just enough when becoming more mobile again.

Recent Changes in Activities

Bed rest due to illness or recovery from recent injury or surgery and even after pregnancy often causes a dramatic change in activities, such that the muscles, especially the calf, tighten up because of the abrupt reduction of otherwise normal mobility. As the gastrocnemius relaxes, it is under little, if any, tension, and according to the law of Davis, the calves get tighter. Then a return to normal activities creates problems solely because of the resulting calf contracture. This is a relatively quick process, taking just weeks to a few months.

Athletes and Increased Activity Situations

On the other end of the spectrum, many athletes, in particular distance runners, seem more at risk for contracture. One would think that athletes should be immune to this phenomenon; however, the repetitive action of running, especially for joggers, raises frequent issues. While running, the gastrocnemius and hamstrings of these athletes are not extended to their full length. In fact, slow motion video shows that the knee only comes to full extension in distance running after toe off and the ankle is plantarflexed as opposed to walking. During a high-mileage run, these muscle groups are overactive, and the opposing muscles, the quadriceps, and the anterior tibialis might get relatively weaker. Over time, the muscles eventually adapt to this shortened position.

PHYSIOLOGIC CHANGES TO MUSCLES AND TENDONS: INTERNAL INFLUENCE

There are definable physiologic changes that take place with aging when it comes to collagen and connective tissue. Cross-linking of collagen increases with age, and connective soft tissues get less compliant and lock the structure in the shortened position if allowed to do so. No doubt this is part of the law of Davis. In addition, the percentage of elastin in connective tissues reduces, which lowers the flexibility of muscles and tendons. This is a fact of aging and is mostly inescapable.

GENETICS

There is no doubt that genetics play, if nothing else, a subtle role in the progressive contracture of connective tissue. This would account for a possible familial proclivity to calf tightness or other muscle groups.

Genetics might also account as to why an individual person might be more prone to muscle contractures that lead to tendon and joint problems in multiple areas of the body or recurrent issues in one location. Some people experience muscle tightness more than others and genetics could be a reason this might occur.

REVERSE EVOLUTION: THE HUMAN INFLUENCE AND THE PREDILECTION PATTERN

Evolution suggests that humans evolved from quadrupeds to a bipedal species, but bipedal gait, as a primary method of locomotion, evolved approximately 2.2 to 3 million years ago.[22,51] Before that time, bipedal gait was used by human ancestors, but only part time. In order for the human foot to adapt to bipedal gait, 2 basic structural changes were required. In the leg, certain muscle groups had to lengthen whereas their opposing muscle groups had to shorten. Simultaneously, the ankle had to unwind and dorsiflex approximately 70°. This dorsiflexion brings the heel down to contact the ground, thus making the foot plantigrade. Additionally, the knee and the hip had to extend to achieve the positioning to allow for a bipedal gait.

There are 2 key lower extremity muscle groups that certainly adapted late in this evolutionary process. In the quadruped, the hamstrings and the triceps surae (gastrocnemius and soleus) are all shortened as the knee is continuously flexed and the ankle joint is in a highly plantar flexed position.

In the course of evolution, these muscle groups (hip flexors, hamstrings, and gastro-csoleus) had to lengthen while the opposing muscle groups (quadriceps and anterior tibialis) had to shorten and gain power. Because these muscle groups adapted later in the evolutionary process, they are the first to move backward and tighten as a person ages, reverting back to their former positions. This is called a predilection pattern, leading to many problems with the calves and the hamstrings. This relative motor imbalance is due, in part, to this evolutionary process and also as a function of the calf, which is required to be stronger for normal human bipedal locomotion. Simultaneous with these muscle changes, to provide a larger weight-bearing base for balance and a lever arm that could adequately propel humans forward in bipedal mode, it was necessary for the foot to drop out of its equinus position, moving the heel to the ground. This rotation of approximately 70° mostly occurs at the ankle joint. This concept can be examined further by looking at the perfect foot.

The Perfect Foot

The perfect foot, from a mechanical standpoint, would be one that evolution left behind long ago, as humans moved away from being quadrupeds. Structurally, a horse or dog has a better foot for wear and abuse than humans. It would be correct to argue that this might be the case because quadrupeds weight bear on 4 legs and, therefore, there is less force exerted on the hind foot. When considering the foot as a biomechanical structure unto itself and the forces humans put on each of theirs through every day, however, it is apparent that the construction of the foot for a quadruped is more mechanically sound; however, the weight-bearing platform of an equinus foot is too small for prolonged maintenance of a bipedal gait. So, the human foot evolved and rotated to place the heel on the ground (described previously). This adaptation provided a much larger plantar surface area for improved force distribution, balance, and necessary leverage for bipedal locomotion. This same new foot position placed the human foot in a biomechanically disadvantaged position, however, due to new leveraged forces it had to withstand.

With weight bearing, the human foot is oriented such that forces shift from a vertical, pure compressive load (perfect foot) to leveraged/bending or vector forces, resulting in higher compressive (dorsal foot and anterior ankle) and tensile forces (plantar foot and posterior ankle). Vector or bending forces clearly produce more asymmetric force on the parts of the system compared with vertical axial loading. Evolution robbed people of stable axial forces, creating bending forces.

The Gastrocnemius: Cause and Effect

If it is believed and accepted that the isolated gastrocnemius contracture is associated with problems in the foot and ankle, there must be a valid reason how this can happen. Nutt described this mechanical linkage in 1913 in the form of Schaeffer's foot.[23] Today, Huerta describes in more detail how a tight gastrocnemius causes plantar fasciitis.

When younger, a flexible, compliant gastrocnemius allows the necessary smoother deceleration of ankle dorsiflexion as the ankle progresses forward late in the ankle rocker phase just as the forefoot rocker begins.[52] The forces are gradual and dampened producing a softer end point, thus a more cushioned force transfer to the foot and ankle.

The damaging forces occur with the isolated gastrocnemius contracture when a tremendous, leveraged force is transmitted to the foot and ankle as the tibia and body pass over the planted or stance foot. Instead of a gradual force transfer, which occurs when younger, there is an abrupt end point in forward progression of necessary ankle dorsiflexion. This effect occurs during the late part of midstance or the ankle rocker phase, just before the heel lifts off the ground. If the calf becomes contracted, this indirect leveraged force is exponentially magnified, creating abnormal, pathologic bending or vector stress to the foot and ankle, thus resulting in stress and strain to the joints and supporting ligaments and tendons. Dorsal compressive and plantar tension forces are magnified. It is also at this point in the gait cycle that individuals who have symptomatic plantar fasciitis demonstrate a characteristic shortened type of antalgic gait as they begin to walk with a characteristic limp. This is the gait of effective pain avoidance until the rest induced by the shortened gastrocnemius can lengthen just enough to allow the forces foot or ankle to reduce, followed by improvement of the gait. Over time, and as a result of taking thousands of steps per day, the foot and ankle succumb to an occult, unrecognized overuse, which ultimately leads to damage.

DISCUSSION

I believe that there is a simple, singular, silent, and remote cause of the many foot and ankle problems, which are mechanically created, leading to incremental damage to the foot and ankle through leveraged forces: the human calf that becomes too tight with age. In short, the isolated gastrocnemius contracture is the common denominator that leads to the many of the human nontraumatic foot and ankle problems. Calves tighten with age: activity changes, physiologic changes in muscles and tendons, genetics, and reverse evolution.

No doubt many more studies will and should emerge that qualify and quantify the role of the tight gastrocnemius on the human foot and ankle. It is likely that study methods, such as high resolution and ultra–high-speed gait laboratory motion analysis, will show this concept to be correct, which, in turn will lead to improved prevention and treatment efforts.

The Silfverskiöld test, in my experience, is only an approximate estimate as a clinical test and is generally only useful for following the results of a particular treatment method. Historically, the Silfverskiöld test, relied on in clinical studies[1,5,20,25,37,38,47,50,53] for the subtle or isolated gastrocnemius contracture, will likely be found to have been a hindrance to understanding. Even though Abbassian and colleagues[1] used the Silfverskiöld test, they were suspicious of its validity. A negative Silfverskiöld test does not exclude the gastrocnemius as a possible cause of the underlying foot or ankle problem. The symptoms and even the diagnosis itself may be the best link to the tight gastrocnemius as the culprit. The classic symptoms, such as start-up pain or stiffness, or even the diagnosis itself, such as posterior tibialis dysfunction or insertional Achilles tendinosis, determine the cause, not this test. In other words, if patients have plantar fasciitis, then by default they have calves that are too tight regardless of what the Silfverskiöld test indicates. Think of it as sort of reverse logic: where there is smoke there is fire, even if the fire cannot be seen.

It has been postulated that epidemiologic factors, such as obesity, sedentary life style, medical comorbities, shoe wear, concrete floors, advanced age, female gender, and overuse issues, to name a few, are responsible for a variety of foot and ankle pathology.[2,16,25,27,28,34,39,41,50,54,55] Although these factors might consistently coexist with a variety of foot and ankle problems and seem to have a causal relationship, it is my assertion that they have little if any direct relationship.

The singular and real association of each of these epidemiologic factors is a contracture of the gastrocnemius muscle, which is camouflaged in this list. Most every other cause of these foot and ankle problems is likely mediated by contributing to the degree and/or rate of an already contracting gastrocnemius. These problems promote gastrocnemius tightness, which in time causes incremental damage to the foot and/or ankle. To put it frankly, the obvious evidence of this is that overweight people with plantar fasciitis stretch and get over their problem and they are still overweight. Women have a calf-lengthening procedure for insertional Achilles tendinosis with resolution of their problem and they are still women. Older people stretch and move on pain-free, yet they do not get magically younger. Gradual, silent calf contracture happens in most people, some less and some more, depending on life choices and circumstances.

SUMMARY

It seems that merely being human places a risk for developing acquired foot and ankle problems. This damage is mediated through the gastrocnemius that tightens for several reasons with age and these same contracted calves do incremental harm to the human foot and ankle. Drs Nutt[23] and Huerta have eloquently described how a silent gastrocnemius contracture, that seemingly has little to do with the foot and ankle, can gradually do so much harm when left undetected and unattended.

Considering this knowledge, I assert, if not challenge, that the calf is a common source of a majority of acquired, nontraumatic adult foot and ankle problems, such as plantar fasciitis, nontraumatic midfoot osteoarthritis, insertional Achilles tendinosis, posterior tibialis tendon dysfunction, and Achilles tendinitis, to name a few. Further investigation should sort out these associations and issues.

As the realization and understanding of the ubiquitous role of the contracted gastrocnemius in many foot and ankle problems move forward, so will the search for optimal treatment: nonoperative and operative.

Controversy, varying opinions, and even urban myth abound when it comes to the best method of calf stretching. No doubt much work remains to sort out the optimal stretch for the calf, whether static, dynamic, eccentric, or other. When it comes to surgical lengthening procedures, whether at the Achilles, at the musculotendinous junction, or more proximal, the search must move on to find the safest, most accurate, and quickest recovery method possible. Of course, prevention, in the form of calf stretching, should be ultimate goal.

Addressing the calf contracture as definitive treatment and, better yet, as prevention, will no doubt become a mainstay of the treatment of many foot and ankle problems. Regardless of whether a preference of treatment is calf stretching or performing lengthening by surgical means, the mission must be to bring awareness of the detrimental role of the gastrocnemius contracture to everyone as soon as possible. It has already been a century since Nutt[23] described much of this the first time; let us not wait too much longer.

ACKNOWLEDGMENTS

My sincerest thanks go to Dr Mark Myerson for his invitation to be a part of this groundbreaking issue of *Foot and Ankle Clinics of North America*. Throughout a 28-year career devoted to the care of the adult foot and ankle, I have been clinically focused on the notion that the human gastrocnemius is the key to much of the foot and ankle pathology we acquire as we age. The concept that we develop calf contractures and, as a result, incremental damage occurs to the foot and ankle, I believe will be brought to the forefront of our basic knowledge, which in turn will result in better patient care. Contained in parts of this overview are my opinions based on experience and a synthesis of the literature, for which I make no apologies. This issue of *Foot and Ankle Clinics of North America* is where we will turn the corner and a new understanding begins.

REFERENCES

1. Abbassian A, Kohls-Gatzoulis J, Solan MC. Proximal medial gastrocnemius release in the treatment of recalcitrant plantar fasciitis. Foot Ankle Int 2012;1:14–9.
2. Aronow MS. Triceps surae contractures associated with posterior tibial tendon dysfunction. Tech Orthop 2000;15:164–73.
3. Aronow MS, Diaz-Doran V, Sullivan RJ, et al. The effect of triceps surae contracture force on plantar foot pressure distribution. Foot Ankle Int 2006;1:43–52.
4. Barrett SL. Understanding and managing equinus deformities. Podiatry Today 2011;24:1–7.
5. Barske HL, DiGiovanni BF, Douglass M, et al. Current concepts review: isolated gastrocnemius contracture and gastrocnemius recession. Foot Ankle Int 2012; 33:915–21.
6. Bolívar YA, Munuera PV, Padillo JP. Relationship between tightness of the posterior muscles of the lower limb and plantar fasciitis. Foot Ankle Int 2013; 1:42–8.
7. DeHeer PA. Understanding equinus. Podiatry Management 2012;157–68.
8. DiGiovanni CW, Kuo R, Tejwani N, et al. Isolated gastrocnemius tightness. J Bone Joint Surg Am 2002;6:962–70.
9. DiGiovanni CW, Langer P. The role of isolated gastrocnemius and combined achilles contractures in the flatfoot. Foot Ankle Clin 2007;2:363–79.
10. Gajdosik RL, Vander Linden DW, McNair PJ, et al. Effects of an eight-week stretching program on the passive-elastic properties and function of the calf muscles of older women. Clin Biomech (Bristol, Avon) 2005;20:973–83.
11. Garrett T, Neibert PJ. The effectiveness of a gastrocnemius/soleus stretching program as a therapeutic treatment of plantar fasciitis. J Sport Rehabil 2013; 22(4):308–12.
12. Gentchos CE, Bohay DR, Anderson JG. Gastrocnemius recession as treatment for refractory achilles tendinopathy: a case report. Foot Ankle Int 2008;6:620–3.

13. Greenhagen RM, Johnson AR, Bevilacqua NJ. Gastrocnemius recession or tendo-achilles lengthening for equinus deformity in the diabetic foot? Clin Podiatr Med Surg 2012;3:413–24.
14. Hill RS. Ankle equinus. Prevalence and linkage to common foot pathology. J Am Podiatr Med Assoc 1995;85:295–300.
15. Kiewiet NJ, Holthusen SM, Bohay DR, et al. Gastrocnemius recession for chronic noninsertional achilles tendinopathy. Foot Ankle Int 2013;4:481–5.
16. League AC. Current concepts review: plantar fasciitis. Foot Ankle Int 2008;3:358–66.
17. Magnussen RA, Dunn WR, Thomson AB. Nonoperative treatment of midportion achilles tendinopathy: a systematic review. Clin J Sport Med 2009;1:54–64.
18. Mahieu NN, Witvrouw E, Stevens V, et al. Intrinsic risk factors for the development of achilles tendon overuse injury: a prospective study. Am J Sports Med 2006;2:226–35.
19. Martin RL, Irrgang JJ, Conti SF. Outcome study of subjects with insertional plantar fasciitis. Foot Ankle Int 1998;12:803–11.
20. Maskill JD, Bohay DR, Anderson JG. Gastrocnemius recession to treat isolated foot pain. Foot Ankle Int 2010;1:19–23.
21. McGlamry ED, Kitting RW. Aquinus foot: an analysis of the etiology, pathology and treatment techniques. J Am Podiatry Assoc 1973;63:165–84.
22. Morton DJ. Evolution of the longitudinal arch of the human foot. J Bone Joint Surg Am 1924;6:56–90.
23. Nutt J. Diseases and deformities of the foot. E.B.Treat & Co; 1913. Google Digital Copy. Available at: books.google.com/books?id=UWgQAAAAYAAJ.
24. Owens BD, Wolf JM, Seelig AD, et al, Risk factors for the Millennium Cohort Study Team. Risk factors for lower extremity tendinopathies in military personnel. Orthopaedic Journal of Sports Medicine 2013;1.
25. Patel A, DiGiovanni B. Association between plantar fasciitis and isolated contracture of the gastrocnemius. Foot Ankle Int 2011;1:5–8.
26. Pfeffer G, Bacchetti P, Deland J, et al. Comparison of custom and prefabricated orthoses in the initial treatment of proximal plantar fasciitis. Foot Ankle Int 1999;20:214–21.
27. Riddle DL, Pulisic M, Pidcoe P, et al. Risk factors for plantar fasciitis: a matched case-control study. J Bone Joint Surg Am 2003;5:872–7.
28. Werner RA, Gell N, Hartigan A, et al. Risk factors for plantar fasciitis among assembly plant workers. PM R 2010;2:110–6.
29. Wolgin M, Cook C, Graham C, et al. Conservative treatment of plantar heel pain: long-term follow-up. Foot Ankle Int 1994;3:97–102.
30. Young R, Nix S, Wholohan A, et al. Interventions for increasing ankle joint dorsiflexion: a systematic review and meta-analysis. J Foot Ankle Res 2013;6:1–10.
31. Tong KB, Furia J. Economic burden of plantar fasciitis treatment in the United States. Am J Orthop 2010;39(5):227–31.
32. Atkins D, Crawford F, Edwards J, et al. A systematic review of treatments for the painful heel. Rheumatology (Oxford) 1999;38:968–73.
33. Crawford F, Thomson C. Interventions for treating plantar heel pain. Cochrane Database Syst Rev 2003;(3):CD000416.
34. Davis PF, Severud E, Baxter DE. Painful heel syndrome: results of nonoperative treatment. Foot Ankle Int 1994;10:531–5.
35. DiGiovanni BF, Moore AM, Zlotnicki JP, et al. Preferred management of recalcitrant plantar fasciitis among orthopaedic foot and ankle surgeons. Foot Ankle Int 2012;6:507–12.

36. Drake M, Bittenbender C, Boyles RE. The short-term effects of treating plantar fasciitis with a temporary custom foot orthosis and stretching. J Orthop Sports Phys Ther 2011;41:221–31.
37. Duthon VB, Lubbeke A, Duc SR, et al. Non-insertional Achilles tendinopathy treated with gastrocnemius lengthening. Foot Ankle Int 2011;32(4):375–9.
38. Gurdezi S, Kohls-Gatzoulis J, Solan MC. Results of proximal medial gastrocnemius release for achilles tendinopathy. Foot Ankle Int 2013;10:1364–9.
39. Holmes GB, Lin J. Etiologic factors associated with symptomatic achilles tendinopathy. Foot Ankle Int 2006;27:952–9.
40. Karagounis P, Tsironi M, Prionas G, et al. Treatment of plantar fasciitis in recreational athletes: two different therapeutic protocols. Foot Ankle Spec 2011;4: 226–34.
41. Riddle DL, Schappert SM. Volume of ambulatory care visits and patterns of care for patients diagnosed with plantar fasciitis: a national study of medical doctors. Foot Ankle Int 2004;5:303–10.
42. Subotnick SI. Equinus deformity as it affects the forefoot. J Am Podiatry Assoc 1971;61:423–7.
43. Tahririan MA, Motififard M, Tahmasebi MN, et al. Plantar fasciitis. J Res Med Sci 2012;8:799–804.
44. Verrall G, Schofield S, Brustad T. Chronic achilles tendinopathy treated with ecentric stretching program. Foot Ankle Int 2011;32:843–9.
45. Wapner KL, Sharkey PF. The use of night splints for treatment of recalcitrant plantar fasciitis. Foot Ankle Int 1991;3:135–7.
46. Macklin K, Healy A, Chockalingam N. The effect of calf muscle stretching exercises on ankle joint dorsiflexion and dynamic foot pressures, force and related temporal parameters. Foot (Edinb) 2012;22:10–7.
47. Porter D, Barrill E, Oneacre K, et al. The effects of duration and frequency of achilles tendon stretching on dorsiflexion and outcome in painful heel syndrome: a randomized, blinded, control study. Foot Ankle Int 2002;7:619–24.
48. Silfverskiöld N. Reduction of the uncrossed two-joints muscles of the leg to one-joint muscles in spastic conditions. Acta Chir Scand 1924;56:315–30.
49. Barouk LB, Toulec E. Resultats de la liberation proximale des gastrocnemius. Med Chir Pied 2006;22:151–6.
50. Harty J, Soffe K, O'Toole G, et al. The role of hamstring tightness in plantar fasciitis. Foot Ankle Int 2005;12:1089–92.
51. Schmidt D. Insights into the evolution of human bipedalism from experimental studies of humans and other primates. J Exp Biol 2003;206(Pt 9):1437–48.
52. Perry J. Gait analysis: normal and abnormal function. SLACK International; 1992.
53. Pinney ST, Hansen ST, Sangeorzan BJ. The effect on ankle dorsiflexion of gastrocnemius recession. Foot Ankle Int 2002;23:26–9.
54. Guyton GP, Mann RA, Kreiger LE, et al. Cumulative industrial trauma as an etiology of seven common disorders in the foot and ankle. What is the evidence? Foot Ankle Int 2000;21:1047–56.
55. Scher DL, Belmont PJ Jr, Bear R, et al. The Incidence of plantar fasciitis in the United States military. J Bone Joint Surg Am 2009;91(12):2867–72.

Effects of Gastrocnemius Tightness on Forefoot During Gait

 CrossMark

Cyrille Cazeau, MD*, Yves Stiglitz, MD

KEYWORDS

- Gastrocnemius muscle • Biomechanics of gait • Gait analysis • Biarticular muscle
- Storage-output principle • Metatarsalgia • Forefoot pathologies

KEY POINTS

- The gastrocnemius muscle has a very specific biomechanical function derived from its biarticular situation crossing knee and ankle.
- In the setting of gastrocnemius tightness, the risk of pain in the forefoot by hyperpressure appears when muscles are maximally stretched.
- Kinematic analysis allows precise identification of the critical phase. It is characterized by the position of the knee in extension and ankle around 0 degrees. It starts approximately in the 60th percentile and ends in the 90th percentile of the stance phase.
- The dynamic results corroborate that the identified phase corresponds to the change in pressure center to the forefoot, under the metatarsal heads. This confirms the idea that surgical release of the gastrocnemius could decrease pressure under the forefoot and in doing so, could minimize or avoid certain surgical interventions distally.
- The optimal site for surgical release has yet to be determined: according to Hill, it seems more coherent to translate the entire elastic model distally by detaching the gastrocnemius at the knee instead of surgically creating a fibrous scar within the muscle belly or calcaneal tendon, thus modifying their elastic properties, even if it would, theoretically, diminish the advantages of a biarticular muscle.

INTRODUCTION

The gastrocnemius muscle has not been studied historically other than in a recent number of investigations. Many publications are available in the medical literature describing its function and the pathologies associated with its dysfunction. This article takes into account the publications focused on its biomechanical features. A synthesis of their conclusions is performed to understand the mechanisms leading to pathology, first and foremost forefoot disorders.

The Authors have nothing to disclose.
Foot and Ankle Department, Clinique Geoffroy Saint Hilaire, 59 rue Geoffroy Saint Hilaire, Paris 75005, France
* Corresponding author.
E-mail address: cyrillecazeau@free.fr

Foot Ankle Clin N Am 19 (2014) 649–657
http://dx.doi.org/10.1016/j.fcl.2014.08.003
1083-7515/14/$ – see front matter © 2014 Elsevier Inc. All rights reserved.

foot.theclinics.com

ANATOMY AND PHYSIOLOGY OF THE GASTROCNEMIUS MUSCLE
Anatomy

The gastrocnemius muscle has two heads: the lateral head originates on the lateral surface of the lateral femoral condyle, whereas the medial head originates from the posterior surface of the medial condyle. The two muscle bellies join in the midline, and distally join the soleus muscle to form the calcaneal tendon. The gastrocnemius therefore belongs to the group of biarticular muscles, which have the singularity of crossing two joints, in this case the knee and the ankle.[1]

Hill Model

A theoretic model of muscle function is useful to understand its physiology and mechanical properties. Hill[2] developed such a model, which is still accepted today and is helpful to understand the involvement of gastrocnemius tightness during gait. According to the model, a muscle is composed of three separate elements: (1) a contractile element, representing muscle actin-myosin crossbridges; (2) a series elastic element, representing actin-myosin bridges and calcaneal tendon (a stiff element, difficult to distend); and (3) a parallel elastic element, representing muscle connective tissues (this element is more compliant and more extensible).

Energy Considerations

Cavagna and colleagues[3] studied the influence of stretching on muscular strength. The contraction of a previously stretched muscle develops a higher force than if the muscle is previously at rest. The stretching of a muscle requires energy, which is stored as elastic energy in the tissue. When the contraction occurs force (and thus their work) is amplified and the mechanical efficiency is increased. The authors named this mechanism "storage-output" principle. In the case of a biarticular muscle stretching varies with the positions of the articulations during movement. Contraction of this type of muscle while in a stretched condition allows a more energy-saving functioning of the system according to the "storage-output" principle.

In relation to Hill's model this prestretching corresponds to an accumulation of elastic energy, the series elastic component. Muscle can therefore generate a greater force per contraction at an equivalent energy cost. Furthermore, calculation of forces and moments based on Newton's mechanical laws demonstrates that a biarticular muscle allows for mechanical energy transfer from one link to another, further minimizing losses.

NORMAL GAIT ANALYSIS
Kinematics of the Stance Phase

Clinical consequences of gastrocnemius tightness are notable during the weight-bearing phase of gait, which is to say during the stance phase. Cappozzo and colleagues[4] studied the simultaneous angular positions of hip, knee, and ankle joints during the stance phase (**Fig. 1**). The numerical values extracted from this work are summarized in **Table 1**.

During the stance phase of gait, the hip, knee, and ankle have various anatomic positions. As with any muscle, the gastrocnemius is tensioned when its attachment is more distant. But as a biarticular muscle this happens when both the knee is in extension and ankle in dorsiflexion (or minimal plantar flexion).[5] We emphasize two significant situations. The first is C zone, a subphase of the stance phase, where the ankle angle is less than 5 degrees (corresponding to a low plantar flexion and a dorsiflexion). This zone ranges from 60% to 88% of the stance phase. Second is X point, defined with the ankle in neutral position. It is located at 70.6% of the stance phase and is a particular position of the C zone.

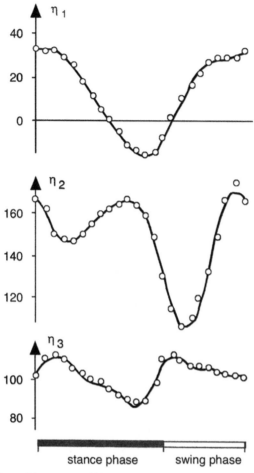

Fig. 1. Plots versus time of the measured kinematic variables (level walking): hip, knee, and ankle angular positions ($\eta 1$, $\eta 2$, $\eta 3$, respectively). (*Adapted from* Cappozzo A, Leo T, Pedotti A. A general computing method for the analysis of human locomotion. J Biomech 1975;8(5):307–20.)

Table 1
Angular values of the hip, knee, and ankle during three moments of the stance phase, and their corresponding anatomic positions

	Heel Strike	Midstance	Preswing (Toe-off)
Hip			
Angle	+30 degrees	−10 degrees	−10 degrees
Position	Flexion	Extension	Extension
Knee			
Angle	+15 degrees	+10 degrees to < +10 degrees	+40 degrees
Position	Extension	Extension	Flexion
Ankle			
Angle	−20 degrees	0 degrees to > +5 degrees	−20 degrees
Position	Plantar flexion	Neutral to dorsal flexion	Plantar flexion

Dynamics of the Stance Phase: Ground Reaction Studies

A force platform is mandatory to study the distribution of the forces applied on the foot during the stance phase. Two forces are involved in this process: weight and ground reaction. They both act on the plantar surface of the foot where they may be linked to clinical symptoms.

The ground reaction force is represented by a vector $\vec{R}$ and has several specifications: a vertical coordinate, which equals the weight and therefore represents the vertical movement of the center of gravity; a sagittal coordinate representing propulsion; and an application point on the plantar surface called "center of pressures."

Eberhart and colleagues[6] described changes in vertical and sagittal coordinates of $\vec{R}$, and in center-of-pressures position during normal walking. Focusing on the previously defined C zone two analyses are performed (**Fig. 2**).

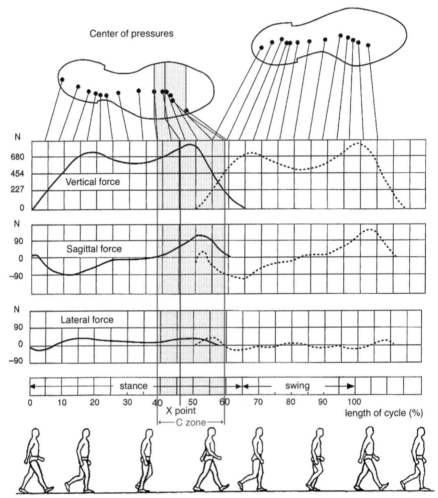

Fig. 2. Combined representations of application point, and vertical, sagittal, and lateral compounds of the reaction vector $\vec{R}$ during gait. (*Adapted from* Eberhart HD, Inman VT, Bresler B. The principal elements in human locomotion. In: Klopsteg PE, Wilson PD, editors. Human limbs and their substitutes. New York: McGraw Hill; 1954. p. 437–71.)

Ground reaction and center of gravity

After the hip crosses vertically over the ankle, the sagittal coordination of $\vec{R}$ rises. This propulsion takes place just before the toe-off. At the same moment the vertical coordination of $\vec{R}$ drops down, signing the falling of the center of gravity preceding the toe-off.

Center of pressures

The center of pressures moves from rear-foot at the beginning of the stance phase to the forefoot at the end. Specifically in the C zone the center of pressure is located under the metatarsal heads. The dynamic study of the stance phase focusing the C zone demonstrates a fall of the center of gravity followed by a propulsion with an application point of these forces located just under the metatarsal heads.

Electromyographic Analysis

Winter and Yack[7] performed an electromyographic (EMG) analysis of several lower limb muscles during normal walking. Six muscles of the leg were studied (**Fig. 3**), divided in two groups regarding their action relative to the gastrocnemius:

- Agonist muscles
  - Gastrocnemius medialis
  - Gastrocnemius lateralis
  - Soleus
  - Peroneus longus
- Antagonist muscles
  - Tibialis anterior
  - Extensor digitorum longus

The EMG analysis in the C zone is described in three parts:

- Beginning of the C zone to the X point: EMG activity of the gastrocnemius muscle is low but rising.
- X point: peak of EMG activity of the gastrocnemius muscle, just after which the activity starts falling.
- End of the C zone: EMG activity of gastrocnemius is still falling while no activity of antagonist muscles is recorded.

Combined Analysis of Kinematics Dynamics and Electromyography

Kinematic and dynamic studies focused the analysis in a narrow period of the stance phase (the C zone defined previously) ranging from 60% to 88% of this phase. During this short time the angular positions of knee and ankle place the gastrocnemius muscle in a stretched situation, when the center of pressure is simultaneously located under the metatarsal heads.

At the beginning of the C zone the lack of EMG activity points out the passive nature of gastrocnemius stretching. The requisite energy is found in the knee extension already noticed in the kinematic study.

Around the X point gastrocnemius reaches its maximal stretching, just after which EMG activity peaks. According to Hill's model the contraction is therefore more efficient and thus energy saving. Because of its biarticular feature the gastrocnemius stores the energy passively transferred by knee extension, and uses this energy for its contraction a few seconds after.

The quick decrease of EMG activity allows the muscle to be passive again when ankle goes toward dorsal flexion. This sequence uses the gravitational potential energy of the center of gravity, which is proved by the dynamics study to be falling and propulsive.

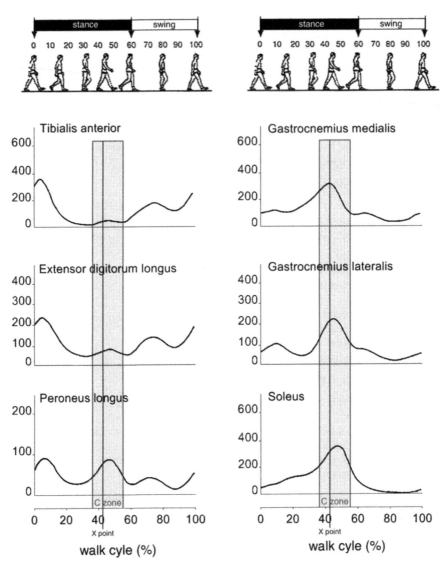

Fig. 3. EMG activity of six muscles of the leg during a walk cycle. (*Adapted from* Winter DA, Yack HJ. EMG profiles during normal human walking: stride-to-stride and inter-subject variability. Electroencephalogr Clin Neurophysiol 1987;67(5):402–11.)

DISCUSSION

The main biomechanical features of the normal gastrocnemius muscle are described previously. They can explain the mechanism of several forefoot pathologies and symptoms, first of which is metatarsalgia. DiGiovanni and colleagues[8] studied and found a link between forefoot and midfoot pain and pathologies but did not clearly explain the pathologic mechanism. According to them, gastrocnemius tightness causes a decrease in ankle dorsiflexion, which we could hypothesize based on the previous kinematics analysis. The dynamic contribution pointed out the position of the center of pressure under the metatarsal head in the C zone, between the 60th and 88th percentile of the stance phase. Combined with the EMG peak of activity at the same moment, it makes three compounds of the link between gastrocnemius tightness and forefoot symptoms.

Theoretically, lengthening the gastrocnemius should decrease the passive stretching during gait but gastrocnemius tightness is a pathologic situation where theory might not be valid. Patients are in pain and have a limited ankle dorsal flexion, which is needed to allow the storage of energy. This explains why patients with gastrocnemius tightness cannot benefit from the "storage-output" principle. Lengthening allows recovering the missing degrees of dorsal flexion and reduces pain. It returns the patient from a pathologic to a more normal situation in which gastrocnemius muscle becomes efficient again. We hypothesize that lengthening is performed by sectioning the fascia represented by the parallel component of Hill's model. Surgery enables the series components to be passively stretched by lengthening the short parallel component.

Exploring normal gait usually implies two main implicit conditions: low walking speed and no slope (ie, on a flat ground surface). These are ideal study conditions, but are not always reflected on day-to-day situations encountered by patients. However, Lichtwark and Wilson[9] demonstrated that gastrocnemius function is very similar in locomotion on a slope whether a decline or incline, and even at different walking speeds. They assumed this stability is caused by its biarticular feature, which would be one more benefit of this kind of muscle.

Spanjaard and colleagues[10,11] have illustrated another example of storage-output property during up and down stairs climbing. A gastrocnemius activity is detected at touch-down of stair descent. The muscle cushions actively the weight of the body going down. Meanwhile, it is passively stretched, which allows storing the energy of the falling body. The output happens the next step with higher efficacy of muscle contraction according to Hill's model.

Thus, from a biomechanical point of view gastrocnemius tightness has undeniable consequences on lower limb joints and the forefoot. Several authors have suggested stretching exercises to correct these disturbances,[12] but this question is still controversial. Johanson and colleagues[13] indeed found no difference in gait analysis between a stretched group and a nonstretched group in a randomized study.

Moreover, various clinical presentations and pathologies are described in which stretching as a single treatment is probably insufficient.[14] An even more confusing and misunderstood association of flatfoot and gastrocnemius tightness was reported with no certainty on pathologic mechanism.[15] If gastrocnemius biomechanics is well documented the consequences of its dysfunction are still to be explored. Recently, two studies demonstrated the highest risk of fall in the elderly with gastrocnemius abnormalities.[16,17]

Stretching must remain a part of treatment protocols even if in our experience clinical improvement happens after a long time and disappears quickly if stretching is discontinued. Surgery is decided with caution and the positive result of a previous nonsurgical option may suggests a success of a lengthening procedure.

SUMMARY

The gastrocnemius muscle has a specific biomechanical function derived from its biarticular situation crossing knee and ankle. In the setting of gastrocnemius tightness, the risk of pain in the forefoot by hyperpressure appears when muscles are maximally stretched. Kinematic analysis allows precise identification of the critical phase. It is characterized by the position of the knee in extension and ankle around 0 degrees. It starts approximately in the 60th percentile and ends in the 90th percentile of the stance phase. The dynamic results corroborate that the identified phase correspond to the change in pressure center to the forefoot, under the metatarsal heads. This confirms the idea that surgical release of the gastrocnemius could decrease pressure under the forefoot, and in doing so could minimize or avoid certain surgical interventions distally.

Comparison between results of the mechanical and EMG studies demonstrates that ankle freedom in dorsiflexion can improve biarticular muscle yield, according to the elastic energy storage-output theory, and diminish cost of movement. Surgical release of the gastrocnemius muscle, useful for increasing dorsiflexion, therefore increases efficiency of gait in terms of performance and energy efficiency.

The optimal site for surgical release has yet to be determined: according to Hill, it seems more coherent to translate the entire elastic model distally by detaching the gastrocnemius at the knee instead of surgically creating a fibrous scar within the muscle belly or calcaneal tendon, thus modifying their elastic properties, even if it would, theoretically, diminish the advantages of a biarticular muscle. This has yet to be corroborated by clinical studies.

REFERENCES

1. Gray H. Anatomy of the human body. Philadelphia: Lea & Febiger; 1918. p. 1396.
2. Hill AV. The heat of shortening and the dynamic constants of the muscle. Proc R Soc Lond B Biol Sci 1938;126:136–95.
3. Cavagna GA, Dusman B, Margaria R. Positive work done by a previously stretched muscle. J Appl Physiol 1968;24(1):21–32.
4. Cappozzo A, Leo T, Pedotti A. A general computing method for the analysis of human locomotion. J Biomech 1975;8(5):307–20.
5. Cazeau C, Stiglitz Y. Analyse des conséquences biomécaniques de la brièveté du gastrocnémien sur l'avant-pied. In: Barouk LS, Barouk P, editors. Brièveté des Gastrocnémiens. Montpellier (France): Sauramps Medical; 2012. p. 79–91.
6. Eberhart HD, Inman VT, Bresler B. The principal elements in human locomotion. In: Klopsteg PE, Wilson PD, editors. Human limbs and their substitutes. New York: McGraw Hill; 1954. p. 437–71.
7. Winter DA, Yack HJ. EMG profiles during normal human walking: stride-to-stride and inter-subject variability. Electroencephalogr Clin Neurophysiol 1987;67(5): 402–11.
8. DiGiovanni CW, Kuo R, Tejwani N, et al. Isolated gastrocnemius tightness. J Bone Joint Surg Am 2002;84-A(6):962–70.
9. Lichtwark GA, Wilson AM. Interactions between the human gastrocnemius muscle and the Achilles tendon during incline, level and decline locomotion. J Exp Biol 2006;209(Pt 21):4379–88.
10. Spanjaard M, Reeves ND, van Dieën JH, et al. Gastrocnemius muscle fascicle behavior during stair negotiation in humans. J Appl Physiol (1985) 2007;102(4): 1618–23.
11. Spanjaard M, Reeves ND, van Dieën JH, et al. Influence of gait velocity on gastrocnemius muscle fascicle behaviour during stair negotiation. J Electromyogr Kinesiol 2009;19(2):304–13.
12. Strehle J. Pain in the sole of the foot. Differential diagnosis and therapy. Praxis (Bern 1994) 1999;88(8):322–7 [in German].
13. Johanson MA, Cuda BJ, Koontz JE, et al. Effect of stretching on ankle and knee angles and gastrocnemius activity during the stance phase of gait. J Sport Rehabil 2009;18(4):521–34.

14. Bowers AL, Castro MD. The mechanics behind the image: foot and ankle pathology associated with gastrocnemius contracture. Semin Musculoskelet Radiol 2007;11(1):83–90.

15. DiGiovanni CW, Langer P. The role of isolated gastrocnemius and combined Achilles contractures in the flatfoot. Foot Ankle Clin 2007;12(2):363–79, viii.

16. Kirkwood RN, Trede RG, Moreira Bde S, et al. Decreased gastrocnemius temporal muscle activation during gait in elderly women with history of recurrent falls. Gait Posture 2011;34(1):60–4.

17. Lee SS, Piazza SJ. Correlation between plantarflexor moment arm and preferred gait velocity in slower elderly men. J Biomech 2012;45(9):1601–6.

Clinical Diagnosis of Gastrocnemius Tightness

Pierre Barouk, MD[a],*, Louis Samuel Barouk, MD[b]

KEYWORDS

- Gastrocnemius • Equinus • Triceps surae

KEY POINTS

- The diagnosis of gastrocnemius tightness is primarily clinical using the Silfverskiold test, which shows an equinus deformity at the ankle with the knee extended but that disappears with the knee flexed.
- The manner in which the Silfverskiold test is performed must be consistent with respect to the applied strength of the maneuver, correction of a flexible hindfoot valgus deformity while performing the test, and reproducibility.
- Additional clinical signs that can help to make the diagnosis when the retraction is not clinically evident include knee recurvatum, hip flexion, lumbar hyperlordosis, and forefoot overload.

INTRODUCTION

The diagnosis of gastrocnemius tightness is based on the clinical examination alone, with an essential point that is common to every examination: the Silfverskiold sign,[1] an equinus of the ankle that is present when the knee is extended but that disappears when the knee is flexed.

Gastrocnemius tightness is also associated with physical signs caused by the equinus, and must be detected during the clinical examination: forefoot overload, knee recurvatum, hip flexion, and hyperlordosis.

CLINICAL EXAMINATION: THE SILFVERSKIOLD TEST

There is gastrocnemius tightness when passive ankle dorsal flexion is negative or at neutral when the knee is in extension, during application of a load using moderate strength under the forefoot; and this loss of dorsiflexion normalizes when the knee is in flexion, with a minimum of 13 degrees of difference (**Fig. 1**A and B).

This passive ankle dorsal flexion difference is common and once identified, it is important to assess the diagnosis. Some elements of this examination must be precise.

---

[a] Foot Surgery Center of the Sport Clinic, 2 Rue Georges Nègrevergne, Merignac 33700, France;
[b] 39 Chemin de la Roche, Yvrac 33370, France
* Corresponding author.
E-mail address: pierre.barouk@wanadoo.fr

Foot Ankle Clin N Am 19 (2014) 659–667
http://dx.doi.org/10.1016/j.fcl.2014.08.004
1083-7515/14/$ – see front matter © 2014 Elsevier Inc. All rights reserved.

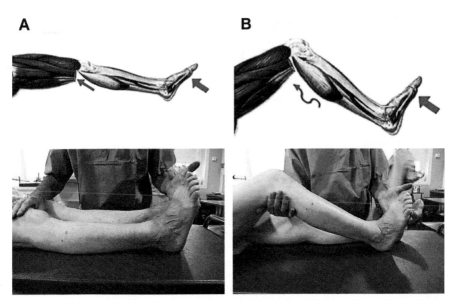

Fig. 1. Gastrocnemius tightness. (*A*) Equinus with knee in extension, but with moderate strength applied. (*B*) Equinus disappears when the knee is flexed. (*Adapted from* Barouk S. Forefoot reconstruction. New York: Springer-Verlag; 2003.)

The Force Under the Foot Is Applied

Force is applied under the head of the second metatarsal, but it can be applied to a larger area under the entire forefoot.

Correction of Hindfoot Valgus Deformity

In the presence of a flexible flatfoot, the heel is usually in a valgus position. When the hindfoot is in valgus, true ankle dorsiflexion does not occur, and most of the dorsiflexion motion occurs in an oblique plane through the transverse tarsal and subtalar joints. To perform the test correctly, the hindfoot must be reduced from valgus into a neutral or varus position. This is only possible to perform if the hindfoot is flexible. We have noted that flexible hindfoot valgus deformity is present in 15% to 25% of the cases when there is gastrocnemius tightness (**Fig. 2**).[2]

Correction of an Eventual Contraction of the Foot Extensors

This occurs essentially when the knee is flexed. The Silfverskiold test is based on passive examination of the foot, and the examiner has to avoid attempted active contraction of the extensors, in particular the tibialis anterior (**Fig. 3**). This commonly occurs when the patient is asked to flex the knee. To avoid this we perform the examination in a prone position, which is more reliable but not as convenient (**Fig. 4**). An alternative method of performing the test is to flex the knee passively and hold it in that position while doing the test (**Fig. 5**).

Strength Applied, and Definition of Gastrocnemius Tightness

The degree of dorsiflexion depends on the strength applied under the forefoot. Although some force has to be exerted under the forefoot when testing for equinus, this should not be more than approximately 2 kg of force. In the example in **Fig. 6**,

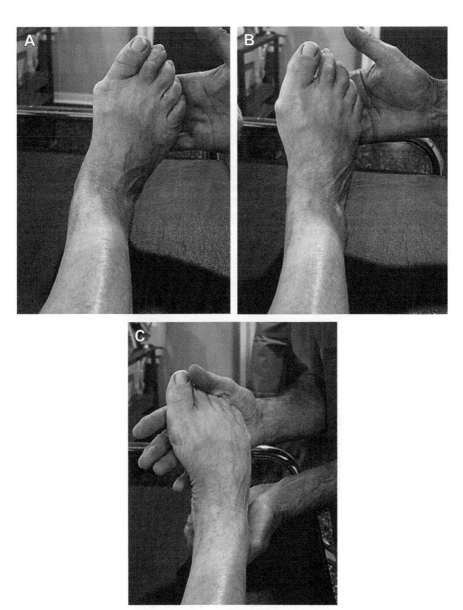

Fig. 2. (*A*) Avoid examination of gastrocnemius tightness with the hindfoot in valgus. The test is performed with the foot in a neutral (*B*) or varus position (*C*).

it seems that there is no equinus but this is because considerable force had to be applied to the foot, which leads to a false-positive result (see **Fig. 6**).

Di Giovanni[3,4] has recommended applying a force no more than 10 nm, which corresponds approximately to 2 kg and can be reliably measured with the equinometer (**Fig. 7**).

Di Giovanni defined subjectively two types of a short gastrocnemius: when the ankle dorsi flexion is equal or inferior to +10 degrees or +5 degrees when the knee is extended, or with a differential when the knee is flexed an average of 11.3 degrees.

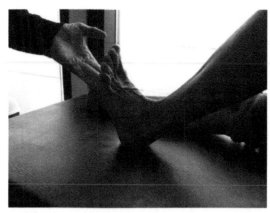

Fig. 3. With the knee flexed note an active contraction of the foot extensors; this leads to a false-positive result.

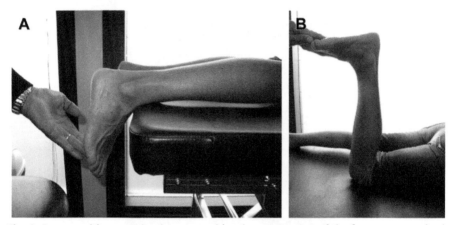

Fig. 4. Prone position examination can avoid active contraction of the foot extensors, both knee extended (*A*), and knee flexed (*B*).

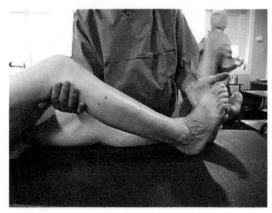

Fig. 5. The best position to avoid foot extensor contraction is when the knee is flexed.

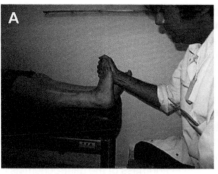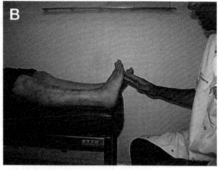

Fig. 6. (*A*) Usually the equinus is tested with a high strength applied under the forefoot. (*B*) For the gastrocnemius examination this strength must be moderate (<2 kg).

It is certain that the measurement with an equinometer is very accurate, and the precision is less than 2 degrees for a trained examiner, but it requires time and special computer equipment, which makes the routine examination difficult. However, it is very useful for experimental investigations in trained hands.

These definitions are quite severe, especially the one that considers a short gastrocnemius when the ankle dorsi flexion is less than +10 degrees, with the knee extended. It is useful for comparative study when the examination is reproducible, but too severe for routine examination.

We started with an examination made in patients with cerebral palsy in whom we determined an angle of dorsiflexion that corresponds to the beginning of the stretching resistance. This degree of dorsiflexion was called "L0" by Tardieu.[5] Our experience[6] gave us the same conclusion as others[7]: the clinical signs (type of walking digitigrade,

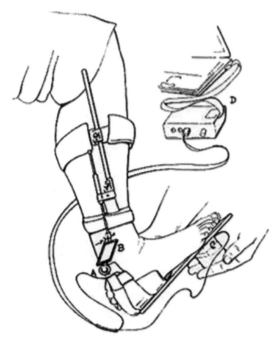

Fig. 7. The equinometer.

appearance of the tonic reflex of stretching) occur when the ankle is at the negative dorsal flexion degree that correspond to the L0.

We applied the principle of the L0 to patients without cerebral palsy because here also the negative effects of the gastrocnemius tightness occur at this level of dorsi flexion, and this resistance to the passive stretching is easy to determine. What is the strength corresponding to an L0 in a nonspastic patient? We could measure this force with a balance: it is approximately 1.7 kg (**Fig. 8**).

With this pressure, in nonspastic patients we obtain in cases of a short gastrocnemius knee extended 13 degrees of dorsal flexion; and knee flexed, + 5 degrees of dorsal flexion. So, the difference is 18 degrees on average, but it can be 13 degrees. With these numbers we consider short gastrocnemius.

For other authors, the pressure used to determine tightness of the gastrocnemius is slightly greater. These authors consider a short gastrocnemius when dorsiflexion with the knee extended is equal or inferior to 0 degrees, and that this difference with flexed knee is 15 degrees.[8–10] These differences are small, but all the authors agree with the principle of a slight pressure of around 1.5 to 2 kg when examining the leg.

In some cases, one has to use the clinical differences of extension and flexion of the knee according to clinical pathology, so that if the dorsiflexion is only slightly positive the differential may then be important. In this case, the lengthening can still be of some benefit, especially in case of metatarsalgia, or plantar fasciitis as observed by Maceira and Orejana.[11]

When there is gastrocnemius and soleus tightness, the dorsiflexion with the knee extended is very limited, and stays negative with the knee flexed. In this case, the surgery has to adapt to the severity and type of contracture of the triceps surae as

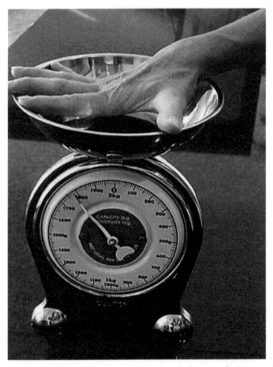

Fig. 8. Common pressure to diagnose gastrocnemius tightness: between 1.7 and 2 kg.

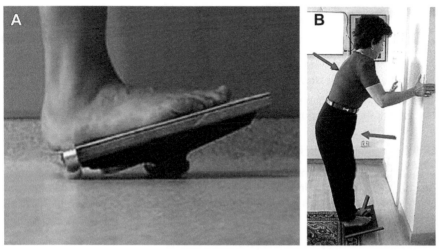

Fig. 9. (*A, B*) Taloche sign. (*Courtesy of* M. Maestro, MD, Nice, France.)

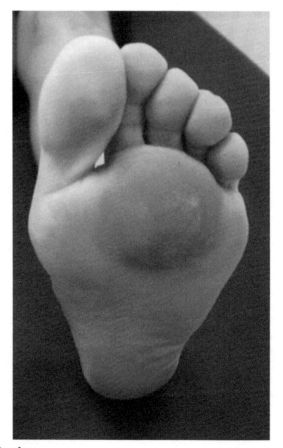

Fig. 10. Round forefoot.

proposed by Rippstein[12]: the lengthening is "global" (ie, just distal to the gastrocnemius-soleus junction [gastrocnemius tendon and soleus aponeurosis], or just on the gastrocnemius [distally to the musculotendinous junction, or at the proximal insertion]).

The Taloche Sign (Maestro)

If a patient with a tight gastrocnemius tries to stand on an inclined plane, it is immediately evident that it is impossible for the patient to be stable in this position (**Fig. 9**).

CLINICAL EXAMINATION: THE ASSOCIATED SIGNS CAUSED BY THE EQUINUS

In forefoot overload the typical sign is the round forefoot, as described by Colombier (**Fig. 10**).[8] Note also on **Fig. 10** the narrow heel. The signs of knee recurvatum, hip flexion, and hyperlordosis are often associated with gastrocnemius tightness as described by Downey and Banks[13] or Kowalski.[14]

SUMMARY

There is a gastrocnemius tightness when on examination there is a negative or neutral ankle dorsiflexion when the knee is extended, with moderate (no more than 2 kg) pressure applied under the forefoot; and there is a differential at least of 13 degrees of dorsiflexion (that becomes positive) when the knee is flexed.

It is necessary during examination to ensure that the heel is reduced, particularly in a flexible flatfoot deformity to reduce hindfoot valgus, and to avoid the contraction of the foot extensors. The assessment with an equinometer is the most accurate way to assess deformity, but this is not clinically practical. The clinical signs caused by equinus must be looked for including forefoot overload, knee recurvatum, hip flexion, and hyperlordosis.

REFERENCES

1. Silfverskiold N. Reduction of the uncrossed two joint muscles of the leg to one joint muscle in spastic conditions. Acta Chir Scand 1924;56:315–30.
2. Barouk LS. Other consequences of short gastrocnemius, that are not the subject of an article in this monograph. In: Brièveté des gastrocnémiens: de l'anatomie au traitement. Montpellier (France): Sauramps; 2012. p. 251–6.
3. DiGiovanni CW, Kuo R, Tejwani N, et al. Isolated gastrocnemius tightness. J Bone Joint Surg Am 2002;84A(6):962–70.
4. Drakos MC, Di Giovanni CW. Importance de la brieveté isolée des gastrocnémiens dans la pathologie du pied. In: Brièveté des gastrocnémiens: de l'anatomie au traitement. Montpellier: Sauramps; 2012. p. 231–41.
5. Tardieu G. Clinical documentation of cerebral palsy. Methods of evaluation and therapeutic applications. Rev Neuropsychiatr Infant 1968;16(1):6–90.
6. Barouk LS. Les brièvetés musculaires postérieures du pied de l'infirme moteur cérébral (IMC). Rev Chir Orthop Reparatrice Appar Mot 1984;70(Suppl 2): 163–6 [in French].
7. Boone DC, Azen SP. Normal range of motion in male subjects. J Bone Joint Surg Am 1979;61 A(5):251–4.
8. Colombier JA. Brièveté des gastrocnémiens dans les métatarsalgies. In: Brièveté des gastrocnémiens: de l'anatomie au traitement. Montpellier (France): Sauramps; 2012. p. 285–94.

9. De Los Santos R. La libération du gastrocnémien médial- Expérience madrilène. In: Brièveté des gastrocnémiens: de l'anatomie au traitement. Montpellier (France): Sauramps; 2012. p. 389–98.
10. Rabat E. Allongement endoscopique du gastrocnémien. In: Brièveté des gastrocnémiens: de l'anatomie au traitement. Montpellier (France): Sauramps; 2012. p. 351–74.
11. Maceira E, Orejana A. Hallux limitus fonctionnel et le système achilléo-calcanéo-plantaire. In: Brièveté des gastrocnémiens: de l'anatomie au traitement. Montpellier (France): Sauramps; 2012. p. 147–95.
12. Rippstein P, editor. Trois localisations de la section distale du triceps, avec leur conséquences, vol. 159. Paris: Maitrise Orthopedique; 2006. p. 26.
13. Downey MS, Banks AS. Gastrocnemius recession in the treatment of nonspastic ankle equinus. A retrospective study. J Am Podiatr Med Assoc 1989;79(4): 159–74.
14. Kowalski C. Le petit livre rouge du pied- Le gastrocourt. Podo 3000, éd. l'académie du pied, Liège 2000.

Functional Hallux Rigidus and the Achilles-Calcaneus-Plantar System

Ernesto Maceira, MD*, Manuel Monteagudo, MD

KEYWORDS

- Functional hallux rigidus • Metatarsophalangeal joint
- Achilles-calcaneus-plantar system

KEY POINTS

- Functional hallux rigidus is a clinical condition in which the mobility of the first metatarsophalangeal (MP) joint is normal under non-weight-bearing conditions, but its dorsiflexion is blocked when first metatarsal is made to support weight.
- In mechanical terms, functional hallux rigidus implies a pattern of interfacial contact through rolling, while in a normal joint contact by gliding is established.
- The windlass mechanism is essential to maintain the plantar vault and is based on the correct functioning of an arch formed by several bony elements, which work through compression, and foot braces, which work through tension, among which the best prepared for its moment arm is the plantar aponeurosis.
- Both the elevation of the head of first metatarsal and the increase in tension in the aponeurosis may alter the joint dynamics in the first MP joint, producing contact by rolling instead of physiologic interfacial contact through gliding.
- Limitation of the dorsiflexion in the ankle or the MP joint blocks the forward movement of the tibia during the stance phase on the sagittal plane, which is compensated through diverse mechanisms that entail abnormal movements on other planes and in other body segments.
- Patients with functional hallux rigidus should only be operated on if the pain or disability makes it necessary. Gastrocnemius release is a beneficial procedure in most patients.

INTRODUCTION

Functional hallux rigidus is a clinical condition in which the first metatarsophalangeal (MP) joint motion is impaired on weight-bearing conditions but not when unloaded.

Disclosures: None.
Foot and Ankle Unit, Department of Orthopaedic Surgery, Hospital Universitario Quirón Madrid, Calle Diego de Velázquez 1, Pozuelo de Alarcón, Madrid 28223, Spain
* Corresponding author.
E-mail address: e.maceira@telefonica.net

foot.theclinics.com
1083-7515/14/$ – see front matter © 2014 Elsevier Inc. All rights reserved.

Weight-bearing motion at the first MP joint depends on structures that are not located at the joint itself, but more proximally. Among these structures, the Achilles-calcaneal-plantar system and the medial column of the foot are mainly responsible for optimally setting the first MP joint to provide for anteromedial support of the foot during the third rocker or propulsive phase of gait; this requires adequate passive dorsiflexion of the joint while the hallux is purchasing the ground and the verticalized first metatarsal is axially loading the hallux-sesamoid complex. Failure to achieve first metatarsal plantarflexion, or an increase on tensile stress at the plantar fascia, will limit passive first MP joint dorsiflexion in the transition from the second rocker (plantigrade support) to the third one (forefoot support). These can impede the ideal gliding contact pattern at the first MP joint, producing rolling contact on the dorsal margin of the joint. Because propulsion takes place in closed kinetic chain conditions, limited passive dorsiflexion of the first MP joint blocks motion in the sagittal plane, which is necessary for the forward progression of the body during gait. Compensatory mechanisms must develop to cope with the lack of motion at the first MP joint. They may or may not lead to the onset of symptoms.

During the second rocker, the tibia must glide forward on the ankle to allow the body's center of mass to progress from an initial position posterior to the supporting foot to a final position anterior to it. A restriction to ankle passive dorsiflexion during the second rocker will increase dorsiflexing moments at the forefoot, thus increasing tensile stress at the plantar soft tissues due to the truss and beam mechanism of the plantar vault support. Contracture of the elastic component of the gastrocnemius muscles will be particularly harmful to ankle kinetics, because the knee must be extended during the second rocker to provide for functional lengthening of the supporting limb while the opposite is swinging. Tension at the soleus muscle is not modified by knee position.

This article focuses on the functional hallux rigidus of biomechanical origin from a clinical and mechanical point of view. Some of the pathologic mechanisms described in this text have not been proven, but are nonetheless very useful to understand the concept of functional hallux rigidus. The role of the Achilles-calcaneal-plantar system is described to provide a wide range of treatments when planning surgical management.

Hallux rigidus of biomechanical origin is the final stage of functional hallux rigidus; both of them are the same disease. When passive dorsiflexion is present in non-weight-bearing conditions, it should be possible to improve motion in weight-bearing conditions, and these cases will respond to joint-preserving surgical procedures. If there is no passive motion at the first MP joint in non-weight-bearing conditions, arthrodesis is the author's preferred procedure regardless of the radiological appearance of the joint. Hallux rigidus of nonmechanical origin, which is not discussed in this article, includes traumatic, metabolic, neuromuscular, rheumatic disease, congenital anomalies, and iatrogenic disorders.

FUNCTIONAL HALLUX RIGIDUS OF BIOMECHANICAL ORIGIN: THE INFLUENCE OF EQUINUS CONTRACTURE

Functional hallux rigidus is a clinical condition in which the first MP joint allows sufficient passive dorsiflexion when the first metatarsal is not bearing weight, but not when it has to support a person's body weight.[1,2] It moves in an open kinetic chain, but not in a closed chain. In a more advanced case of hallux rigidus, complete passive dorsiflexion even when not bearing any weight is not possible; this is referred to as a structural hallux rigidus. In hallux rigidus, the capacity for passive dorsiflexion of the first MP joint is practically canceled. Examination of the mobility of the first MP joint exclusively while not bearing weight does not provide information on its behavior during the gait cycle.[3,4]

How much passive dorsiflexion is necessary to be considered normal? In this aspect, there is notable discrepancy between different authors. It can be assumed that the minimum first MP joint dorsiflexion to achieve a normal third rocker is 60°.[5] In mechanical terms, the distinction between functional hallux rigidus and an ideal first MP joint is simpler: under ideal conditions, the pattern of contact is pure gliding, while hallux rigidus produces an evident rolling contact of the joint.

An elevated position of the head of the first metatarsal with respect to the proximal phalanx of the hallux, or an increase in tension in the plantar aponeurosis, would induce a tendency toward rolling contact pattern in the first MP joint during the transition from the second to the third rocker. It has been widely debated whether the elevation of the head of the first metatarsal is the primary mechanical anomaly or whether the increase in tension in the plantar aponeurosis is the culprit.[1] In the presence of either alteration, the other may end up occurring: an elevation of the head of first metatarsal will increase the tension in the plantar aponeurosis by reducing the vault's anticollapse moment arm, while an abnormal increase in the tension of the aponeurosis will impede the gliding contact in the first MP joint, increasing the dorsal compressive forces in the joint.

In a pattern of rolling interfacial contact, the instant center of rotation (the point with the least movement in an infinitesimal amount of time) is located on the surface of the convex element where it contacts with the concave surface, while in gliding contact, the instant center of rotation is located in the geometric center of the convex element (**Fig. 1**).[6] Although in most patients with hallux rigidus it may be possible to objectively detect an elevation of the first metatarsal with respect to the second metatarsal in a lateral weight-bearing radiograph, in others this is not possible. In some cases, there is evidence of instability of the first metatarsocuneiform joint on the sagittal plane during clinical examination, but this may not be evident radiographically. Hallux rigidus may occur in a patient without evidence of relative dorsiflexion of the first metatarsal on the radiograph. However, the author has never seen hallux rigidus *of biomechanical origin* in a patient with an increase in the inclination of the first metatarsal in the lateral weight-bearing projection (ie a cavus forefoot), nor a case with marked elevation of the first metatarsal and normal first MP joint mobility in weight-bearing conditions.

The diagnosis of functional hallux rigidus should be established on the basis of clinical examination. The test for functional hallux rigidus is performed with the patient lying in a supine position (**Fig. 2**).[7] When the first metatarsal is brought to plantar flexion, at least 60° of passive dorsiflexion should be attained; if not, this is a case of hallux rigidus that is either progressing or fully developed (hallux rigidus). To simulate the conditions of weight-bearing (closed kinetic chain) in the patient, the head of the first metatarsal is pushed upward, until the ankle enters its neutral position. At that point, passive extension of the first MP joint by applying a dorsiflexion force to the distal end of the proximal phalanx of the hallux should be attempted. If the foot has adequate function, applying this force creates a dorsiflexion of 90° (at least superior to 60°) and the examiner perfectly notes how the head of the first metatarsal moves to plantar flexion, increasing the height of the medial arch (**Fig. 3**).[4,7,8]

Samuel Barouk (Personal communication) showed that on performing the test for functional hallux rigidus with the knee in flexion, in some patients the windlass mechanism becomes normalized, allowing adequate passive mobilization of the first MP joint in dorsiflexion (**Fig. 4**). The only structures that negatively influence the windlass mechanism with the knee in extension, but which cease to do so with the knee flexed, is the gastrocnemius. Actually, this phenomenon displays the correlation between the

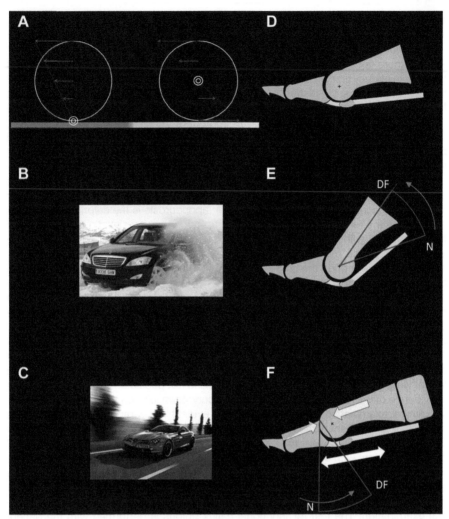

Fig. 1. Patterns of interfacial contact in the first MP joint. From a mechanical point of view, the pattern of interfacial contact between 2 surfaces, of which one is convex, can be through rolling (*A, left*) or sliding (*A, right*), depending on the location of the instant center of rotation (the point with the least movement in an infinitesimal amount of time). Under normal conditions, the contact of the first MP joint during the transition from the second to the third rocker should be made through gliding, which means that the instant center of rotation will be in the geometric center of the convex surface. This is what is produced when the wheel of a car is unable to grip the road surface because of ice (*B, E*). In functional hallux rigidus, a pattern of rolling contact appears, with the instant center of rotation in the point of contact of both surfaces. This is what is produced when the wheel of a car moves normally along an asphalt surface (*C, F*). A relative elevation of the head of first metatarsal with respect to the proximal phalanx of the hallux and an increase in the tensile stresses are 2 of the causes that can lead to the establishment of a pattern of contact by rolling in the first MP joint: one may end up causing the other. There does not necessarily need to be radiological evidence of the elevation of the head of first metatarsal in the lateral weight-bearing radiograph. DF, dorsiflexion; N, neutral position. (*D*) Normal static first MP joint is depicted in its neutral position; the relative elevation of the head, or the increase of tensile stresses of the aponeurosis, may give rise to the situation presented in (*F*).

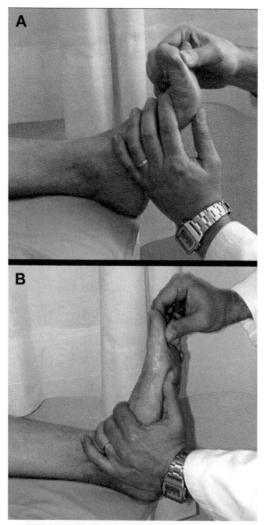

Fig. 2. Test for functional hallux rigidus. With the patient in a supine position, the mobility is first tested in passive dorsiflexion of the first MP joint, bringing the first metatarsal to plantarflexion (*A*). Under normal conditions, dorsiflexion of the first MP joint to 90° is easily reached. Subsequently, the first metatarsal is brought to dorsal flexion, until the point at which the sole of the foot is placed at a right angle with the axis of the leg, maintaining neutral alignment of the foot on the coronal plane. In a normal foot, as a result of the windlass mechanism, it is noted how the first metatarsal tends toward plantar flexion, allowing 90° of passive dorsiflexion in the first MP joint. A case of functional hallux rigidus is considered to be present when upon simulating the closed kinetic chain the first MP joint does not reach 60° (*B*). If non-weight-bearing mobilization does not reach 60°, it is thought that there is an early stage case of hallux rigidus. In degenerative hallux rigidus, non-weight-bearing passive dorsiflexion is practically or totally blocked. In either form of hallux rigidus, if the proximal phalanx of the hallux is pushed further to create passive dorsiflexion, the movement will not be produced in the first MP joint, but rather in the ankle.

biarticular component of the triceps surae and the plantar aponeurosis. The positive Barouk maneuver (test showing anomalous functional hallux rigidus with the knee extended, but normal function with the knee flexed) is simply the combination of the Silfverskjold test for gastrocnemius contracture with the test for functional hallux rigidus.

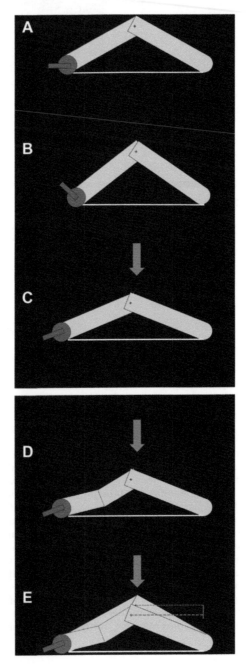

The plantar fascia should not only be understood as an anatomic structure that passively contributes to the movement of the inner longitudinal arch during the stance phase of the foot but also that among its functions is that of contributing to the maintenance of the inner longitudinal arch during stance (see **Fig. 3**). Transection of the aponeurosis or resection of a heel spur may produce overload injuries, especially in the fourth and third metatarsals (which in feet with an intact aponeurosis fracture less frequently than the second metatarsal) and collapse of the plantar vault (**Fig. 5**).

The term equinus initially referred to walking like horses, and most quadrupeds, do, with the ankle in plantar flexion. In the clinically evident equinus deformity, the patient is unable to make his or her heel contact with the ground. In subclinical or nonevident equinus, there is increased plantar flexion moment at the ankle but the heel can contact the ground.

Sagittal Plane Block and Compensatory Mechanisms

It is evident that the widest range of joint movements of the lower limbs during the gait cycle is produced in the sagittal plane. The *blockage* of any of these joints in the *sagittal plane* will require compensatory mechanisms to allow progression.[7] The compensation must occur in the sagittal plane, but may impose changes or the appearance of abnormal movement elsewhere. For example, a lack of dorsiflexion in the ankle may be compensated for by an intrinsic dorsiflexion of the foot, but this will entail pronation; it takes place at the expense of pronation.[7,9] The problem is that the consequences of compensation can cease to be tolerated well, thus becoming a clinically significant condition.

Equinus may be considered to be vestigial, thus resulting in the frequency of its subclinical presentations.[9] It can be present in normal, healthy subjects, who have an anatomic variation such as a reduction in the length ratios of the triceps/tibia. If the ankle does not provide adequate passive dorsiflexion during the second rocker and the transition to the third rocker, its blockage on the sagittal plane can be compensated in various manners: lifting the heel earlier (thus shortening the second rocker), pronating the foot, hyperextending the knee, externally rotating the leg, and so on.[7] In each case, the *compensatory mechanism* will be conditioned by anatomic factors, diseases, and habits, and these can be considered particular to each individual. They may be clinically pathologic, or never become a consideration if they do not cause any pain or disability. Nevertheless, subclinical equinus, a rather frequent variation among the healthy population, can eventually cause a problem as a side effect of various

---

Fig. 3. The windlass mechanism. The plantar arch remains in the same form as a truss; it is a structure formed by several elements that work through compressive stress, and the beams, which join together in the apex and are solidified at the base by a brace, which works through tensile stress. In the case of the foot, the beams are the bones and the brace is the plantar aponeurosis. It is, however, a dynamic truss because of the presence of the hallux, which is what is really joined to the brace by one of its ends (*A*). Dorsiflexion of the toe tenses the aponeurosis, which translates to an increase in the height of the arch and brings the plantar ends of the beams closer to each other, the same as a windlass would do (*B*). Conversely, the load on the arch would tense the brace, which would cause plantar flexion of the toe (reverse windlass) (*C*). This mechanism is the most important in the stabilization of the toes against the ground when the foot bears weight. The elevation of the head of the first metatarsal, whether due to a bodily deformity such as flat feet, acquired instability of the joints that incorporate the inner arch, or a surgical procedure that causes the head of first metatarsal to rise (*D*) will produce an increase in the tensile stress in the aponeurosis, resulting in the toe tending to remain in plantar flexion; due to the reduction in the anticollapse moment arm of the aponeurosis (*E*).

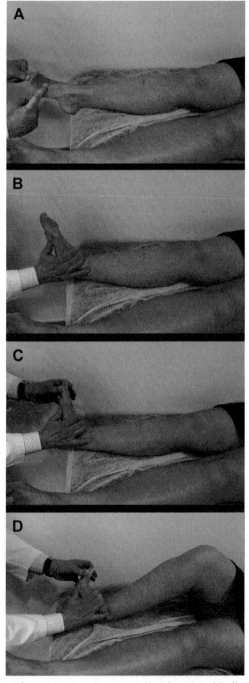

Fig. 4. The Barouk test for gastrocnemius-dependent functional hallux rigidus. It is a combination of the test for functional hallux rigidus (*A–C*) with the Silfverskjold maneuver (*D*). If the test is repeated in a patient with functional hallux rigidus with the knee in flexion (ie, if the involvement of the gastrocnemius is removed), the test for functional hallux rigidus is normal (*D*). In later stages of rigidus, the test will no longer give a normal result even with knee flexed.

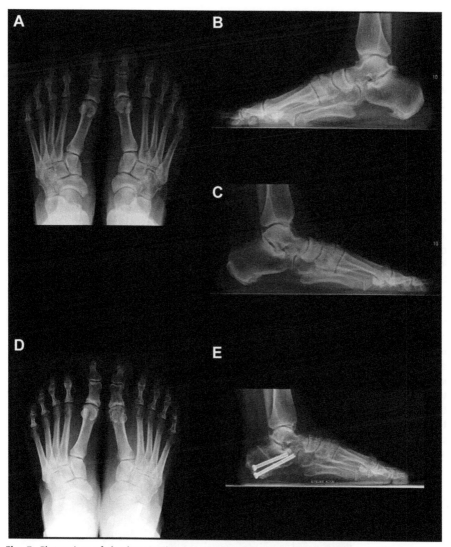

Fig. 5. Flattening of the longitudinal arch after the removal of a heel spur. Note that the foot had a cavus configuration. After the exeresis of the spur, flattening of the plantar arch occurred. (*A*) It can be appreciated how the right foot improves its alignment after the spur removal since the talocalcaneal divergence increased; however, the discomfort became incapacitating and did not improve with orthopedic treatment. (*C*) A lateral projection of the operated foot; its arch appears more normal than the one visible in (*B*), but the foot initially was cavus, whereas now the foot is flattened to a normal arch, but painful. Observe the diastasis of the first tarsometatarsal joint in its plantar portion. The performance of a medialization osteotomy of the calcaneal tuberosity reduces the pronating moment arm of the ground reaction force after initial contact, which reduces the external moments that the plantar soft tissues must withstand. The procedure was completed with lengthening of the Achilles tendon. The final result was a more cavus foot, with the disappearance of the previous symptoms (*D, E*).

compensatory mechanisms, or as a result of the tissue stress that equinus itself cause.[7,9,10]

The Achilles-Calcaneus-Plantar System During the Gait Cycle

The functional connection between the triceps surae and the soft tissue of the plantar arch was made by Arandes and Viladot,[10] who described the Achilles-calcaneal-plantar system based on the studies of Sieberg. In this system, the bony intermediate portion, the posterior tuberosity of the calcaneus, would be considered a large sesamoid, which would transmit the flexor power of the triceps surae to the forefoot.[10] It also transmits the effects of a shortening of the triceps to the plantar system (**Fig. 6**). The enthesis/enthetic organ of the heel is the archetype of fibrocartilaginous enthesis and guarantees the functional continuity of the Achilles-calcaneal-plantar system.[11]

In which periods of the gait cycle can equinus be responsible for overloading of the foot? Overloading of the foot will be most evident when extension of the knee and dorsiflexion of the ankle are simultaneously required of the supporting limb (**Fig. 7**). This instant corresponds to the transition of the second rocker to the third rocker.[12–14] As discussed above, during the second rocker, the knee must be extended to functionally lengthen the stance limb. The shortening of the elastic component of the calves may begin to overload the foot from the instant in which the tibia exceeds the vertical plane of the talus. In fact, this moment marks the beginning of the powerful eccentric action of the soleus.[13] Successively, while the knee remains extended, the ankle will be required to perform passive dorsiflexion. Under normal conditions, during the second rocker, the position of the foot must change from pronation to supination; from a relaxed and cushioning conformation to a rigid and propulsive one.[10] If the ankle is unable to provide the necessary passive dorsiflexion for the center of mass to be placed in front of its vertical plane, one of the ways to achieve these degrees of dorsiflexion is the pronation of the foot. Clinically, this phenomenon must be looked for by observing the patient walking barefoot to estimate whether the pronation, something normal after the initial contact is made, is prolonged excessively and reaches the end of the second rocker. During the second half of the second rocker, the foot must be clearly supinated. If not, it will be impossible to place the internal column above the external

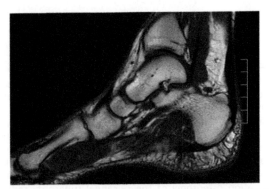

Fig. 6. NMR image of a patient with clinical diagnosis of mechanical talalgia due to plantar fasciitis, functional hallux rigidus, and shortening of the calf muscles. Furthermore, it should be observed that in addition to thickening of the proximal plantar aponeurosis, there is also (nonsymptomatic) thickening of the Achilles tendon. The posteroinferior trabecular system of the calcaneus assures functional continuity between the tendon and the aponeurosis. Continuity in the periosteum is also visible, relatively swollen. Note the instability of the first tarsometatarsal joint, which may be the cause or consequence of functional hallux rigidus.

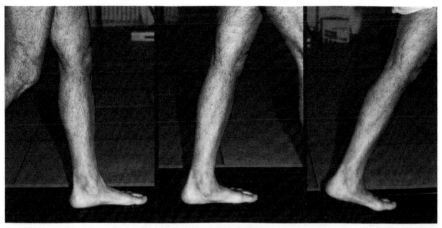

Fig. 7. During the second rocker, the stance knee must be extended to functionally lengthen the extremity. The truly tense instant for the Achilles-calcaneal-plantar system is the transition from the second to the third rocker as extension of the knee and passive dorsiflexion of the ankle are simultaneously required. In gastrocnemius-dependent equinus, given that the ankle does not exceed the neutral position (90° leg-sole of the foot), the progression of the anterograde rotation of the tibia would be blocked. To compensate this blockage of the heel on the sagittal plane, this patient resorts to constant pronation of the foot from the time the tibia exceeds a vertical position. This case is a functional hallux rigidus mediated by a shortening of the calves. Observe several clinical stigmata of hallux rigidus-rigidus: the dorsal prominence of the head of first metatarsal and increased interphalangeal joint dorsiflexion.

column at the proximal level (midtarsal joint), which will effectively turn the foot into a bag of loose bones.[15,16] The flattening of the longitudinal arch and the elevation of the head of the first metatarsal bone may be the consequence of this pronation.[7,9]

Relationship Between the Degree of Equinnus and the Resulting Pathology

There is not a direct correlation between the degree of equinnus and its harmful effect on the plantar fascia and the windlass mechanism. Furthermore, a restraint of additional passive dorsiflexion from the neutral ankle position at 90° represents a longer lever arm for tensioning of the plantar fascia, thus producing limited dorsiflexion at the metatarso-phalangeal joint and symptoms of plantar fasciitis. But direct equinnus with ankle block in plantar flexion results in increased axial compressive stress underneath the metatarsal heads but less plantar fascia tensioning. The restraint in ankle dorsiflexion with the ankle around its neutral position increases tensile stress in the plantar aponeurosis while the restraint in ankle dorsiflexion when the ankle is plantar-flexed produces higher compressive stress at the ball of the foot but less tensile stress on the plantar fascia.

During clinical examination of patients, various signs suggestive of gastrocnemius-dependent equinus may be present. The presence of extensor overactivity and second rocker keratosis in the forefoot are clinical signs frequently apparent in patients with shortening of the calf muscles (**Fig. 8**). Mixed keratoses with combined stigmata of the second and third rockers are also highly suggestive of gastrocnemius shortening.[16] The presence of pure third rocker keratoses ought to cause doubt that the gastrocnemius muscles are responsible; direct equinus through the shortening of the whole triceps, or through ankle joint blockage of dorsiflexion, may limit foot

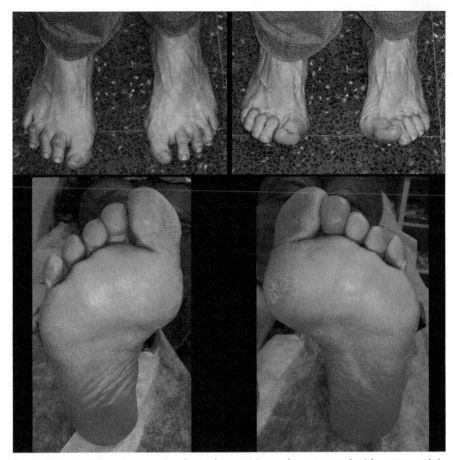

Fig. 8. Patient with gastrocnemius-dependent equinus who presented with metatarsalgia. The patient exhibits keratosic lesions of the second rocker; there is no tendency to extend toward the toe nor to the neighboring keratoses, strictly plantar to the head of each overloaded metatarsal bone during the plantigrade stance. In this case, there is no problem with dorsiflexion of the first MP joint nor with pronation of the foot; in fact, there is supination. The lesser digits have a claw deformity due to overrecruitment of the long extensors. Although the tibialis anterior functions normally, it is unable to cope with the excessive plantarflexing moment produced by the gastrocnemius. If the patient is asked to stand on his heels, the long extensors are excessively active, yet he is barely able to lift the forefoot from the ground.

support to a single third rocker, but in this case, the problem is not solved by a gastrocnemius release. On the other hand, the absence of keratoses on the forefoot in no way excludes the presence of equinus. A reduction or annulment of the first rocker or early performance of the third rocker can also be clinical signs that lead to the discovery of subclinical equinus.[5] The Silfverskjold test is a specific examination to determine whether the individual case of equinus depends exclusively on the gastrocnemius muscles or not.[17] It is important to recognize the role of shortening of the gastrocnemius in a pathologic situation in order not to overprescribe surgical treatment. Shortening of the elastic component of the gastrocnemius will increase passive dorsiflexing moments at the forefoot because of the ground reaction force. The plantar vault will flatten, thus increasing tension in the plantar fascia.

CLINICAL EXAMINATION AND DIAGNOSIS

Hallux rigidus of mechanical origin is the final stage in the evolution of functional hallux rigidus. It is, therefore, the same condition, in different evolutionary phases and with different radiological findings. Its signs and symptoms are similar. It should be taken into account that there is no direct correlation between the radiological findings and the clinical signs and symptoms in a patient with hallux rigidus. Several different attempts have been made to classify hallux rigidus, mainly based on the radiological appearance. Regnauld proposed a 3-stage classification from mild osteoarthritic changes to severe ankylosis.[18] A fourth initial stage has been added, characterized by the absence of osteoarthritic changes at the first MP joint.[19,20] It must be pointed out that a stage 1 hallux rigidus may be painful or produce transfer metatarsalgia, whereas a stage 4 ankylotic patient may be asymptomatic.

A simple inspection may prove conclusive when diagnosing the most typical cases. With the foot not bearing weight, the prominence of the back of the first MP joint and the spoonlike shape of the first ray are pathognomonic of a blockage in dorsiflexion of the first MP joint during the third rocker (**Fig. 9**).[21] The dorsal prominence of the head of

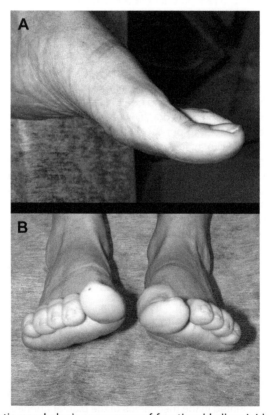

Fig. 9. Characteristic morphologic appearance of functional hallux rigidus. Not all cases of functional hallux rigidus present thus, but this morphology indicates that the first MP joint cannot dorsiflex, at least when bearing weight. The spoonlike appearance of the first ray is due to the dorsiflexion of the first metatarsal and the plantar flexion of the first MP joint with dorsiflexion of the interphalangeal joint (*A*, medial view of the left foot; *B*, anterior view of both feet, the right one being normal).

the first metatarsal is not always associated with the presence of an osteophytic growth. In time, degenerative osteoarthritis will probably develop, but in the initial phases of functional hallux rigidus, the articular surfaces are completely normal. In this joint, the articular blockage precedes the arthritic changes. The dorsal prominence appears when there is significant elevation of the head of the first metatarsal even while not bearing weight. Furthermore, the proximal phalanx is in plantar flexion and the interphalangeal joint is in dorsal flexion. However, in some patients with functional hallux rigidus, the appearance of the toe is completely normal. Usually a keratosis appears under the plantar aspect of the interphalangeal joint of the first toe, due to the hyperpressure and shearing forces, which it is subjected to during the third rocker. The passive mobility of the first MP joint while not bearing weight may be completely normal, the same as its active non-weight-bearing mobility, but both are impaired in stage 1 hallux rigidus when the first metatarsal is loaded: the test for functional hallux rigidus exposes the prevention of dorsiflexion when first metatarsal is bearing weight. Unfortunately, it is not known exactly how much force should be applied when performing the test. The force to be applied cannot be quantified, but in practice dorsal flexion is applied to the foot, and the head of the first metatarsal is pushed in a cephalad direction until the ankle is in a neutral position, maintaining neutral alignment in the coronal plane (see **Fig. 2**). It must be taken into account that the force that the forefoot withstands in the first part of the third rocker is superior to the subject's body weight, thus being much higher than that performed during the test. Once the load has been simulated on the first ray, passive dorsiflexion of the first MP joint from the end of the proximal phalanx is attempted. The test is considered positive, indicating the presence of functional hallux rigidus when the ankle is what moves upon pushing the phalanx up and not the first MP joint. Under ideal conditions, the first MP joint will reach complete dorsiflexion and the effects of the windlass mechanism will be noted as described previously (see **Fig. 3**).[8] The author considers that a diagnosis of functional hallux rigidus cannot be established if 60° of dorsiflexion are exceeded on performing the test. If this degree of dorsiflexion is not attained while plantar-flexing the first metatarsal and while the patient is not bearing weight, it can be said that structural hallux rigidus is developing. As mentioned above, the combination of the Silfverskjold test and the test for functional hallux rigidus led Barouk to describe the phenomenon of normalization of the kinematics of the first MP joint when the passive action of shortening of the calf muscles is canceled out. A positive result in the Barouk test indicates that in the case in question, the shortening of the elastic component of the gastrocnemius is a determining factor in the dynamic locking of the first MP joint (see **Fig. 4**). As such, selective release of the calf muscles could be considered as a treatment of functional hallux rigidus in the patient, but those patients usually improve satisfactorily with the use of Dananberg-style orthotics or with anterolateral wedges, together with gastrocnemius stretching exercises. These patients frequently have other alterations such as the elevation of the head of the first metatarsal, such that if an operation becomes necessary, this usually involves a bony procedure in addition to the gastrocnemius release (**Fig. 10**).

Associated morphologic and functional alterations should be looked for, such as the presence of pronation of the foot, the dysfunction of the peroneus longus muscle, and equinus.[9] As was presented in the mechanics of the plantar aponeurosis and the inner arch, the clinical signs that are classically described to explore the function of the posterior tibial tendon actually explore the integrity of the windlass mechanism: single and double heel-rise tests. Hintermann's test (first metatarsal rise test)[22] exposes the functional canceling out of the peroneus longus when the subtalar joint is pronated (**Fig. 11**). The mechanical explanation of this phenomenon is due to the loss in the

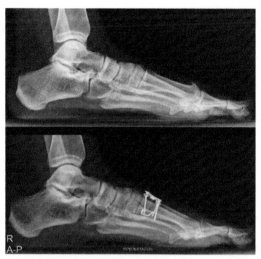

Fig. 10. Proximal opening wedge plantar flexing osteotomy of the first metatarsal. An incomplete osteotomy (spanning approximately three-fourths of the thickness of the bone) was performed with the addition of a dorsal wedge, in this case fixed with a spacer plate. On the plantar aspect of the metatarsal, a staple is placed beforehand to attempt to avoid breaking the fulcrum, which would entail an undesired effect of extension with loss of the capacity for plantar flexion of the osteotomy. The gap is filled with an autologous graft originating from the cheilectomy. Medial gastrocnemius lengthening after Barouk was performed as well. This treatment is the author's treatment of choice when the first metatarsal is not long, because it is the only procedure with which passive dorsiflexion of the first MP joint was markedly and durably improved in a patient with functional hallux rigidus.

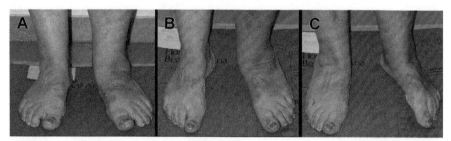

Fig. 11. First metatarsal rise sign, by Hintermann, described for the diagnosis of posterior tibial claudication. The pronation of the foot nullifies the capacity of the peroneus longus tendon to stabilize the first metatarsal against the ground. When the subtalar joint is pronated, the necessary difference in level between the cuboid and the first metatarsal for the peroneus longus tendon to have a component of first metatarsal plantar flexion is lost. On rotating the leg externally in a stationary stance, or passively placing the heel in varus, the head of first metatarsal of the affected foot is not capable of remaining on the ground. (*A*) Patient in bipedal static stance; observe the pronation of the pathologic left foot. On requesting the patient to turn to the right with her soles on the ground, the left foot pronates even more, but the right foot brings the heel into varus and is able to hold the first metatarsal on the ground (*B*). However, on requesting that she turn toward the left, the head of the left first metatarsal cannot remain in contact with the ground and rises (*C*).

difference in height between the cuboid bone and the first metatarsal base. Thanks to this difference in height, the peroneus longus is able to pull the first metatarsal toward the ground, stabilizing it in plantar flexion. With rear-foot pronation, the cuboid tends to rise and the first metatarsocuneiform joint tends to descend, which cancels out the stabilizing moment arm of the peroneus longus over the first metatarsal.[23]

The stability of the internal column against passive dorsiflexion should be specifically explored, as was indicated earlier, but furthermore, the level or levels at which it is located should be found: the fault may be located at the level of the first tarsometatarsal joint, but may also be in the naviculo-cunneiform, the talonavicular joint, or several of these. The fault point or points can usually be well felt on palpation (**Fig. 12**). The planning of surgical treatment may be incorrect if the level of instability is not determined. Fusion at the level of the tarsometatarsal joints placing first metatarsal in plantar flexion is a useful intervention to re-establish the joint dynamics of the first MP joint.[9,24,25]

The most frequent locations for pain are the first MP joint and the interphalangeal joint of the big toe, typically with discomfort on the dorsal aspect of the MP joint.[26] The pain may radiate along the dorsal surface of the first ray and frequently is misdiagnosed as tendinitis. Sesamoiditis may cause plantar pain because of traction. The interphalangeal joint may be painful, and occasionally nail problems due to hyperextension of the hallux may cause friction with the shoe. Cases of transfer metatarsalgia

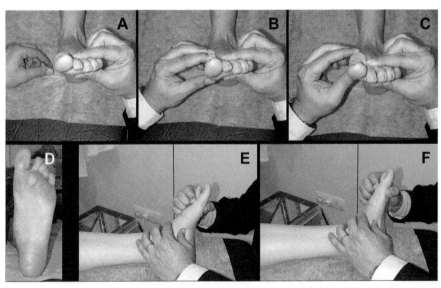

Fig. 12. Exploration of the stability of the first ray on the sagittal plane. With the patient lying supine, the metatarsal palette between the second and fifth digits is firmly held with one hand (A). With the other hand, the head of first metatarsal is passively led toward plantar (B) and dorsal flexion. The dorsiflexion of first metatarsal is considered to be excessive when its head dorsally exceeds the level of the back of the fingers of the hand, which is holding the minor toes (C). On the other hand, inspection and palpation allow one to estimate in which joint or joints of the inner arch dorsal inflexion is occurring (E, F). This patient corresponds to a typical case of functional hallux rigidus because of the instability of the internal column with shortening or the calf muscles; observe the second rocker keratosis under the second metatarsal head, as well as the plantar surface of the interphalangeal joint of the big toe (D).

are frequent, related to walking with increased supination during the third rocker or with elevation of the first metatarsal (relative lowering of the second metatarsal).

As was mentioned earlier, one of the mechanisms that can compensate for functional hallux rigidus is increased supination of the forefoot during the third rocker.[2,27] Once the first MP joint is blocked, the third rocker can no longer take place over the hallux MP joint, but rather over the interphalangeal joint of the first toe. Furthermore, the metatarsal parabola will no longer be anatomic, but rather it will be a straight line connecting the interphalangeal of the hallux with the head of the fifth metatarsal.

The most frequent symptom is transfer metatarsalgia in the minor rays, particularly the fourth and fifth. When keratoses appear, they present the typical stigmata of third rocker overload: a clear distal extension of the keratosis, which continues along the external and distal aspect of the head of the fifth metatarsal. These keratoses are very different than the ones that appear in subtalar joint varus (stigmata of the second rocker), which are strictly plantar to the head of the metatarsal, without distal extension, isolated, and narrower (**Fig. 13**).[16]

Adduction of the lesser toes may be another of the consequences of functional hallux rigidus when the compensatory mechanism is final supination of the forefoot.

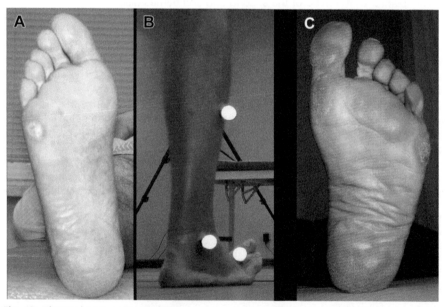

Fig. 13. Plantar keratoses in the fifth metatarsal. These keratoses may be of the second or third rocker, as in the rest of the rays. Those produced during the second rocker (*A*) are strictly plantar to the head of the fifth metatarsal, without distal extension, limited, and usually due to subtalar joint varus. They may be associated with keratoses at the base of the fifth metatarsal. They are unrelated to functional hallux rigidus. Note the hyperactivity of the extensors, from the swinging motion to the second rocker, the phase during which (*B*) was taken, in an attempt to help achieve eversion of the foot. Third rocker keratoses (*C*) have distal extension to the toe and are wider. These keratoses may be due to the supination compensating for the limitation of the dorsiflexion of the hallux during the third rocker. In (*C*), apart from the third rocker keratoses, other stigmata of hallux rigidus are present, such as the keratosis in the interphalangeal joint of the hallux and the second rocker lesions under the second and third metatarsals related to the relative lowering of these bones with respect to the first metatarsal, which is raised.

Whenever all the lesser toes are in adduction at the level of the MP joints, it is almost certain that the first MP joint will not dorsiflex under weight-bearing conditions (**Fig. 14**).

At times, only the second toe is involved, and it is highly probable that there exists a relative protrusion of the second metatarsal on the first and/or the third one causing what is referred to as a second space syndrome occurs (painful divergence of toes 2 and 3 in the second space and the second MP joint).[28] This syndrome may present with a normally functioning first MP joint, but when it occurs in conjunction with hallux rigidus, the second toe may end up mounted on top of the first, giving a crossover toe, independently of whether the first toe is adducted or not (see **Fig. 14**). It is understood that adduction of the minor toes is rarely due to a primary fault in the external collateral ligaments of the MP joints, but rather it is supination/external rotation of the forefoot during the third rocker, which medially diverts the toe, in the long term distending the lateral articular soft tissues.

During the plantigrade stance, the elevation of the first metatarsal head entails a relative descent of the head of the second metatarsal. Transfer metatarsalgia in the second ray is thus a consequence of the elevation of the first metatarsal and therefore the overloading occurs during the second rocker.[16] The keratosis will therefore be strictly plantar at the head of the second and sometimes also the third metatarsals, without spreading toward the toe, restricted and without being joined to the keratoses of the neighboring metatarsals when these are present. Faced with a foot such as the one pictured in **Fig. 15**, an alteration of the metatarsal parabola can be discarded as the cause of the overloading; a thorough inspection will reveal that the big toe is in plantar flexion and the underlying skin of the head of first metatarsal is practically un-used. In these patients, osteotomies of pure shortening of the second metatarsal should not be used. Osteotomies will only move the problem, in terms of its location, to a more proximal one.[16,28] Gastrocnemius release and stabilization of the first metatarsal in plantar flexion may provide highly beneficial mechanical effects for these patients.[9]

The plantar skin represents the best baro-pographic record of a foot. A keratosis is usually the response of normal skin to abnormal loading (shear, compression), although they may be absent in mechanically abnormal feet, and occasionally, they

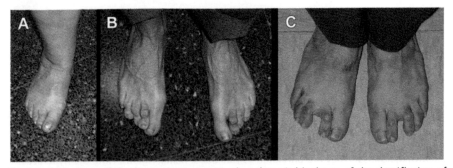

Fig. 14. Adduction of the lesser toes suggests that there is blockage of the dorsiflexion of the first MP joint during the third rocker (*A, B*), which is another of the effects derived from the compensatory mechanisms of hallux rigidus. It is a presentation of propulsive metatarsalgia and there is almost invariably an appreciable relative protrusion of the second metatarsal over the first and/or the third metatarsals. When the second space syndrome is established in a foot with blockage of dorsiflexion of the first MP joint, the second toe ends up mounted on top of the first, independently of whether there is an existing associated deformity in the form of hallux valgus (*C*). The result will be a crossover toe.

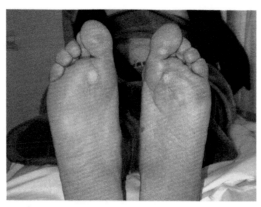

Fig. 15. The presence of clear second rocker keratosis is a contraindication for metatarsal shortening, regardless of the type of metatarsal parabola. A keratosis clearly produced during the second rocker does not bear any relationship to the length of the overloaded metatarsal, but rather its anatomic or functional angle. In this case, there are 2 additional details, which direct one to the origin of the lesion: the smoothness of the underlying skin of the head of the first metatarsal and the plantar flexion of the big toe. This case may have been resolved with a procedure of plantar flexion and stabilization of the first metatarsal. Selective lengthening of the triceps surae could help as well. However, the multiple interventions on the plantar skin under which the patient underwent, and the simple Weil osteotomies that were performed afterward, did not improve the metatarsalgia related to the elevation of first metatarsal. During the second rocker, elevation of first metatarsal is equivalent to a lowering of the second one.

may be due to dermatologic disease. When the skin under the first metatarsal head shows no signs of wear while the rest of the forefoot sole presents with keratoses, there is evidence of first metatarsal rise regardless of the radiological appearance of that foot.

In many patients with hallux valgus, the movement on the sagittal plane is good when it is examined with the toe adducted, but on attempting to align it on the transverse plane, dorsiflexion is blocked. Abduction of the big toe may be a compensatory mechanism in some cases of hallux rigidus. In this instance, it is hallux valgus rigidus, and in the case of surgical treatment being required, the lowering of the head of first metatarsal should somehow be associated with the lateralization of its head (**Fig. 16**).

Frequently, patients with hallux rigidus present other signs and symptoms related to an increase in the tensile stresses in the Achilles-calcaneal-plantar system. Rochera and López-Laserna noted the frequency of association of hallux rigidus with plantar fasciitis and the appearance of calcaneal spurs.[16] **Fig. 17** shows a lateral weight-bearing radiograph of a case of hallux rigidus, in which the arthritic changes in the first MP joint are added to the frank elevation of first metatarsal and the ossification of the enthesic organ of the heel. Achillodynia, calf muscle pain, and difficulty ascending slopes are also frequent in patients with shortening of the calf muscles.[29]

In the initial phases of functional hallux rigidus, the radiological appearance of the articular surfaces and the sesamoids of the first MP joint are normal (stage 1 hallux rigidus). The elevation of the first metatarsal should be evaluated, not by the impression of the position of its head with respect to the second metatarsal head, as this may vary significantly depending on the level and angle of the incident ray, but rather by focusing on the parallelism or divergence of the dorsal diaphyseal cortices of the second and first metatarsals (**Fig. 18**). If the difference in apparent height of both

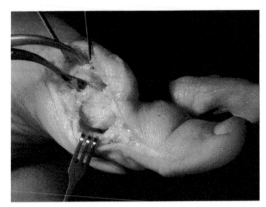

Fig. 16. In hallux rigidus/valgus, in addition to its lateralization, the head of first metatarsal must be lowered, or at least be prevented from rising more. Many surgical techniques can provide both effects simultaneously. In the image, there is a scarf osteotomy with the associated effect of head lowering.

metatarsals alone is focused on, some of the normally aligned feet will be considered as having an elevated first metatarsal. The dorsal cortices are easy to identify and they can be representative of the axes of the 2 metatarsals. If they diverge in such a way that the first metatarsal is in a more horizontal position than the second metatarsal, it can be certain that there is a relative elevation of first metatarsal during the second rocker (forefoot varus; pronated foot), in the same way that if the first metatarsal is more inclined, it can be affirmed that it is plantarflexed (forefoot valgus; supinated foot).[5] We will not come across a case of hallux rigidus *of biomechanical origin* in the latter case: there may be a limitation of first MP joint mobility, but this is not primarily mechanical in origin.

However, the cortices may be seen parallel in the lateral weight-bearing radiograph and nevertheless show clinical evidence of instability of the first ray on dorsiflexion (**Fig. 19**). The Meary-Tomeno line, established by the axes of the first metatarsal and the talus in the lateral weight-bearing projection, is very useful to investigate where the instability of the inner arch is located.[30] In the first tarsometatarsal joint, the instability is present and radiologically evident when there is a diastasis of the

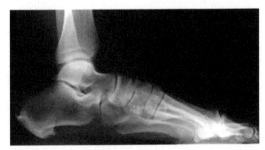

Fig. 17. Lateral weight-bearing radiograph of a patient with signs of overloading of the Achilles-calcaneal-plantar system and hallux rigidus. Note the elevation of first metatarsal (cortical divergences of the first and second metatarsals) and osteoarthritis of the first MP joint. Rochera and López-Laserna observed a close relationship between hallux rigidus and the ossification of the entheses in the Achilles-calcaneal-plantar system. Here the naviculo-cuneiform and the first tarsometatarsal joints appear to be at fault.

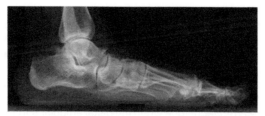

Fig. 18. The radiological evidence of the relative elevation of first metatarsal with respect to the second metatarsal is taken from the divergence of the dorsal diaphyseal cortices of both bones (not from the apparent distance between the first and second metatarsal heads). In this patient, hallux rigidus presents together with instability in all segments of the medial arch. Although frank osteoarthritis is absent at the level of the first MP joint, it is in plantar flexion and the interphalangeal joint of the big toe is in dorsal flexion. The subtalar joint remained pronated since early age, presenting with bone adaptation changes in the talonavicular joint, attempting to appear similar to a calcaneocuboid joint: the talar beak appears with or without tarsal coalition as long as subtalar pronation is early onset. The big toe of this patient moves perfectly while not bearing weight, but as soon as it must support weight, or is subjected to the test for functional hallux rigidus, dorsiflexion of the first MP joint is completely blocked. The main complaint of this patient is pain at the first MP joint. Most of the alterations leading to this patient's symptoms are located away from the painful joint itself.

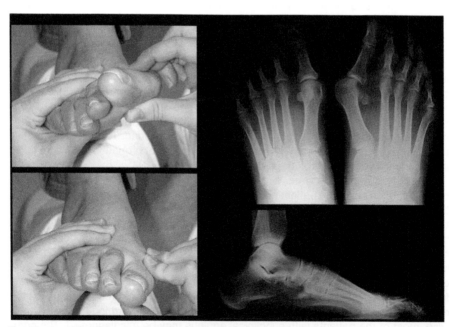

Fig. 19. Example of frank instability of the first metatarsal in a patient with hallux rigidus/ valgus. Clinical exploration and the dorsoplantar radiograph are suggestive of instability, but in the lateral projection, elevation of first metatarsal is not observable. Instability with a normal or minimally altered lateral radiograph may exist, such as the slight first cuneometatarsal plantar diastasis that can be observed in this case, without divergence of the dorsal cortices of the 2 first metatarsals.

plantar margins of the joint, or when a misalignment of the dorsal edges of the base of first metatarsal and the first cuneiform can be observed (subluxation). Dorsiflexion at the talo-navicular or cunneo-navicular joints may not be accompanied by plantar diastasis and only be appreciable because of the misalignment of the different segments. The angle of each one of the joints with respect to the ground and to the talo-first metatarsal axis must be observed. For instance, opening dorsal wedge plantarflexion osteotomy of the medial cuneiform after Cotton,[31] in order to plantarflex the first metatarsal, will be the preferred technique when the distal articular surface of the first cuneiform is closer to vertical.

The appearance of osteoarthritic changes in the first MP joint indicates a developed case of hallux rigidus. Once more, it should be pointed out that the loss of movement in closed kinetic chain precedes the appearance of radiological changes in hallux rigidus.

TREATMENT OF FUNCTIONAL HALLUX RIGIDUS

The author is not in favor of surgically operating on patients with nonsymptomatic functional hallux rigidus.[32] As in any other mechanical impairment of the foot, the author considers that a deformity or functional alteration should only be operated on if it produces pain and/or disability. The disease will probably progress once the mechanical impairment is present at early stages, but surgery cannot provide predictable results. On the other hand, many patients do well with nonoperative management or even with no treatment at all.[32]

Noninvasive treatment should include a range of options, from devices that some patients themselves place in their footwear to rehabilitative treatment, to various types of orthoses that may alleviate the symptoms and assist in functioning. Among these orthoses, the kinetic wedge designed by Dananberg[33] **(Fig. 20)**, based on the principles of facilitating movement on the sagittal plane, can be useful for some patients, just as other anterolateral solid wedges may also be useful.[34] There is no consensus on the most suitable type of orthosis. The use of the shoes with rocker bottom soles allows the patient to move the tibia forward, even though the second rocker (ankle block) and third rocker (first MP joint block) are altered. The forward movement is not made over the foot. It is made with the shoe on the ground. The patient response to this footwear is highly variable. The presence of rear-foot pronation should be taken into account when designing the orthotics.[35,36]

The surgical intervention must be planned based on the hierarchy of the deformities present in each case; the patient may consult for various reasons, among which functional hallux rigidus may or may not have been noticed by the patient. For example, transfer metatarsalgia may be due to functional hallux rigidus and not be accompanied by pain in the first ray. If functional hallux rigidus is not identified in this case as the origin of the lateral pain, and the intervention is performed directly on the minor rays, the clinical result will be unpredictable. The involvement of the Achilles-calcaneal-plantar system in the pathogenesis of functional hallux rigidus is very frequent. The Silfverskjold test must be performed after locking the midtarsal joint: it must be asssured that the subtalar joint is inverted while performing the test. Otherwise, most of the patients with subclinical equinus may be misdiagnosed. The complete or selective lengthening of the triceps surae is included as part of the surgery for functional hallux rigidus if there is evidence of equinus. For the complete lengthening of the triceps, the author prefers partial percutaneous tenotomies of the Achilles according to Hoke.[37] When this procedure is performed, the patient must remain immobilized for 6 weeks. Currently, for selective lengthening of the calf muscles, the

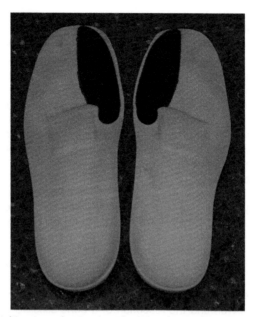

Fig. 20. Dananberg's kinetic wedge insoles. These insoles are basically the incorporation of a low-density element under the head of the first metatarsal with the aim of facilitating plantar flexion. Their use is still controversial compared with the use of other orthoses, but they are tried before considering surgical treatment of functional hallux rigidus because they are well tolerated and are inexpensive. In structural deformities, it may be useful to use rocker bottom shoes, which allow the tibia to perform in the third rocker what the first MP joint is incapable of doing.

author uses the Silfverskjold-Barouk technique, which allows the safe transsectioning of the soft fibers (tendinous, aponeurotic, and muscular).[38] The author has abandoned procedures on the junction of the calf muscles and the soleus because of the cosmetic problems from central approaches, excessive power loss, and the risk of injury of the sural nerve. Furthermore, the release to the medial gastrocnemius is limited, according to Barouk and Barouk.[29]

The author has not performed an isolated gastrocnemius release as a surgical treatment of functional hallux rigidus as opposed to cases of plantar fasciitis or Achilles tendinopathy. Until now, it has always formed part of an intervention involving bony procedures when managing hallux rigidus.[9] Medial gastrocnemius release could be performed as a single procedure in patients with a positive Barouk test (absence of hallux rigidus when performing the test with the knee flexed) (see **Fig. 4**), and who do not display elevation of the head of first metatarsal, but in these patients, pain is rarely significant.

Dorsiflexing osteotomies of the proximal phalanx of the hallux by means of the removal of a dorsal wedge (Moeberg effect) do not increase first MP joint range of motion, but set it at a more effective interval providing for additional dorsiflexion of the joint.[39] Even in severe cases, it may lead to satisfactory results when fixed plantarflexion of the first MP joint is present. This osteotomy is commonly associated with other bony and soft tissue procedures in the management of hallux rigidus.

Cheilectomy is a popular technique in the management of stage 1 and 2 hallux rigidus among some surgeons as an isolated operation.[40] The author prefers to use it in conjunction with other surgical procedures. The operation consists of the removal of the dorsal exostosis of the first metatarsal head together with a variable amount of the articular surface (20%–30%). It is a simple procedure that usually leaves a stable joint and may preserve motion and strength.[41,42]

As long as some painless passive motion in the first MP joint is preserved in non-weight-bearing conditions, joint-preserving procedures should be attempted. First metatarsal osteotomies are currently commonly used in those cases of hallux rigidus of biomechanical origin. Both an elevated first metatarsal and gastrocnemius contracture may play an important role in the production of hallux rigidus; whenever these conditions are present in a patient with hallux rigidus, the author aims to address them as long as the joint is still flexible in non-weight-bearing conditions. If the joint shows no passive motion when unloaded, or the available passive motion is painful, arthrodesis will probably be the preferred option.[43–45]

In all the cases of functional hallux rigidus that the author has treated, a mechanical effect that has always figured among the objectives has been the lowering of the head of the first metatarsal. If the metatarsal formula is of the type index plus (ie with a slightly longer first metatarsal), the procedure of choice is a simple Weil-type osteotomy (**Fig. 21**),[46–48] which provides for simultaneous metatarsal head lowering and shortening. Several osteotomies had been described to achieve simultaneous shortening and lowering of the first metatarsal, most of them based on a chevron-type osteotomy.[49–51] The mechanical effects they produce depend on the inclination of the 2 cuts of the chevron and the resection of a bone slice from the dorsal margin of the proximal fragment.

In those cases of hallux rigidus in which the first metatarsal is shorter or equal in length to the second one and there is evidence of metatarsus primus elevatus, the author prefers plantarflexing osteotomies with an opening dorsal wedge at

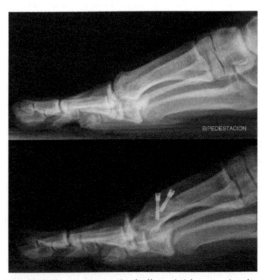

Fig. 21. First metatarsal Weil osteotomy in hallux rigidus to simultaneously lower and shorten the head of first metatarsal. It is used in patients with a metatarsal formula of index plus or plus-minus. It is usually associated with a cheilectomy; first metatarsal head lowering, as small as it might be, assists in improving the dynamics of the first MP joint. This particular case is a Paralympics runner who improved his status for ordinary activities but was unable to return to high-level competition. No gastrocnemius lengthening was associated to preserve propulsive power.

the base of first metatarsal (see **Fig. 10**). A technical inconvenience of the latter is the risk of complete interruption of the proximal end of the bone by its plantar cortex, meaning that head lowering will not be achieved, but rather a lengthening of the metatarsal, and therefore, the functional disorder of the first MP joint will not be corrected; it will continue to present a pattern of contact through rolling and not gliding (**Fig. 22**).

Before performing the partial osteotomy of the base of the metatarsal on its dorsal surface (spanning approximately two-thirds to three-fourths of the dorsoplantar width), a plantar staple is placed centered on the projection of the osteotomy, to have a fulcrum protected from breakage. However, despite this, the plantar cortex may be broken, meaning the first metatarsal will be lengthened instead of lowered (**Fig. 23**). The width of the additional dorsal wedge can be estimated on the lateral weight-bearing radiograph, whether by tracing an outline or through a process of quantization in digital radiographs: the millimeters of dorsal distraction are measured and need to be given to the osteotomy to make the dorsal cortices of the diaphyses of first and second metatarsals remain parallel.

Frequently, functional hallux rigidus is associated with pronation of the foot. In these cases, a necessary mechanical effect to achieve this is to reduce heel valgus, for which the author prefers osteotomies of medial displacement of the tuberosity (Koutsogiannis procedure).[52] The main mechanical effect of the osteotomy is to reduce the moment arm of the ground reaction forces acting on the subtalar joint. The closer the tuberosity of the calcaneus is placed to the projection of the axis of the tibia, the less pronation the foot will have to support after the initial contact. Lengthening osteotomies of the calcaneus may be advisable in addition to the medial translation of the

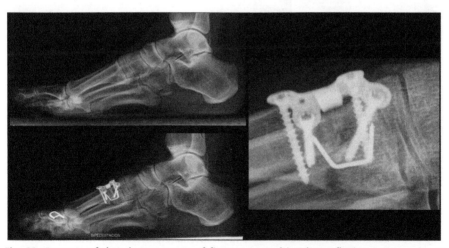

Fig. 22. Fracture of the plantar cortex of first metatarsal in plantarflexing osteotomies at the base of the first metatarsal is a technically unresolved problem. Despite not bearing weight for 6 weeks and the placement of a plantar staple, a diastasis may result that causes the action of plantar flexion to become a lengthening of the metatarsal, which will not improve the joint dynamics. The combination of other procedures, such as gastrocnemius release and the Moeberg procedure in this case, may improve the symptoms, but does not address the mechanical problem and therefore their future is uncertain. The placement of the staple is difficult, if, as the author has done, a single medial approach is used; its excessively dorsal location can be observed in this instance. Other times, the staple itself may cause the fracture.

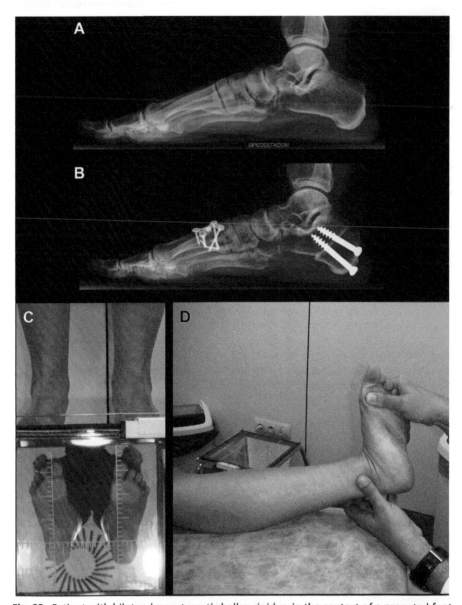

Fig. 23. Patient with bilateral symptomatic hallux rigidus, in the context of a pronated foot with shortening of the triceps surae at the expense of the calf muscles. A reconstruction was considered at multiple levels, including medial gastrocnemius release, medial glide osteotomy of the tuberosity of the calcaneus, and an incomplete osteotomy with an additional dorsal wedge at the base of the first metatarsal. In this case, the effect of the lowering of first metatarsal was insufficient. Even so, the windlass mechanism became reasonably restored, probably because of the associated surgical procedures. (A) Lateral preoperative radiograph; (B) lateral radiograph 11 months postoperatively, in which the tarsal alignment is satisfactory, but elevation of first metatarsal persists. (C) Preoperative clinical image on the podoscope, in which a cavovalgus foot with a medial transfer of the weight can be observed. The medial toes, especially the big toe, are blocked in plantar flexion on supporting weight. (D) Clinical image at 11 months with passive dorsiflexion of the heel superior to the neutral position with the knee extended after the selective release of the medial gastrocnemius.

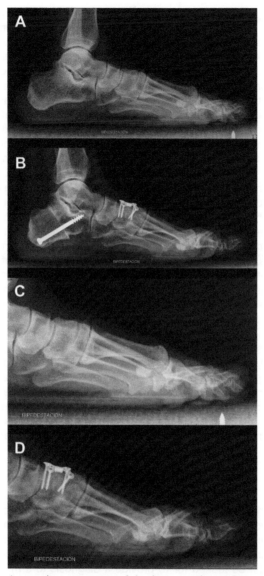

Fig. 24. Dorsal opening wedge osteotomy of the first cuneiform after Cotton is particularly useful in the case of a vertically aligned first tarso-metatarsal joint. This technique is frequently used in combination with other procedures used in the management of the pronated foot with first ray elevation. In this particular case both medial gastrocnemius release and calcaneal osteotomy were performed together with the Cotton procedure. Preoperative general (A), postoperative general (B). Note the preoperative divergence of the dorsal cortices of M1 and M2, in the preoperative close-up view (C). At follow-up, the first and second metatarsals are parallel to each other and the first metatarso-phalangeal joint shows adequate alignment (D).

tuberosity if there is midtarsal abduction.[53] In the author's practice, it is common to perform a combination of selective lengthening of the triceps surae, medialization osteotomy of the calcaneus, and lowering of the head of the first metatarsal, whether with a dorsal opening wedge osteotomy at the base of the first metatarsal, a first tarsometatarsal fusion with plantar flexion of the first metatarsal, or a Cotton osteotomy with plantar flexion in the first cuneiform (**Fig. 24**).[9,25,31] To choose the most appropriate procedure to descend and stabilize the first metatarsal head, the location of the inner arch center of rotation angulation (CORA) must be paid attention to: it may be placed at any of the joints of the medial column or at the bones themselves. The author reserves the Lapidus procedure for the cases in which foot pronation is the main landmark of the impairment with demonstrated instability at the first tarsometatarsal joint.

Given that it is understood that the cause of the limitation of movement in the first MP joint in hallux rigidus of mechanical origin is rarely situated in the joint itself, its replacement with a prosthesis would not be very effective. The current designs of these implants only allow replacement of the articular surfaces. The author has seen subjects with perfectly normal radiographs and complete passive mobility in the first MP joint who, nevertheless, are incapable of allowing passive dorsiflexion of the joint on subjecting the first metatarsal to light dorsiflexion. If the best articular surfaces do not allow dorsiflexion, a prosthesis will not either, unless the conditions of functioning of the internal column as a whole are simultaneously changed or an implant is designed that is not limited to the replacement of the facet joints. The first MP joint prostheses that appear to last longest are those in which the movement continues to be blocked, meaning they are similar to an arthrodesis, but more expensive and slightly more risky. On the other hand, when the rigidity of the first MP joint is not mechanical in origin, but rather biological (gout, rheumatic disease, connective tissue disease) or a result of trauma, the implants have much higher probabilities of being successful.

From a theoretic point of view, plantar fascia release may improve passive dorsiflexion at the first MP joint, but it increases the risk of medial arch breakdown. The author would not recommend this procedure, although renowned surgeons are currently performing it.

SUMMARY

Functional hallux rigidus is a clinical condition in which the mobility of the first MP joint is normal under non-weight-bearing conditions, but its dorsiflexion is blocked when the first metatarsal is made to support weight. It may be present in asymptomatic subjects or become incapacitating. Throughout its evolution, it goes from being a phenomenon that must be looked for to provide a diagnosis to a medical condition of florid arthrosis of the first MP joint. The author thinks that it is at the origin of mechanical hallux rigidus and is considered different phases of the same condition.

In mechanical terms, functional hallux rigidus implies a pattern of interfacial contact through rolling, while in a normal joint contact by gliding is established. The windlass mechanism is essential to maintain the plantar vault and is based on the correct functioning of an arch formed by several bony elements that work through compression and foot braces, which work through tension, among which the best prepared for its moment arm is the plantar aponeurosis. This forms a functional unit with the Achilles-calcaneal-plantar system, thanks to the enthesis/enthetic organ of the heel, meaning excessive traction of the triceps will be transmitted directly or indirectly to the fascia. Pronation of the foot and blockage of heel dorsiflexion may increase the tension in the aponeurosis. Both the elevation of the head of first metatarsal and the increase in tension in the aponeurosis may alter the joint dynamics in the first MP joint, producing contact by rolling instead of physiologic interfacial contact through gliding. Furthermore, each one of these alterations may give rise to the other. Equinus due to the shortening of the elastic component of the calf muscles is a frequent finding among the general population, probably as a vestige of what our foot was millions of years ago. Limitation of the dorsiflexion in the ankle or the MP joint blocks the forward movement of the tibia during the stance phase on the sagittal plane, which is compensated through diverse mechanisms that entail abnormal movements on other planes and in other body segments. The compensatory mechanisms are usually tolerated well, but they may also produce pain or impairment, thus becoming medical conditions. Orthopedic and surgical measures are at our disposition to treat the blockage of movement on the sagittal plane. Among the latter, the lowering and stabilizing of the head of first metatarsal and the lengthening of all or part of the triceps are favorable mechanical procedures to resolve the blockage. Patients with functional hallux rigidus should only be operated on if the pain or disability makes it necessary. Gastrocnemius release is a beneficial procedure in most patients.

REFERENCES

1. Roukis TS. Metatarsus primus elevatus in hallux rigidus. Fact or fiction? J Am Podiatr Med Assoc 2005;95(3):221–8.
2. Dananberg HJ. Functional hallux limitus and its relationship to gait efficiency. J Am Podiatr Med Assoc 1986;76(12):648–52.
3. Roukis TS, Scherer PR, Anderson CF. Position of the first ray and motion of the first metatarsophalangeal joint. J Am Podiatr Med Assoc 1996;86:538.
4. Kirby KA. Foot and lower extremity biomechanics II: Precision Intricast Newsletters, 1997-2002. Payson (AZ): Precision Intricast Inc; 2002.
5. Seibel MO. Foot function. A programmed text. Baltimore (MD): Williams & Wilkins; 1988.
6. Nordin M, Frankel VH. Biomecánica básica del sistema musculoesquelético. México: McGraw-Hill-Interamericana; 2005.
7. Dananberg HJ. Gait style as an etiology to chronic postural pain. Part I: functional hallux limitus. J Am Podiatr Med Assoc 1993;83(11):433.
8. Hicks JH. The mechanics of the foot. II. The plantar aponeurosis and the arch. J Anat 1954;88(1):25–30.
9. Hansen ST. Functional reconstruction of the foot and ankle. Philadelphia: Lippincott Williams & Wilkins; 2000.
10. Viladot A. Quince lecciones sobre patología del pie. 2nd edition. Barcelona (Spain): Springer-Verlag Ibérica; 2000.
11. Shaw HM, Vázquez-Osorio T, McGonagle D, et al. Development of the human Achilles tendon enthesis organ. J Anat 2008;213:718–24.
12. Perry J. Gait analysis. Normal and pathological function. Thorofare (NJ): Slack Inc; 1992.
13. Kirtley C. Clinical gait analysis. Theory and practice. New York: Churchill Livingstone Elsevier; 2006.
14. Gage JR, Schwartz MH, Koop SE, et al. The identification and treatment of gait problems in cerebral palsy. 2nd edition. London: Mac Keith Press; 2009.
15. Maceira E. Análisis cinemático y cinético de la marcha humana. Revista del Pie y Tobillo 2003;17(1):29–37.
16. Maceira E. Aproximación al estudio del paciente con metatarsalgia. Revista del Pie y Tobillo 2003;17(2):14–29.

17. Silfverskjold N. Reduction of the uncrossed two-joint muscles of the leg to one-joint muscles in spastic conditions. Acta Chir Scand 1924;56:315–30.

18. Regnauld B. The foot. Pathology, aetiology, semiology, clinical investigation and therapy. Berlin: Springer-Verlag; 1986.

19. Drago JJ, Oloff L, Jacobs AM. A comprehensive review of hallux limitus. J Foot Surg 1984;23(3):213–20.

20. Vanore JV, Christensen JC, Kravitz SR, et al. Diagnosis and treatment of first metatarsophalangeal joint disorders. Section 2: hallux rigidus. J Foot Ankle Surg 2003;42(3):124–36.

21. Kowalski C. La rétraction du tríceps sural et ses consequences sur l'avant pied. Montpellier: Sauramps Médical; 2005.

22. Hintermann B, Gächter A. The first metatarsal rise sign: a simple, sensitive sign of tibialis posterior tendon dysfunction. Foot Ankle Int 1996;17(4):236–41.

23. Donatelli RA. Biomechanics of the foot and ankle. 2nd edition. Philadelphia: F.A. Davis Co; 1995.

24. Jack EA. Naviculo-cuneiform fusion in the treatment of flat foot. J Bone Joint Surg Br 1953;35(1):75–82.

25. Lapidus PW. A quarter of a century of experience with the operative correction of the metatarsus varus primus in hallux valgus. Bull Hosp Joint Dis 1956;17(2): 404–21.

26. Munuera PV, Trujillo P, Güiza I. Hallux interphalangeal joint range of motion in feet with and without limited first metatarsophalangeal joint dorsiflexion. J Am Podiatr Med Assoc 2012;102(1):47–53.

27. Giannini S, Ceccarelli F, Faldini C, et al. What's new in surgical options for hallux rigidus? J Bone Joint Surg Am 2004;86(Suppl 2):72–83.

28. Espinosa N, Brodsky JW, Maceira E. Metatarsalgia. J Am Acad Orthop Surg 2010;18(8):474–85.

29. Barouk LS, Barouk P. Compte rendu symposium gastrocnémien court. Toulouse 2006. Maitrise Orthopédique 2006;159:21–8.

30. Montagne J, Chevrot A, Calmiche JM. Atlas de radiología del pie. Barcelona: Masson; 1980.

31. Cotton FJ. Foot static and surgery. N Engl J Med 1936;214(8):353–62.

32. Smith RW, Katchis SD, Ayson LC. Outcomes in hallux rigidus patients treated nonoperatively: a long-term follow-up study. Foot Ankle Int 2000;21(11):906–13.

33. Dananberg HJ. The kinetic wedge. J Am Podiatr Med Assoc 1988;78(2): 98–9.

34. Scherer PR, Sanders J, Eldredge DE, et al. Effect of functional foot orthoses on first metatarsophalangeal joint dorsiflexion in stance and gait. J Am Podiatr Med Assoc 2006;96(6):474–81.

35. Munuera PV, Domínguez G, Palomo IC, et al. Effects of rearfoot-controlling orthotic treatment on dorsiflexion of the hallux in feet with abnormal subtalar pronation. J Am Podiatr Med Assoc 2006;96(4):283–9.

36. Shrader JA, Siegel KL. Nonoperative management of functional hallux limitus in a patient with rheumatoid arthritis. Phys Ther 2003;83:831–43.

37. Hatt RN, Lamphier TA. Triple hemisection: a simplified procedure for lengthening the Achilles tendon. N Engl J Med 1947;236:166–9.

38. Barouk LS. Forefoot reconstruction. Paris: Springer; 2003.

39. Citron N, Neil M. Dorsal wedge osteotomy of the proximal phalanx for hallux rigidus. Long-term results. J Bone Joint Surg Br 1987;69(5):835–7.

40. Roukis TS. The need for surgical revision after isolated cheilectomy for hallux rigidus: a systematic review. J Foot Ankle Surg 2010;49(5):465–70.

41. Smith SM, Coleman SC, Bacon SA, et al. Improved ankle push-off power following cheilectomy for hallux rigidus: a prospective gait analysis study. Foot Ankle Int 2012;33(6):457–61.

42. Easley ME, Davis WH, Anderson RB. Intermediate to long-term follow-up of medial-approach dorsal cheilectomy for hallux rigidus. Foot Ankle Int 1999; 20(3):147–52.

43. Shereff MJ, Baumhauer JF. Current concepts review. Hallux rigidus and osteo-arthrosis of the first metatarsophalangeal joint. J Bone Joint Surg Am 1998; 80(6):898–908.

44. Coughlin MJ, Shurnas PS. Hallux rigidus: demographics, etiology, and radio-graphic assessment. Foot Ankle Int 2003;24(10):731–43.

45. Horton GA, Park YW, Myerson MS. Role of metatarsus primus elevatus in the pathogenesis of hallux rigidus. Foot Ankle Int 1999;20(12):777–80.

46. Barouk LS. The Weil first metatarsal decompression osteotomy. In: Forefoot reconstruction. 2nd edition. Paris: Springer; 2005. p. 115–38.

47. Ronconi P, Monachino P, Baleanu PM, et al. Distal oblique osteotomy of the first metatarsal for the correction of hallux limitus and rigidus deformity. J Foot Ankle Surg 2000;39(3):154–60.

48. Malerba F, Milani R, Sartorelli E, et al. Distal oblique first metatarsal osteotomy in grade 3 hallux rigidus: a long-term followup. Foot Ankle Int 2008;29(7):677–82.

49. Youngswick FD. Modifications of the Austin bunionectomy for treatment of meta-tarsus primus elevatus associated with hallux limitus. J Foot Surg 1982;21(2): 114–6.

50. Dickerson JB, Green R, Green DR. Long-term follow-up of the Green-Watermann osteotomy for hallux limitus. J Am Podiatr Med Assoc 2002; 92(10):543–54.

51. Radovic P, Yadav-Shah E, Choe K. Modified Youngswick procedure for hallux limitus. J Am Podiatr Med Assoc 2007;97(5):420–3.

52. Koutsogiannis E. Treatment of mobile flat foot by displacement osteotomy of the calcaneus. J Bone Joint Surg Br 1971;53(1):96–100.

53. Evans D. Calcaneo-valgus deformity. J Bone Joint Surg Br 1975;57(3):270–8.

The Effect of the Gastrocnemius on the Plantar Fascia

Javier Pascual Huerta, PhD

KEYWORDS

- Gastrocnemius muscle • Plantar fascia • Achilles tendon • Sagittal foot mechanics
- Gastrocnemius tightness • Plantar fasciitis • Ankle dorsiflexion stiffness

KEY POINTS

- The exact role that gastrocnemius tightness has on the plantar fascia has been a topic of discussion for many years and remains incompletely understood.
- The anatomic connection between the gastrocnemius muscle and the plantar fascia is disputable and seems to vary with age.
- The relationship between gastrocnemius tension and the plantar fascia during weight-bearing activities can be explained from a mechanical view of the foot in the sagittal plane.
- Gastrocnemius tightness increases Achilles tendon tension and increases dorsiflexion stiffness of the ankle joint during weight-bearing activities, which also increase plantar fascia tension during weight-bearing.

INTRODUCTION

The gastrocnemius (both the medial and lateral heads) and soleus muscles work through the Achilles tendon in their posterior insertion on the calcaneus.[1] The Achilles tendon is the largest and most powerful tendon of the ankle and its tensional force is transmitted to its insertion by active contraction of the gastrocnemius and/or soleus muscles or by passive tension of the musculotendinous unit of these muscles. Passive tension can occur because of an increase in dorsiflexion of the foot or because of gastrocnemius and/or soleus tightness. The tensional force (active or passive) in the Achilles tendon produces a plantarflexion moment at the ankle joint. In weight-bearing conditions, a plantarflexion moment at the ankle joint can decelerate dorsiflexion movement of the ankle during the stance phase of the gait cycle, accelerate plantarflexion movement of the ankle during the propulsive phase of the gait cycle, and stabilize ankle joint over dorsiflexion moments during weight-bearing, balancing the foot in the sagittal plane.[2,3]

Conflict of Interests: Author declares he has no conflict of interests.
Private Practice, Clínica del Pie Embajadores, C/ Embajadores, 183, Madrid 28045, Spain
E-mail address: javier.pascual@hotmail.com

Foot Ankle Clin N Am 19 (2014) 701–718
http://dx.doi.org/10.1016/j.fcl.2014.08.011
1083-7515/14/$ – see front matter © 2014 Elsevier Inc. All rights reserved.

The plantar fascia is a dense band of connective tissue that originates in the plantar tuberosity of calcaneus and courses along the plantar foot dividing into 5 slips that insert in the base of the proximal phalanges of the toes by the plantar plate and in the plantar skin by superficial extensions of the plantar fascia.[4–6] Hicks[7,8] compared foot function with the engineering structures of an arched beam and a truss, and explained nicely how the foot can work variably as one of these structures during weight bearing conditions. In the truss model, the bones of the foot represent an arch structure with the plantar fascia working at the bottom as a resistive tie. Because of its material properties and mechanical behavior, it is accepted that the plantar fascia can be viewed as a representative tendinous/ligamentous structure in the sole of the foot that plays an important role in foot stability.[9–11] Nowadays, there is a considerable amount of evidence, by means of in vitro studies, of the importance of the plantar fascia as stabilizer of the foot in static[12–17] and simulated dynamic walking conditions.[18,19] All of these studies have pointed to the plantar fascia as a major contributor of 3-plane stability of different tarsal joints,[20] although its contribution to arch stability seems to be more substantial in some feet than others.[21] Additionally, computational models developed have predicted a variable decrease in arch height after plantar fasciotomy in static conditions accompanied by a dramatic increase of tensile forces on plantar ligaments and internal stresses of the foot.[22–25]

ACHILLES–CALCANEUS–PLANTAR SYSTEM

In 1953, Arandes and Viladot, 2 Spanish orthopedic surgeons, published a paper that linked the structures of Achilles tendon and plantar fascia into an independent functional unit named the "Achilles–calcaneus–plantar System" (ACPS; in Spanish, *sistema aquileo–calcáneo–plantar*). They described a functional connection between the Achilles tendon, the plantar fascia, and short flexors of the foot by means of the posterior trabecular system of calcaneus that would work as a big sesamoid transmitting the force from the Achilles tendon to the intrinsic muscles of the sole of the foot. They stated that "linking these structures (Achilles tendon and plantar aponeurosis and short muscles of the sole) it is found the posterior portion of the calcaneus as a big sesamoid such as the patella with the patellar tendon."[26] This concept of functional connection reinforced early anatomic textbooks that had described an anatomic link from Achilles tendon to the plantar fascia through a continuity of the fibers in the posterior tuberosity of the calcaneus.[27,28] Arandes and Viladot described ACPS as "an independent functional unit that connects both structures."[26]

The authors justified this concept by means of ontogenic and phylogenic anatomic observations. From an ontogenic view, they observed a marked anatomic continuity between Achilles tendon and plantar aponeurosis in histologic sections of embriogenic specimens. This observation has been supported recently in a study of the embryologic development of Achilles tendon in fetuses in which the authors remarked a surprising continuity of fibers between Achilles tendon and plantar fascia through a thickened perichondrium in the posterior part of the main body of the calcaneus.[29] Arandes and Viladot pointed that this continuity would be maintained until the age of 7, when the secondary ossification center appears inside these fibers that connect the Achilles tendon to the plantar fascia. Ultimately, it fuses with the main body of the calcaneus to form the posterior tuberosity at the age of 9 or 10. From a phylogenetic view, they observed that in some animals the gastrocnemius muscle expands from the femur to the metatarsals, but in humans bipedal adaptation would have bent the Achilles tendon in a 90°, fashion putting the calcaneus under the talus. The posterior tuberosity of calcaneus then acquired great importance in the weight-bearing position touching the ground and starting to support high compressive forces. With these ideas in mind, Arandes and Viladot theorized that the system was the final result of the ossification of the gastrocnemius muscle with its supposed sesamoid bone over the posterior calcaneus to form the posterior calcaneal tuberosity. Then, a unique Achilles tendon (from the femur to the metatarsals) would have been converted into 2 different structures: The Achilles tendon (from femur to calcaneus) and the plantar fascia (from calcaneus to metatarsals). If this idea were correct, it would be reasonable that histologic and mechanical properties of the plantar fascia would be quite similar to that of tendinous tissues, especially the Achilles tendon. Although the author has been unable to find studies comparing these 2 structures, recent studies on histologic[6] and mechanical properties[9] of the plantar fascia have shown reasonable similarities to the histologic and mechanical properties of tendons.[30–32]

By this explanation, the plantar fascia could be viewed as a continuation of the Achilles tendon into the sole of the foot. That idea led Arandes and Viladot to think that Achilles forces would be transmitted in some way to the plantar fascia through the posterior calcaneal tuberosity as they were initially connected: "main function of this system is to transmit Achilles tendon force to distal structures that will add to short flexors. These actions are clear is the equinus position of gait and would explain the heel raising mechanism for dynamic activities."[26]

The ACPS concept became very popular in the European Orthopedic community. Clinicians had long suspected that gastrocnemius tightness increased tension in the plantar fascia, although the exact mechanism of this clinical finding was not completely clear. In this context, the idea of a kind of anatomic and functional connection between the Achilles tendon and plantar fascia by means of ACPS was well accepted. The idea has been referenced in many textbooks as a keystone of the mechanical behavior of the foot and lower extremity. It has been used to explain the heel rise mechanism during propulsion, running, jumping or dancing for >50 years in the European literature.[33–36]

However, although the idea of ACPS has some merit, the exact mode of connection of these structures is not completely clear. On the one hand, the exact anatomic connection of Achilles tendon and plantar fascia remains debatable. Some studies have specifically investigated the anatomic relationship of the Achilles tendon and the plantar fascia in cadaver specimens[6,37,38] and magnetic resonance images of in vivo patients.[39] The results of these studies have shown that this connection occurs in a minority of specimens or subjects. They also give some evidence that supports the idea that this anatomic connection could vary with the plantar fascia in neonates, which is lost in adults and absent in the elderly.[37,38] At older ages, the plantar fascia seems to continue proximally with a thin band corresponding with the periosteum of the calcaneus in continuity with a thin paratenon of the Achilles tendon.[6,37] On the other hand, although tensional forces in the plantar fascia are mainly in a longitudinal direction,[40] there is no evidence that the trabecular system of the calcaneus can transmit tensional forces from Achilles tendon to the plantar fascia longitudinally and vice versa, as Arandes and Viladot proposed.

MODELING THE FOOT IN THE SAGITTAL PLANE

In the last decade, a mechanical connection of the gastrocnemius muscle, by means of the Achilles tendon, and plantar fascia has been demonstrated.[41–44] This connection can be explained by a mechanical model of the foot and ankle in the sagittal plane that allows a better understanding of the mechanical relationship between these structures (**Fig. 1**). Models are frequently used in biomechanics as a simplified

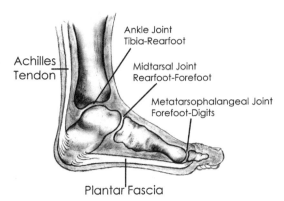

Fig. 1. Sagittal model of the foot. The foot is modeled into hind foot, forefoot, and digits with joints between the tibia and hind foot at the ankle, hind foot, and forefoot in the mid-tarsal joint and forefoot and digits in the metatarsophalangeal joints. Internal structures of the model are Achilles tendon and plantar fascia. (*Adapted from* Kirby KA. Foot and lower extremity biomechanics II: precision intricast newsletters 1997–2002. Payson (AZ): Precision Intricast Inc; 2002. p. 141; with permission.)

representation of reality that increases our understanding of the mechanical behavior of the anatomic structures represented.[45] Internal tensional forces of the Achilles tendon and plantar fascia can be studied by the modeling technique of free body diagram analysis. A free body diagram is a graphic representation commonly used by physics and engineering to analyze the forces and moments acting on the object of study. This is done by defining and modeling the shape of the object or group of objects of study and adding the known external forces acting on it. Afterward, Newton's laws of motion are used to calculate internal forces and moments within that structure.[46,47] Its main utility in the foot and ankle is to predict internal forces and moments in internal structures just by studying the known external forces and moments applied to it.[48,49] This technique is extremely helpful to understand how the tension or tightening in 1 structure of the foot and ankle can influence the mechanical behavior of other parts or structures of the foot. They also help to predict the mechanical response of some treatments, such as surgery in the Achilles tendon or gastrocnemius muscle and the effect of conservative treatments such us braces, shoes, or insoles.

The model presented in **Fig. 1** simplifies foot structure by dividing the foot into the hind foot, forefoot, and digits with joints between the tibia and hind foot at the ankle, hind foot, and forefoot at the midtarsal joint and forefoot and digits at the metatarsophalangeal joints. The Achilles tendon and plantar fascia are also represented in the model. With these anatomic parts, a free body diagram can be represented by adding the external forces acting on the foot and the internal force generated by the gastrocnemius muscle to predict the mechanical response of the plantar fascia in different situations. This model has been described previously by Kevin Kirby, DPM and can be used to explain the mechanical behavior of the foot and ankle in the sagittal plane.[49–51]

The main external force acting on the foot is gravity. This force is interpreted as body mass acceleration toward the center of the earth, namely weight. Weight is counteracted by ground reaction forces, which maintain the body weight in equilibrium on the ground surface. Weight force acts toward the tibia vertically in a downward direction, whereas ground reaction forces act in the plantar foot (mainly calcaneus and metatarsals) vertically in an upward direction. When these forces are equal (sum of forces equals zero), the object is in equilibrium and there is no linear acceleration of the object (**Fig. 2**).[52] The main internal forces represented in the model are the Achilles tendon and the plantar fascia tensional forces.

In non–weight-bearing conditions and with no contraction of the anterior muscle group, an increase in Achilles tendon tension produces a plantarflexion movement of the ankle joint. However, in static weight-bearing conditions Achilles tension produces a plantarflexion moment at the ankle joint without movement as long as the foot remains in static equilibrium. This plantarflexion moment at the hind foot decreases ground reaction forces in the calcaneus and increases ground reaction forces in the forefoot displacing the center of pressure of the foot anteriorly to the forefoot (**Fig. 3**). The increase in ground reaction forces in the forefoot produces an increase of ankle joint dorsiflexion moments that counteract the plantarflexion moment at the ankle joint created by the increase in Achilles tendon tension. If the dorsiflexion moment produced by the ground reaction forces of the forefoot is of the same magnitude as the plantarflexion moment produced by the Achilles tendon tensional force, the ankle joint will not move and will stay in static equilibrium.[53]

The increase in ground reaction forces in the forefoot also produces an increase in dorsiflexion moments of the forefoot to the hind foot at the midfoot joints (midtarsal, cuneonavicular, and Lisfranc joints) that are simplified in the model as 1 simple midtarsal joint. The combination of hind foot plantarflexion moments and forefoot dorsiflexion moments created by Achilles tendon tension tends to flatten the arch of the foot. This flattening force on the arch is counteracted by tension of the plantar structures, such as the plantar fascia that produces a dorsiflexion moment of the hind foot

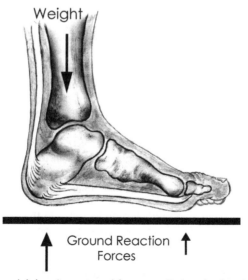

Fig. 2. Sagittal foot model showing external forces applied to the foot in the sagittal plane. Body weight acts from tibia vertically in downward direction. Body weight force is counteracted by ground reaction forces in the calcaneus and metatarsals that act vertically in an upward direction. Note that the sum of these forces (body weight and ground reaction forces) is zero, which makes the whole system to stay in equilibrium (no upward or downward acceleration of the system). (*Adapted from* Kirby KA. Foot and lower extremity biomechanics II: precision intricast newsletters 1997–2002. Payson (AZ): Precision Intricast Inc; 2002. p. 145; with permission.)

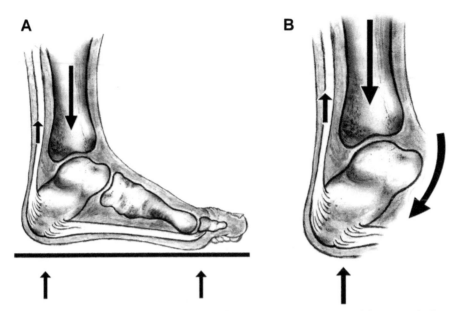

Fig. 3. (*A*) Free body diagram in the sagittal foot model showing external forces applied on the foot and internal forces generated by Achilles tendon. Tension of Achilles tendon produces a plantarflexion moment of the hind foot (*B*), which increases ground reaction forces on the forefoot. Note that as body weight is transferred through the tibia into the talus, there is an increased ground reaction forces in the hind foot compared forefoot (see **Fig. 2**). With Achilles tendon tension ground reaction forces in hind foot tend to decrease and ground reaction forces in the forefoot tend to increase moving the center of pressure anteriorly. (*Adapted from* Kirby KA. Foot and lower extremity biomechanics II: precision intricast newsletters 1997–2002. Payson (AZ): Precision Intricast Inc; 2002. p. 146; with permission.)

to forefoot and a plantarflexion moment of the forefoot (**Fig. 4**). Although there are several plantar structures to avoid arch flattening, cadaveric studies have consistently shown that the plantar fascia is more important to prevent arch collapse than other plantar ligaments, such as the spring ligament, dorsal calcaneonavicular ligament, or the long and short calcaneocuboid ligaments.[12,16,25] Moreover, plantar fascia section has been shown to produce a dramatic increase in tension of plantar ligaments especially short and long calcaneocuboid ligaments that can vary from 47 to 200%.[22–25,54] It is evident that, after plantar fascia disruption, the tensional force exerted by the plantar fascia has to be shared by other structures to avoid arch flattening. These studies have also predicted an increase in the stress of compressive forces in the dorsal aspect of midfoot bones that could be responsible for stress lesions in this area that has been described as possible complications after plantar fasciotomy or in chronic plantar fasciitis patients.[55–58]

In summary, it can be noted that the more the tension in Achilles tendon in weight-bearing conditions, the more the plantarflexion moment at the hind foot, the more the ground reaction forces on the forefoot and also the more dorsiflexion moments of the forefoot to hind foot. It is the combination of hindfoot plantarflexion moments and forefoot dorsiflexion moments that increase the tendency to arch flattening and collapse in midfoot joints. These collapsing forces are counteracted passively by tension of the plantar fascia. Plantar fascia tension in weight-bearing conditions produce dorsiflexion moments of the hind foot to forefoot and plantarflexion moments of the forefoot

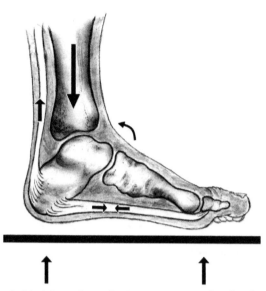

Fig. 4. The increase in hind foot plantarflexion moments and in forefoot ground reaction forces produce a tendency of the arch to flatten. This is counteracted by a plantarflexion moment of the forefoot on the hind foot exerted by tension in the plantar fascia. (*Adapted from* Kirby KA. Foot and lower extremity biomechanics II: precision intricast newsletters 1997–2002. Payson (AZ): Precision Intricast Inc; 2002. p. 147; with permission.)

to hind foot as a passive mechanical response for the increase in Achilles tendon tension and ground reaction forces in the forefoot (**Fig. 5**). Conversely, a decrease of Achilles tendon tension reduces the plantarflexion moments of the hind foot, the amount of ground reaction forces in the forefoot, and the passive tension of plantar fascia during weight-bearing activities.

This model has been fully supported by several studies performed on cadaveric specimens and finite element analysis. First, studies that measured the effect of Achilles tendon on plantar pressure distribution in cadaver feet have reported gradual decrease in hind foot plantar pressure and gradual increase in forefoot plantar pressure with Achilles tendon tensional force in static situations[59,60] accompanied by an anterior displacement of the center of pressure.[61] Second, Thordason and colleagues[17] and Blackman and colleagues[62] noted an arch deforming effect of Achilles tendon overpull in cadaveric specimens. The paper from Blackman and colleagues[62] simulated a flatfoot deformity by previous attenuation of plantar ligaments and noted that the increase in Achilles tendon tension produced movement in midfoot joints that had been previously attenuated. These movements tended to flatten the arch and were very important in the talonavicular joint, calcaneal inclination angle and talus-first metatarsal angle in the sagittal plane showing the arch-deforming effect that Achilles tendon overpull has in these feet. Third, cadaveric and finite element studies have shown that tension in Achilles tendon increases plantar fascia tension in static weight-bearing conditions. Carlson and colleagues[41] studied 8 lower limb specimens subjected to static load and measured plantar fascia tension at different Achilles tendon loads (0–500 N) and at different angulations of the first metatarsophalangeal joint. Results showed that tension in the plantar fascia has a direct relationship with Achilles tendon load and that first metatarsophalangeal joint dorsiflexion increased

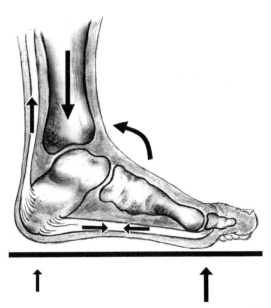

Fig. 5. Increased tension of Achilles tendon (active or passive) produces an increase of ground reaction forces under the forefoot in weight-bearing. That increase in ground reaction forces under the forefoot produces a dorsiflexion moment of the forefoot on the hind foot with a tendency to arch flattening. Under this circumstances, tensional force in the plantar fascia increase counteracting the arch-flattening effect. (*Adapted from* Kirby KA. Foot and lower extremity biomechanics II: precision intricast newsletters 1997–2002. Payson (AZ): Precision Intricast Inc; 2002. p. 147; with permission.)

the effect of tension in the plantar fascia made by Achilles load. Cheng and colleagues[43] used the same design with a finite element analysis model of the foot modeling the plantar fascia as a nonlinear elastic material and obtained identical results that those reported by Carlson and colleagues.[41] Cheung and colleagues[42] studied the effect of Achilles tendon tension in plantar fascia in another finite element analysis in conditions of vertical compression forces in the plantar foot and in vertical compression forces in the plantar foot plus Achilles tendon tension. Although tension in the plantar fascia increased with the increase of vertical compression forces alone, Achilles tendon loading was found to produce greater straining effect on plantar fascia than those produced by vertical compression forces alone. They predicted that increase in Achilles tendon tension reduces calcaneal inclination angle and shifts the center of pressure anteriorly and laterally from the hind foot to the forefoot increasing tension in plantar fascia.

Although this model has been presented in static conditions, the same principles can be applied to dynamic situations, such us walking. During heel strike, ground reaction forces are acting mainly on the hind foot and little or no ground reaction forces are acting in the forefoot. The gastrocnemius muscle is relaxed, and the Achilles tendon and plantar fascia has little or no tension (**Fig. 6**A). As the foot progresses to the stance phase, the gastrocnemius muscle starts to fire actively, the Achilles tendon exerts tensional force in calcaneus and ground reaction forces appear in the forefoot. This tensional force of Achilles tendon produces a plantarflexion moment at the ankle joint, which tends to decelerate the anterior displacement of the tibia on the foot (opposing the dorsiflexion movement of the ankle joint). As a consequence, there is

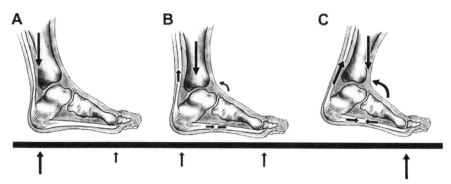

Fig. 6. Free body diagram of the foot in the sagittal plane during stance phase of the gait cycle under normal conditions. (*A*) Contact period: At heel strike, there is little or no load in the forefoot and Achilles tendon tension and plantar fascia tension are minimal. Weight is acting on the heel. (*B*) Midstance: At this moment, weight is acting on the foot in a more anterior area and the forefoot is getting a determined amount of load. Achilles tendon starts to have tensional force by active contraction of gastrocnemius and soleus that decelerate the anterior movement of the shank. Plantar fascia tension is medium. (*C*) Propulsion: At this time, Achilles tendon tension and forefoot pressure are greatest. Hind foot plantarflexion moments and forefoot dorsiflexion moments are highest and are counteracted by plantar fascia tension that is also highest at that instant. (*Adapted from* Kirby KA. Foot and lower extremity biomechanics II: precision intricast newsletters 1997–2002. Payson (AZ): Precision Intricast Inc; 2002. p. 147; with permission.)

a plantarflexion moment on the hind foot and an increase in pressure of the forefoot, which increase the dorsiflexion moments of the forefoot to hind foot. The plantar fascia starts to increase its tensional force to counteract the flattening arch force, limiting foot collapse (see **Fig. 6**B). As the gait cycle continues and foot enters the propulsive phase, the heel starts to lift up off the ground and all ground reaction forces are concentrated in the forefoot. At that moment, gastrocnemius muscle contraction is at its maximum, hind foot plantarflexion moments are highest, and ground reaction forces in the forefoot are also the highest, creating maximum dorsiflexion moments of the forefoot. It is at this specific time when the plantar fascia acquires its maximum tensional force during the gait cycle, stabilizing the foot arch (see **Fig. 6**C). It is when the foot enters the propulsive phase that the mechanical connection of the gastrocnemius muscle and plantar fascia is more evident (**Fig. 7**).

Erdemir and colleagues[44] studied the dynamic relationship of the Achilles tendon and plantar fascia in 7 specimens making a dynamic simulation of the stance phase of gait. They measured plantar fascia tension by means of a fiberoptic cable at different moments of the stance phase. Their results showed very good correlation between Achilles tendon force and plantar fascia tension dynamically ($r = 0.76$). They found that plantar fascia tension increases gradually during the stance phase of the gait cycle as Achilles tendon tension increase with its maximum value at 80% of stance phase reaching 96% ± 36% of estimated body weight. Interestingly, in the paper described by Cheung and colleagues,[42] Achilles tendon tension produced a decrease in calcaneal inclination angle before lifting the heel. It could be reasonable to think that the foot increases its stiffness (working as a beam) before heel lifts by maximum tension in the plantar fascia produced by maximal Achilles tendon tensional force at that moment.

All these studies give credit to the indirect effect that gastrocnemius muscle has on plantar fascia tension in weight-bearing conditions by a combination effect of

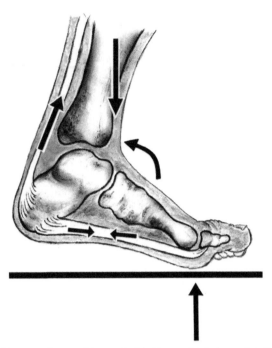

Fig. 7. Free body diagram of propulsive period in the sagittal plane. Achilles tendon tension is increased by contraction of gastrocnemius–soleus muscles, which creates a hind foot plantarflexion moment. Heel is off the ground and all pressure is in the forefoot, which creates a forefoot dorsiflexion moment. Plantar fascia increases its passive tension counteracting the increase in hind foot plantarflexion moments and forefoot dorsiflexion moments. (*Adapted from* Kirby KA. Foot and lower extremity biomechanics II: precision intricast newsletters 1997–2002. Payson (AZ): Precision Intricast Inc; 2002. p. 147; with permission.)

increased hind foot plantarflexion moments and increased forefoot dorsiflexion moments. They support the predictions of the model presented and confirm the idea that Achilles tendon and plantar fascia have a functional relationship that goes beyond further a simple anatomic connection. However, it is important to note that although the model presented is helpful to understand the mechanical behavior of the gastrocnemius muscle and plantar fascia in the sagittal plane, it has some limitations and one should be cautious to draw multiple conclusions. Oversimplification of the foot joints can lead to some inaccuracies of foot behavior as a rigid beam when in reality it would probably store some energy of Achilles tendon force through its midfoot joints to function as a rigid beam before heel lifts. So, transmission of forces in the model would be no ideal and magnitude of forces presented in the figures could vary substantially from some feet to others.

GASTROCNEMIUS TIGHTNESS AND CLINICAL APPLICATIONS

Ankle equinus can be described as a plantarflexion deformity of the foot with the inability to dorsiflex it beyond 90°, producing characteristic gait abnormalities traditionally associated with neurologic disorders such as cerebral palsy. However, it was during the second half of the twentieth century when other forms of nonspastic equinus were initially recognized. These cases presented limitation of dorsiflexion at the ankle joint during non–weight-bearing examination in normal neurologic patients with no spastic classical signs and were attributed to congenital shortening of gastrocnemius, soleus, or Achilles tendon.[63,64] Focus was then placed on limited ankle joint dorsiflexion during non–weight-bearing examination as a key point for normal function during gait. It then evolved into a theoretic biomechanical framework encompassing the gait cycle and was also related to different foot disorders of the foot and lower extremity.[65–67]

Shortening of the gastrocnemius muscle, congenital or acquired, is the most common cause for the lack of ankle joint dorsiflexion range of motion.[67,68] It is believed that sitting for long periods, sleeping in supine/prone position, and the continuous use of high heels can allow the gastrocnemius accommodate to a shortened position. Without regular stretching, the gastrocnemius can progressively shorten and develop a progressive stiffness with aging. Moreover, some authors have argued that from an evolutionary view, an elongated Achilles tendon was a crucial adaptation that contributed to human bipedalism.[69–71]

Even though it is difficult to establish a normal ankle joint dorsiflexion range for a normal gait, normalcy has been widely discussed by different authors proposing different ranges that could be considered normal varying from 5° to 10° as a cutoff value to diagnose a decrease in ankle joint dorsiflexion.[68,72–77] However, 1 problem associated with the concept of ankle joint dorsiflexion range of motion is that range is usually measured clinically with little or no attention placed to the forces needed to achieve that particular range. It is impossible to measure the forces during clinical examination, such that the examination varies among different clinicians, leading to high interobserver variability.[78–80] In the biomechanics field the term *stiffness* is used to describe the ability of a structure to resist changes in its initial shape.[81] Stiffness is defined as the amount of force required to produce a measurable amount of deformation in a structure or material.[82] This concept of stiffness can be applied to joint mechanics in the study of the range of motion of the ankle joint giving a more precise idea of the mechanical behavior that gastrocnemius tightness has on forefoot pressures and plantar fascia tension. The advantage of this definition is that it does not rely only in the amount of dorsiflexion achieved during the examination of gastrocnemius tightness patients, but in the amount of force needed to achieve a specific range of dorsiflexion.

Gastrocnemius tightness can be viewed mechanically as an increase of the stiffness of the ankle joint in a dorsiflexion direction. With gastrocnemius tightness, the clinician should not only be thinking in the range of motion of the ankle joint, but in the forces needed to achieve a particular range of ankle joint dorsiflexion. Moreover, it has been recently shown that dorsiflexion ankle range of motion and ankle joint stiffness are poorly correlated in normal subjects.[83] In the context of the modeling behavior described herein, the idea for the clinicians to take account the individual force needed to achieve a particular range of ankle joint dorsiflexion could be useful for a better understanding of the mechanical relationship of gastrocnemius and plantar fascia in the clinical setting.

In the model presented, Achilles tension was modeled as gastrocnemius and or soleus contraction. However, it is important to note that the gastrocnemius muscle can make its tensional force into Achilles tendon actively by gastrocnemius muscle contraction or passively by excessive ankle dorsiflexion and/or shortening–tightening of the musculotendinous unit. Gastrocnemius shortening increases Achilles tendon tension during weight-bearing with knee fully extended increasing the stiffness of ankle joint in dorsiflexion. During normal weight-bearing activities, individuals with gastrocnemius tightness have increased passive tension of Achilles tendon compared with individuals with no gastrocnemius tightness, which accelerates the mechanical events described. In static weight-bearing, an ankle joint with increased dorsiflexion stiffness, because of gastrocnemius tightness, has a great amount of Achilles tendon tension (just by putting the ankle at 90° during static stance with knee extended) compared to an ankle joint with decreased dorsiflexion stiffness. The increase of Achilles tendon tensional forces in weight-bearing increases plantar-flexion moments at the hind foot and simultaneously increase ground reaction forces at the forefoot increasing dorsiflexion moments of the forefoot to hind foot. So, in an individual with gastrocnemius tightness the combination of hind foot plantarflexion moments and forefoot dorsiflexion moments exerted by the muscle tension increases plantar fascia passive tension compared with an individual without gastrocnemius tightness (**Fig. 8**).

These ideas give a mechanically coherent explanation of several foot disorders such as plantar fasciitis,[84] metatarsalgia,[68,85] and dorsal midfoot compression pain[58,68] seen in patients with gastrocnemius tightness. Riddle and colleagues[86] and Patel and DiGiovanni[84] established a clear relationship between limited ankle joint dorsiflexion of the ankle measured clinically and plantar fasciitis. Riddle and colleagues[86] in a case-control study design found that cases with ankle joint dorsiflexion less than 0° had an odds ratio of 23.3 for plantar fasciitis compared with individuals with 10° of dorsiflexion. Patel and DiGiovanni[84] found that, in a sample of 254 patients with plantar fasciitis, 83% had a limitation of ankle joint dorsiflexion because of gastrocnemius and/or gastrocnemius-soleus tightness. Only 17% of plantar fasciitis patients had normal ankle dorsiflexion range of motion.[84] This connection would also explain the beneficial effect of calf stretching and night splints in the treatment of plantar fasciitis, which has been shown to be effective in randomized, controlled studies.[87–89]

As has been described, ankle joint dorsiflexion stiffness is also important in plantar pressures of the forefoot and in the pathogenesis of forefoot ulcerations in neuropathic

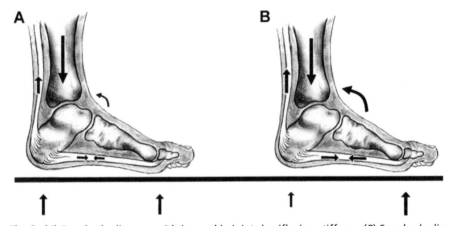

Fig. 8. (A) Free body diagram with low ankle joint dorsiflexion stiffness. (B) Free body diagram with high ankle joint dorsiflexion stiffness. The increase of stiffness in ankle joint dorsiflexion is mediated by increase in passive Achilles tendon tension in weight-bearing. This increase in tension during weight-bearing increases plantarflexion moments of the hind foot, ground reaction forces in the forefoot, dorsiflexion moments of the forefoot to hind foot, and passive plantar fascia tension in weight-bearing. (*Adapted from* Kirby KA. Foot and lower extremity biomechanics II: precision intricast newsletters 1997–2002. Payson (AZ): Precision Intricast Inc; 2002. p. 147; with permission.)

patients. In patients with diabetic neuropathy, limited ankle joint dorsiflexion correlates well with forefoot plantar pressures during gait. Lavery and colleagues[90] showed that diabetic patients with limited ankle joint dorsiflexion ($\leq 0°$) had a significant increase in plantar pressures in the forefoot during gait compared to those with ankle joint dorsiflexion greater than $0°$. Equally, Orendurff and colleagues[91] found that peak plantar pressure in the forefoot in diabetics during gait was greater in patients with ankle joint dorsiflexion limitation. Their results showed that the greater the limitation of ankle joint dorsiflexion, the greater the peak plantar pressure in the forefoot in those patients. It would also explain the beneficial effect of Achilles lengthening or gastrocnemius recession in neuropathic patients with forefoot ulcers.[92–95] Armstrong and colleagues[92] showed that percutaneous lengthening of the Achilles tendon reduced plantar pressures in the forefoot by a mean of 86 N after 8 weeks in diabetic patients with risk of forefoot plantar ulceration. Müeller and colleagues[93] in a randomized, controlled study compared the effect of combined treatment of total contact cast with percutaneous Achilles tendon lengthening with total contact cast alone in healing and recurrences. Although wound healing rate was similar in both cases, after 2 years there was a recurrence rate of ulcerations of 81% in the group that was treated in total contact cast alone by a 38% of recurrence in the group of total contact cast plus percutaneous Achilles tendon lengthening.

SUMMARY

In this article, a functional relationship has been proposed between both structures that goes beyond a simple anatomic relationship. From the model presented herein, tightness of the gastrocnemius muscle produces an increase in Achilles tendon tension during weight-bearing activities and increasing dorsiflexion stiffness of the ankle joint. Increased tension in the Achilles tendon during weight-bearing produces plantarflexion moments at the hind foot and an increase in forefoot plantar pressure with an anterior displacement of center of pressure. The combination of hind foot plantarflexion moments and forefoot dorsiflexion moments tend to collapse the arch, and the plantar fascia increases its passive mechanical longitudinal tension counteracting the arch flattening effect of gastrocnemius tightness. With these ideas in mind, the relationship between the gastrocnemius muscle and the plantar fascia could be considered as a relationship derived from the mechanical behavior of the foot in weight-bearing conditions instead of direct transmission of tension through the calcaneal trabecular system. Although the model presented has some limitations, such as the effect of intrinsic foot and deep posterior calf muscle contraction, it can serve for a better understanding of the effect of gastrocnemius tightness in specific foot disorders. These ideas can also help to explain clinical findings of patients with gastrocnemius tightness and open new possibilities of treatment for specific foot problems, such as plantar fasciitis, metatarsalgia, midfoot dorsal pain, and forefoot ulcerations of neuropathic patients.

ACKNOWLEDGMENTS

The authors thank Ramón Vaillo for his work in the figures presented in this article.

REFERENCES

1. Cohen JC. Anatomy and biomechanical aspects of the gastrosoleus complex. Foot Ankle Clin 2009;14:617–26.

2. Kirby KA. Biomechanics of gastrocnemius-soleus complex. In: Foot and lower extremity biomechanics III: precision intricast newsletters, 2002-2008. Payson (AZ): Precision Intricast, Inc; 2009. p. 85–92.

3. Whittle MW. Normal gait. In: Gait analysis: an introduction. 4th edition. Oxford (United Kingdom): Butterworth-Heinemann Elsevier; 2007. p. 47–100.

4. Sarrafian SK. Retaining systems and compartments. In: Anatomy of the foot and ankle. Descriptive, topographic, functional. 2nd edition. Philadelphia: JB Lippincott Company; 1993. p. 113–58.

5. Deland JT, Lee KT, Sobel M, et al. Anatomy of the plantar plate and its attachments in the lesser metatarsophalangeal joint. Foot Ankle Int 1995;16:480–6.

6. Stecco C, Corradin M, Macchi V, et al. Plantar fascia anatomy and its relationship with Achilles tendón and paratenon. J Anat 2013;223:66576. http://dx.doi.org/10.1111/joa.12111.

7. Hicks JH. The foot as a support. Acta Anat (Basel) 1955;25(1):34–45.

8. Hicks JH. The three weight bearing mechanisms of the foot. In: Evans FG, editor. Biomechanical studies of the musculoskeletal system. Springfield (IL): CC Thomas Co; 1961. p. 161–91.

9. Kitaoka HB, Luo ZP, Growney ES, et al. Material properties of the plantar aponeurosis. Foot Ankle 1994;15:557–60.

10. Wright DG, Rennels DC. A Study of the elastic properties of plantar fascia. J Bone Joint Surg Am 1964;46:482–92.

11. Pavan PG, Stecco C, Darwish S, et al. Investigation of the mechanical properties of the plantar aponeurosis. Surg Radiol Anat 2011;33:905–11.

12. Huang CK, Kitaoka HB, An KN, et al. Biomechanical evaluation of longitudinal arch stability. Foot Ankle 1993;14:353–7.

13. Kitaoka HB, Luo ZP, An KN. Mechanical behavior of the foot and ankle after plantar fascia release in the unstable foot. Foot Ankle Int 1997;18:8–15.

14. Kitaoka HB, Luo ZP, An KN. Effect of plantar fasciotomy on stability of arch of foot. Clin Orthop Relat Res 1997;344:307–12.

15. Murphy GA, Pneumaticos SG, Kamaric E, et al. Biomechanical consequences of sequential plantar fascia release. Foot Ankle Int 1998;19:149–52.

16. Liang J, Yang YF, Yu GR, et al. Deformation and stress distribution of the human foot after plantar ligaments release: a cadaveric study and finite element analysis. Sci China Life Sci 2011;54:267–71.

17. Thordason DB, Schmotzer H, Chon J, et al. Dynamic support of the human longitudinal arch: a biomechanical evaluation. Clin Orthop 1995;316:165–72.

18. Ward ED, Smith KM, Cocheba JR, et al. In vivo forces in the plantar fascia during the stance phase of gait. J Am Podiatr Med Assoc 2003;93:429–42.

19. Sharkey NA, Ferris L, Donahue SW. Biomechanical consequences of plantar fascial release or rupture during gait. Part I: disruptions in longitudinal arch conformation. Foot Ankle Int 1998;19:812–20.

20. Tweed JL, Barnes MR, Aleen MJ, et al. Biomechanical consequences of total plantar fasciotomy. A review of the literature. J Am Podiatr Med Assoc 2009; 99:422–30.

21. Kitaoka HB, Ann TK, Luo AP, et al. Stability of the arch of the foot. Foot Ankle Int 1997;18:644–8.

22. Gefen A. Stress analysis of the standing foot following surgical plantar fascia release. J Biomech 2002;35:629–37.

23. Cheung JTM, Zhang M, An KN. Effects of plantar fascia stiffness on the biomechanical responses of the ankle-foot complex. Clin Biomech 2004;19: 839–46.

24. Wu L. Nonlinear finite element analysis for musculoskeletal biomechanics of medial and lateral plantar longitudinal arch of Virtual Chinese Human after plantar ligamentous structure failures. Clin Biomech 2007;22:221–9.
25. Tao K, Ji WT, Wang DM, et al. Relative contributions of plantar fascia and ligaments on the arch static stability: a finite element study. Biomed Tech (Berl) 2010;55:265–71.
26. Arandes R, Viladot A. Biomecánica del calcaneo. Med Clin (Barc) 1953;21:25–34.
27. Jones FW. Structure and function as seen in the foot. 2nd edition. London (United Kingdom): Bailliére: Tindall & Cos; 1944. p. 60.
28. Poirier P. Myologie. In: Poirier P, Charpy A, editors. Traite d'Anatomie Humain, vol. 2. Paris: Maison et Cie; 1901. p. 298.
29. Shaw HM, Vázquez Osorio T, McGonagle D, et al. Development of the human Achilles tendon enthesis organ. J Anat 2008;213:718–24.
30. Nordin M, Lorenz T, Campello M. Biomechanics of tendons and ligaments. In: Nordin M, Frankel VH, editors. Basic biomechanics of the musculoskeletal system. Baltimore (MD): Lippincott Williams & Wilkins; 2001. p. 102–25.
31. Wang JH. Mechanobiology of tendon. J Biomech 2006;39:1563–82.
32. Wren TAL, Yerby SA, Beaupré GS, et al. Mechanical properties of the human Achilles tendon. Clin Biomech 2001;16:245–51.
33. Llanos Alcázar LF, Maceira Suarez E. Biomorfología. In: Núñez-Samper Pizarroso M, Llanos Alcázar LF, editors. Biomecánica, Medicina y Cirugía del Pie. Barcelona (Spain): Masson SA; 2007. p. 49–66.
34. Henríquez A, Ripollés JV, Roger LL. Traumatismos del retropie. In: Viladot Pericé A, editor. Quince Lecciones sobre Patología del Pie. Barcelona (Spain): Springer-Verlag Ibérica; 2000. p. 233–50.
35. Miralles Marrero RC, Miralles Rull I, Llusa Pérez M, et al. Biomecánica de los sistemas extensores de las extremidades. In: Miralles Marrero MC, Miralles Rull I, editors. Biomecánica Clínica de las Patologías del Aparato Locomotor. Barcelona (Spain): Masson SA; 2007. p. 109–37.
36. De Palma L, Coletti V, Santucci A, et al. Embriogenesi del sistema Achilleo-calcaneo-plantare. Arch Putti Chir Organi Mov 1985;35:135–41.
37. Snow SW, Bohne WH, DiCarlo E, et al. Anatomy of the Achilles tendon and plantar fascia in relation to the calcaneus in various age groups. Foot Ankle Int 1995;16:418–21.
38. Kim PJ, Richey JM, Wissman LR, et al. The variability of the Achilles tendon insertion: a cadaveric examination. J Foot Ankle Surg 2010;49:417–20.
39. Kim PJ, Martin E, Ballehr L, et al. Variability of insertion of the Achilles tendon on the calcaneus: an MRI study of younger subjects. J Foot Ankle Surg 2011;50:41–3.
40. Clark RA, Franklyn-Miller A, Falvey E, et al. Assessment of mechanical strain in the intact plantar fascia. Foot (Edinb) 2009;19:161–4.
41. Carlson RE, Fleming LL, Hutton WG. The biomechanical relationship between the tendoachilles, plantar fascia and metatarsophalangeal joint dorsiflexion angle. Foot Ankle Int 2000;21:18–25.
42. Cheung JTK, Zhang M, An KN. Effect of Achilles tendon loading on plantar fascia tension in the standing foot. Clin Biomech 2006;21:194–203.
43. Cheng HY, Lin CL, Wang HW, et al. Finite element analysis of plantar fascia under stretch-the relative contribution of windlass mechanism and Achilles tendon force. J Biomech 2008;41:1937–44.
44. Erdemir A, Hamel AJ, Fauth AR, et al. Dynamic loading of the plantar aponeurosis in walking. J Bone Joint Surg Am 2004;86-A:546–52.

45. Nigg BM. Force system analysis. In: Nigg BM, Herzog W, editors. Biomechanics of the musculo-skeletal system. 2nd edition. West Sussex (United Kingdom): John Wiley & Sons; 1999. p. 446–57.
46. Bansal RK. Conditions of equilibrium. In: A textbook of engineering mechanics engeneerings. 4th edition. New Delhi (India): Laxmi Publications; 2002. p. 61–91.
47. Özcaya N, Nordin M. Statics: analyses of system in equilibrium. In: Fundamentals of biomechanics. Equilibrium, motion and deformation. 2nd edition. New York: Springer Science; 1999. p. 49–80.
48. Fuller EA. The Windlass mechanism of the foot: a mechanical model to explain pathology. J Am Podiatr Med Assoc 2000;90:35–46.
49. Fuller EA, Kirby KA. Subtalar joint equilibrium and tissue stress approach to biomechanical therapy of the foot and lower extremity. In: Albert SF, Curran SA, editors. Lower extremity biomechanics: theory and practice, vol. 1. Denver (CO): Dipedmed, LLC; 2013. p. 205–64.
50. Kirby KA. Biomechanics of functional hallux limitus. In: Foot and lower extremity biomechanics ii: precision intricast newsletters, 1997-2002. Payson (AZ): Precision Intricast, Inc; 2002. p. 137–52.
51. Kirby KA. Plantar fascia biomechanics. In: Foot and lower extremity biomechanics III: precision intricast newsletters, 2002-2008. Payson (AZ): Precision Intricast, Inc; 2009. p. 93–104.
52. Enoka RM. Movement forces. In: Enoka RM, editor. Neuromechanics of human movement. 3rd edition. Champaign (IL): Hemoan Kinetics; 2002. p. 57–118.
53. Fuller EA. Center of pressure and its theoretical relationship to foot pathology. J Am Podiatr Med Assoc 1999;89:278–91.
54. Crary JL, Hollins JM, Manoli A. The effect of plantar fascia release on strain in the spring and long plantar ligaments. Foot Ankle Int 2003;24:245–50.
55. Bui-Mansfield LT, Thomas WR. Magnetic resonance imaging of stress injury of the cuneiform bones in patients with plantar fasciitis. J Comput Assist Tomogr 2009;33:593–6.
56. Sharkey NA, Donahue SW, Ferris L. Biomechanical consequences of plantar fascial release or rupture during gait. Part II: alterations in forefoot loading. Foot Ankle Int 1999;20:86–96.
57. Yu JS, Solmen J. Stress fractures associated with plantar fascia disruption: two case reports involving the cuboid. J Comput Assist Tomogr 2001;25:971–4.
58. Kirby KA. Orthosis treatment of forefoot and midfoot pathology. In: Foot and lower extremity biomechanics: a ten year collection of precision intricast newsletters. Payson (AZ): Precision Intricast, Inc; 1997. p. 147–68.
59. Ward ED, Phillips RD, Patterson PE, et al. The effects of extrinsic muscle forces on the forefoot-to-rearfoot relationship in vitro. Tibia and Achilles tendon. J Am Podiatr Med Assoc 1998;10:471–82.
60. Aronow MS, Diaz-Doran V, Sullivan RJ, et al. The effect of triceps surae contracture force on plantar foot pressure distribution. Foot Ankle Int 2006;27:43–52.
61. Kim KJ, Uchiyama E, Kitaoka HB, et al. An in vitro study of individual ankle muscle actions on the center of pressure. Gait Posture 2003;17:125–31.
62. Blackman AJ, Blevins JJ, Sangeorzan BJ, et al. Cadaveric flatfoot model: ligament attenuation and Achilles tendon overpull. J Orthop Res 2009;27:1547–54.
63. Levine MS. Congenital short tendo calcaneus. Report of a family. Am J Dis Child 1973;125:858–9.
64. Hall JE, Salter RB, Bhalla SK. Congenital short tendo calcaneus. J Bone Joint Surg Br 1967;49:695–7.

65. Root ML, Orion WP, Weed JH. Abnormal motion of the foot. In: Normal and abnormal function of the foot, vol. II. Los Angeles (CA): Clinical Biomechanics Corp; 1977. p. 295–348.
66. Sgarlato TE, Morgan J, Shane HS, et al. Tendo Achillis lengthening and its effect on foot disorders. J Am Podiatry Assoc 1975;65(9):849–71.
67. Downey MS. Ankle equinus. In: Banks AS, Downey MS, Martin DE, et al, editors. McGlamry's comprehensive textbook of foot and ankle surgery, vol. 1, 2nd edition. Philadelphia: Lippincott Williams & Wilkins; 2001. p. 715–60.
68. DiGiovanni CW, Kuo R, Tejwani N, et al. Isolated gastrocnemius tightness. J Bone Joint Surg Am 2002;84-A:962–70.
69. Sellers W, Pataky TC, Caravaggi P, et al. Evolutionary robotic approaches in primate gait analysis. Int J Primatol 2010;31:321–38.
70. Bramble DM, Lieberman DE. Endurance running and the evolution of Homo. Science 2004;432:345–52.
71. Kuo S, Desilva JM, Devlin MJ, et al. The effect of the Achilles tendon on trabecular structure in the primate calcaneus. Anat Rec (Hoboken) 2013;296: 1509–17.
72. Charles J, Scutter SD, Buckley J. Static ankle joint equinus. Toward a standard definition and diagnosis. J Am Podiatr Med Assoc 2010;100:195–203.
73. Baggett BD, Young G. Ankle joint dorsiflexion: establishment of a normal range. J Am Podiatr Med Assoc 1993;83:251–4.
74. Lindsjo U, Danckwardt-Lilliestrom G, Sahlstedt B. Measurement of the motion range in the loaded ankle. Clin Orthop 1985;199:68–71.
75. Saxena A, Kim W. Ankle dorsiflexion in adolescent athletes. J Am Podiatr Med Assoc 2003;93:312–4.
76. Tabrizi P, McIntyre WM, Quesnel MB, et al. Limited dorsiflexion predisposes to injuries of the ankle in children. J Bone Joint Surg 2000;82-B:1103–6.
77. Rome K. Ankle Joint dorsiflexion measurement studies. A review of the literature. J Am Podiatr Med Assoc 1996;86:205–11.
78. Kim PJ, Peace R, Mieras J. Interrater and intrarrater reliability in the measurement of ankle joint dorsiflexion is independent of examiner experience and technique used. J Am Podiatr Med Assoc 2011;101:407–14.
79. Meyer DC, Werner CM, Wyss T, et al. A mechanical equinometer to measure the range of motion of the ankle joint: interobserver and intraobserver reliability. Foot Ankle Int 2006;27:202–5.
80. Martin RL, McPoil TG. Reliability of ankle goniometric measurements: a literature review. J Am Podiatr Med Assoc 2005;95:564–72.
81. Baumgart E. Stiffness – an unknown world of mechanical science? Injury 2000; 31(S-2):14–23.
82. Özcaya N, Nordin M. Stress and strain. In: Özcaya N, Nordin M, editors. Fundamentals of biomechanics. Equilibrium, motion and deformation. 2nd edition. New York: Springer Science; 1999. p. 127–51.
83. Whitting JW, Steele JR, McGhee DE, et al. Passive dorsiflexion stiffness is poorly correlated with passive dorsiflexion range of motion. J Sci Med Sport 2013;16: 157–61.
84. Patel A, Digiovanni B. Association between plantar fasciitis and isolated contracture of the gastrocnemius. Foot Ankle Int 2001;32:5–8.
85. Hill RS. Ankle Equinus. Prevalence and linkage to common foot pathology. J Am Podiatr Med Assoc 1995;85:295–300.
86. Riddle DL, Pulistic M, Pidcoe P, et al. Risk factors for plantar fasciitis: a matched case-control study. J Bone Joint Surg Am 2003;85:872–7.

87. Probe RA, Baca M, Adams R, et al. Night splint treatment for plantar fasciitis. A prospective randomized study. Clin Orthop 1999;368:190–5.
88. Barry LD, Barry AN, Chen Y. A retrospective study of standing gastrocnemius-soleus stretching versus night splinting in the treatment of plantar fasciitis. J Foot Ankle Surg 2002;41:221–7.
89. DiGiovanni BF, Nawoczenski DA, Lintal ME, et al. Tissue-specific plantar fascia-stretching exercise enhances outcomes in patients with chronic heel pain: a prospective, randomized study. J Bone Joint Surg Am 2003;88:1775–81.
90. Lavery LA, Armstrong DG, Boulton AJ. Ankle Equinus deformity and its relationship to high plantar pressure in a large population with diabetes mellitus. J Am Podiatr Med Assoc 2002;92:479–82.
91. Orendurff MS, Rohr ES, Sangeorzan BJ, et al. An equinus deformity of the ankle accounts for only small amount of the increased forefoot plantar pressure in patients with diabetes. J Bone Joint Surg Br 2006;88:65–8.
92. Armstrong DG, Stacpoole-Shea Nguyen H, Harkless LB. Lengthening of the Achilles tendón in diabetic patients who are at high risk for ulceration of the foot? J Bone Joint Surg 1999;81-A:535–8.
93. Müeller MJ, Sinacore DR, Hastings MK, et al. Effect of Achilles tendon lengthening on neuropathic plantar ulcers. A randomized clinical trial. J Bone Joint Surg Am 2003;85-A:1436–45.
94. Frykberg RG, Bevilacqua NJ, Habershaw G. Surgical off-loading of the diabetic foot. J Am Podiatr Med Assoc 2010;100:369–84.
95. Cunha M, Faul J, Steinberg J, et al. Forefoot ulcer recurrence following partial first ray amputation. The role of tendo-Achilles lengthening. J Am Podiatr Med Assoc 2010;100:80–1.

Gastrocnemius Shortening and Heel Pain

Matthew C. Solan, FRCS (Tr&Orth)[a,b,c,d,*], Andrew Carne, FRCR[a],
Mark S. Davies, FRCS (Tr&Orth)[d]

KEYWORDS

- Gastrocnemius • Shortening • Contracture • Heel pain

KEY POINTS

- Pain and reduced function caused by disorders of either the plantar fascia or the Achilles tendon are common.
- Although heel pain is not a major public health problem it affects millions of people each year.
- For most patients, time and first-line treatments allow symptoms to resolve. A proportion of patients have resistant symptoms. Managing these recalcitrant cases is a challenge.
- Gastrocnemius contracture produces increased strain in both the Achilles tendon and the plantar fascia. This biomechanical feature must be properly assessed otherwise treatment is compromised.

BACKGROUND

Heel pain is very prevalent.[1,2] Pain, especially after a period of rest, is the main symptom. Reduced ability to walk long distances and inability to participate in exercise and sport are other complaints. Heel pain is classified clinically as either posterior or plantar.[3] Posterior heel pain is most commonly caused by tendinopathy of the noninsertional portion of the Achilles tendon. This pain is associated with sport and is becoming an increasingly common complaint as people continue to exercise into older age.[4–9] Plantar heel pain is most commonly caused by plantar fasciitis. In the

The Authors have nothing to disclose.
This article would not be possible without the inspiration of both L.S. Barouk and P. Barouk. Like so many surgeons in Europe, M.C. Solan and M.S. Davies both learned their forefoot surgery skills in Bordeaux, France. It was here that M.C. Solan was so impressed with the proximal medial gastrocnemius release technique that he extended its use to the management of recalcitrant heel pain.
[a] Department of Trauma and Orthopaedic Surgery, Royal Surrey County Hospital, Egerton Road, Guildford, Surrey GU2 5XX, UK; [b] University of Surrey, Guildford, UK; [c] Surrey Foot and Ankle Clinic, Guildford, UK; [d] London Foot and Ankle Centre, London, UK
* Corresponding author. Department of Trauma and Orthopaedic Surgery, Royal Surrey County Hospital, Egerton Road, Guildford, Surrey GU2 5XX, UK.
E-mail address: matthewsolan1@aol.com

United States more than 1 million people seek help for this each year.[10] Most cases never come to hospital and are managed in primary care.

There are many different treatments that are used for both plantar fasciitis and noninsertional Achilles tendinopathy. The evidence for many forms of treatment is weak.[1,2] At present the use of formal calf stretching programs is widely considered to be the best first-line treatment of both plantar fasciitis and noninsertional Achilles tendinopathy.[1,11–26] The Achilles has even been shown to recover its normal structure after eccentric stretching.[27] For plantar fasciitis there are additional benefits with stretches to the fascia.[28,29] The mechanism by which these stretches help have not been fully elucidated. What is well established is that calf contracture is associated with a variety of clinical problems in the foot and ankle.[30,31] Laboratory evidence also supports the commonsense assumption that increased plantar fascia strain is seen with increased calf muscle tension.[32] Reducing a calf contracture therefore improves biomechanics.[33,34] For most patients, stretching with physiotherapy supervision is sufficient. If this fails, surgery to address the gastrocnemius contracture has been used in refractory cases of heel pain with good effect.[3,35]

MANAGEMENT OF HEEL PAIN

Optimum management of both plantar fascia pain and disorders of the Achilles tendon requires a thorough clinical assessment and appropriate radiological investigation. Many patients with recalcitrant heel pain have had the condition for years while unsuccessfully trying to improve their symptoms. The patients referred to our Heel Pain Clinic are assessed and most commonly investigated by ultrasonography scan, with color-Doppler capability. A critical part of the clinical assessment is physical examination of the calf muscle complex. There is a strong association between complaints of plantar fasciitis or Achilles tendinopathy and calf contracture. Gastrocnemius contracture in isolation is particularly important in this respect. Once assessed, patients can be divided into groups from their biomechanical profiles and the exact nature of the tendinopathy/fasciopathy. Treatment can be tailored accordingly. Many patients are evaluated, scanned, classified, and then begin their individualized treatment all at the first appointment in this 1-stop clinic.

The first distinction to make clinically is between plantar heel pain and posterior heel pain. The former is commonly caused by plantar fasciitis. Other orthopedic causes include a stress fracture of the os calcis or, less commonly, tarsal tunnel syndrome (**Box 1**). Inflammatory, neurologic, and rare neoplastic disorders must be borne in mind, especially if first-line treatments fail to improve symptoms.

Box 1
Guildford classification of heel pain

1. Posterior heel pain
   a. Tendinopathy of the main body of the Achilles
   b. Insertional tendinopathy
2. Plantar heel pain
   a. Plantar fasciopathy of the calcaneal insertion
   b. Atypical fasciopathy (distal/fibroma)

ACHILLES TENDINOPATHY

Posterior heel pain most commonly arises from the Achilles tendon. Clain and Baxter[36] classified Achilles pain as arising from the insertional portion of the tendon or from the noninsertional region. The distinction is helpful clinically.

Noninsertional Achilles tendon disorder is much more common than insertional tendinopathy. Like tendinopathies around the knee, shoulder, and hip there is degenerative change within the substance of the tendon, thickening of the paratenon, or a combination of the two. Contemporary research emphasizes that tendinopathy is a failed healing response rather than an acute inflammation.

TERMINOLOGY IN ACHILLES TENDON PAIN

Maffulli and colleagues[37] have proposed a logical nomenclature for describing Achilles tendon disorders.[38–40] This nomenclature has reduced the use of many synonyms that have confused the literature. The emphasis is on tendon degeneration and not inflammation (**Box 2**). The clinical presentation of pain, swelling, and impaired function is referred to as Achilles tendinopathy.[37] This terminology may also be used for the rotator cuff, patellar tendon, and other tendons that have painful overuse symptoms.[37,41] The term tendinopathy does not define the underlying pathologic processes causing the symptoms. In a chronic tendinopathy there is no inflammatory response and granulation tissue is rarely seen when tissues are examined in the laboratory. It is for this reason that the term tendinitis should be abandoned.[38]

The molecular biology of tendinopathy is gradually becoming better understood. It is the focus of much ongoing research.[42] Histology studies of tissue from the insertion of the tendon show necrosis and mucoid degeneration rather than inflammatory infiltration.[7,43]

LOCAL ANATOMY

To diagnose the cause of posterior heel pain or swelling arising in the region of the Achilles tendon insertion it is essential to have a thorough understanding of the anatomy (**Fig. 1**).

DEMOGRAPHICS

Achilles tendinopathy is common, but reliable epidemiologic data are not available.[44] An association with athletic training suggests that overuse is one principal cause.[43,45]

Box 2
Nomenclature in Achilles tendon pain

Terminology of Achilles tendon pain

Clinical

1. Tendinopathy: pain, swelling, and reduced function

2. Paratenonopathy: affects paratenon clinically

3. Panatendinopathy: affects both tendon and paratenon clinically

Histologic

1. Tendinosis: mucoid degeneration and collagen disorganization

2. Paratenonitis: hyperemia and inflammatory cells. Fibrosis and thickening. Most common in specimens from younger patients

---

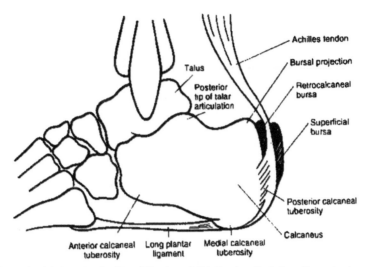

Fig. 1. Posterior heel anatomy. (*From* Stephens MM. Haglund's deformity and retrocalcaneal bursitis. Orthop Clin North Am 1994;25:41–6.)

Young athletes have a lower incidence of Achilles pain than older individuals participating in the same sport.[15,46] However, posterior heel pain can affect sedentary individuals as well.[47,48] It has been noted that older athletes have a higher prevalence of insertional tendinopathy than their younger counterparts.[48] Studies consistently show that noninsertional tendinopathy is 4 times more prevalent than symptomatic insertional tendinopathy (**Fig. 2**).[43,45]

EXAMINATION

Excessive heel valgus with a low medial longitudinal arch and forefoot varus causes overpronation of the foot and secondary Achilles tendon injury.[49] Patients with this planovalgus foot posture invariably have adaptive shortening of the gastrocnemius in isolation, demonstrable using the Silfverskiöld test. This test must be performed with the forefoot held in a position to ensure reduction of the talonavicular joint. If this joint is not reduced then false-negative findings occur, because the heel escapes

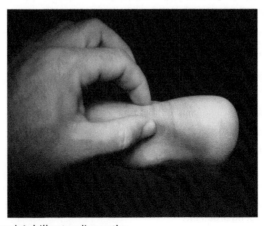

Fig. 2. Noninsertional Achilles tendinopathy.

into valgus, which masks the gastrocnemius contracture by shortening the distance between the knee and the Achilles insertion.[50]

INSERTIONAL TENDINOPATHY

This is characterized by posterior heel pain, with tenderness that is maximal in the center of the insertion of the tendon. There is often calcification within the central portion of the tendon and a spur may be seen arising from the middle one-third of the calcaneus on a lateral radiograph.

RETROCALCANEAL BURSITIS

In cases in which there is swelling and the maximal tenderness away from the midline of the heel, most commonly on the posterolateral aspect, then inflammation within the retrocalcaneal bursa is the likely cause. This condition is well shown on MRI scan or ultrasonography.

NONINSERTIONAL TENDINOPATHY

The main body of the Achilles tendon is assessed for thickening and tenderness. In rare cases of true paratendinopathy the location of the tender area does not alter with movement of the ankle. By contrast, the focal area of tendinosis moves proximal to distal as the ankle is put through a range of dorsiflexion and plantar flexion.

IMAGING

Plain radiographs are useful to assess the overall structure of the foot. They should include a lateral weight-bearing view of the foot an ankle. Anteroposterior (AP) weight-bearing views of both feet and an oblique view supplement the weight-bearing lateral film for the assessment of planovalgus deformity. For a foot with cavus deformity an additional weight-bearing AP ankle film and mortise view of the ankle are recommended.

Calcification in the insertional portion of the tendon is well shown with plain radiographs and is less well seen on MRI.

In cases of noninsertional Achilles tendinopathy the initial choice of imaging is ultrasonography.

Ultrasonography provides useful information about the tendon and bursae.[51] The principal disadvantage of ultrasonography is the absence of a permanent image to which the treating surgeon can usefully refer. This point is not relevant if surgeon and radiologist are present together at the time of the scan. The advantages of a dynamic assessment and the option to proceed to injection treatment mean that ultrasonography is the investigation of choice for Achilles problems.

Doppler ultrasonography can be used to identify associated neovascularization. Identification of hypervascularity on the anterior surface of the tendon allows sclerosant injection prolotherapy treatment (**Fig. 3**).

TREATMENT
Nonoperative Treatment

Stretching
Stretching regimens for noninsertional tendinopathy are extremely effective, with up to 90% of patients responding when the stretches are performed properly.[15] The results in cases of insertional tendinopathy are less good, with only one-third of patients

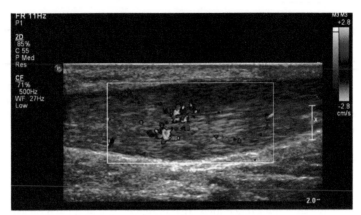

Fig. 3. Neovascularity of the main body of the Achilles tendon.

responding.[15] Stretches are still worth pursuing, particularly if adaptive shortening of the gastrocnemius is pronounced. If the hamstrings are tight with a large popliteal angle then stretches for this muscle group should be added to the regimen.[52]

Accurate assessment to identify the source of the pain guides treatment. Nonoperative treatment is preferred initially. Steroid injection is avoided wherever possible, and if performed ultrasonography guidance is used. The patient is counseled regarding the risk of rupture. For recalcitrant cases surgery has good results.[3] If an isolated gastrocnemius contracture cannot be corrected by physiotherapy then gastrocnemius release is considered.

Physiotherapy stretches for insertional tendinopathy are less reliable than when used for the treatment of noninsertional tendinopathy. For this reason gastrocnemius lengthening surgery is less frequently indicated in insertional Achilles disorders.

PLANTAR FASCIOPATHY

Plantar heel pain is most commonly caused by plantar fasciitis. This term implies acute inflammation and is therefore a misnomer. We prefer the term plantar fasciopathy, which is consistent with the current nomenclature used for disorders of the Achilles tendon. In the United States more than 1 million people seek help for this pain every year.[10] We see approximately 250 cases of recalcitrant heel pain in the Heel Pain Clinic each year. However, most cases never come to hospital and are managed in primary care (1500 cases/y in podiatry service alone).

EXAMINATION

Patients with recalcitrant plantar fasciopathy are either sedentary and overweight, often with a very high body mass index, or extremely athletic (**Fig. 4**). Long distance runners form a significant proportion of the patients in our Heel Pain Clinic. An assessment of the overall foot shape, when standing, is important. There is a strong association between planovalgus foot posture, gastrocnemius contracture, and heel pain. Hallux valgus and the adverse influence that this has on the stability of the medial column of the foot should also be noted. Careful examination of the plantar fascia is imperative. The site of maximal tenderness is usually at the medial calcaneal tuberosity. Any tenderness more distally in the fascia is relevant. Pulses and sensation should be documented, paying particular attention to the presence of any altered sensation or

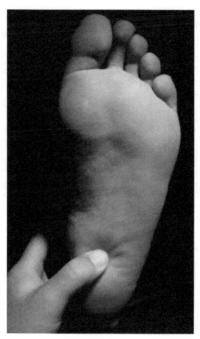

Fig. 4. Plantar fasciopathy at the calcaneal origin.

positive Tinel sign behind the medial malleolus. These features may suggest the (rare) diagnosis of tarsal tunnel syndrome. A calcaneal squeeze test, if very tender, may indicate a calcaneal stress fracture, which is most likely in runners who have increased their training or in older female patients.

IMAGING

Intractable cases can prove difficult to treat. In current standard care plantar fasciopathy is not routinely imaged and treatment is empirical. This treatment is inadequate for stubborn cases.

In our Heel Pain Clinic, patients with intractable plantar heel pain undergo routine ultrasonography scanning. Our findings have led to an improved ability to distinguish between plantar fasciopathy that affects the insertion of the fascia at the os calcis and patients with atypical findings.

Patients referred to the clinic were prospectively followed. Their ultrasonography scans were reviewed to determine the characteristics of their plantar fascia disease (**Fig. 5**).

One-hundred and twenty-five feet (120 patients) were included. Sixty-four percent had typical insertional disorders only on ultrasonography scanning. The remaining 36% had atypical distal fascia disease or a combination of insertional and distal disease. Patients with distal disease had either distal thickening or discrete fibromas (**Fig. 6**).[53]

The high proportion of atypical noninsertional disease indicates that ultrasonography scanning is valuable in determining location and characterizing the disorders in the plantar fascia. Atypical characteristics, in this cohort of recalcitrant plantar fasciopathy, would otherwise not be detected.

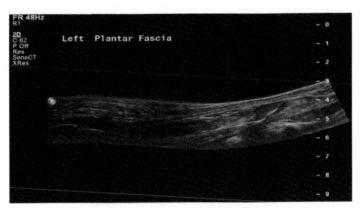

Fig. 5. Ultrasound scan (USS) of plantar fascia.

We advocate the classification of plantar fasciopathies into insertional fasciopathy or noninsertional fasciopathy. This system is in keeping with current classification of Achilles tendinopathy, which is particularly relevant because therapies for insertional disease are more predictable and reliable than the same treatments when used for noninsertional fasciopathy. Empirical treatment is not adequate for recalcitrant cases of plantar fasciopathy.

TREATMENT

There are many different treatments that are used for plantar fasciitis. The evidence for many forms of treatment is weak.[1,2] Steroid injections, either blind or under ultrasonography control, are still widely used. However, there is good evidence that they are of limited value.[54] The risks of fat pad atrophy and fascia rupture are both of concern, and we do not recommend routine use of steroid injections.

At present the use of formal calf stretching with additional stretches for the plantar fascia is widely considered to be the best first-line treatment.[28,29] The mechanism by which these stretches help is not well established.[18,55–57] However, calf contracture is

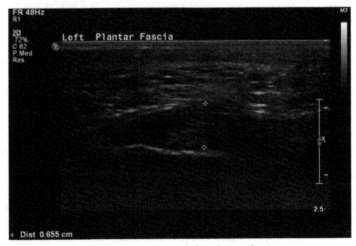

Fig. 6. Thickening of the calcaneal insertion of the plantar fascia.

associated with a variety of clinical problems in the foot and ankle.[30,31] There is also laboratory evidence that increased plantar fascia strain is seen with increased calf muscle tension.[32] Extracorporeal shockwave lithotripsy (ESWL) is a noninvasive treatment that administers pulsed, radial waves of energy that penetrate body tissues. In its original form it was used to break up kidney stones. Lower-dose treatments have been used with varying success to treat calcific tendinitis of the shoulder, tennis elbow, plantar fasciitis, and Achilles tendinopathy (both insertional and noninsertional).[58–67] There have been several modifications of the technology and this has led to confusion within the literature regarding the effectiveness of ESWL for treating musculoskeletal complaints.

Recently published, well-designed studies have shown that radial ESWL is useful in the management of patients with Achilles tendinopathy (both insertional and noninsertional) and plantar fasciitis.[68–70]

The UK National Institute for Clinical Excellence has reviewed the available evidence for the use of ESWL in plantar fasciitis and in Achilles tendinopathy. For both of these conditions the recommendation is that further high-quality research is required.

Our experience has been favorable when using ESWL for the treatment of plantar fasciopathy affecting the insertion of the fascia onto the calcaneum. However, if there is persistent biomechanical imbalance (contracture of the gastrocnemius) there is a much lower success rate. Patients who have gastrocnemius shortening are likely to fail to improve with ESWL, but the same patient is greatly improved after surgical gastrocnemius release. For this reason we advocate that gastrocnemius contracture that persists after 3 months of proper stretching, supervised by specialist physiotherapists, should be treated surgically (**Fig. 7**).

GASTROCNEMIUS CONTRACTURE
Pathomechanics of Calf Contracture

A precise figure for the amount of ankle dorsiflexion that is required for normal gait is controversial because of the difficulty in achieving reliable measurements. It is agreed that ankle dorsiflexion beyond neutral is required. At the end of the stance phase of gait, maximal ankle dorsiflexion occurs just before the heel lifts from the ground. At this moment of maximal ankle dorsiflexion the knee is in full extension (with the gastrocnemius at full stretch). The foot is supinated to create a rigid structure, largely through the action of the tibialis posterior.

In the presence of a tight calf, gait is affected in several ways. Early heel lift leads to increased pressure under the forefoot. The center of mass moves forward relative to the foot and allows the heel to reach the ground, which is achieved through compensatory lumbar lordosis, hip flexion, or knee recurvatum. Subtalar joint pronation and unlocking of the transverse tarsal joint permit dorsiflexion through the talonavicular and calcaneocuboid joints. Increased strain in the tibialis posterior tendon and spring ligament results and gastrocnemius contracture has been implicated in the cause of tibialis posterior dysfunction.[71] Isolated gastrocnemius tightness can increase midfoot and forefoot pressure during stance phase and causes the same degree of change as combined gastrocnemius-soleus tightness.[71]

The Silfverskiöld test is used clinically to distinguish between contractures that are predominantly in the gastrocnemius and those that affect both gastrocnemius and soleus. The proximal attachment of the gastrocnemius to the posterior surface of the femoral condyles means that this muscle is tight when the knee is extended. When the knee is flexed there is relaxation of the gastrocnemius. Thus a loss of ankle dorsiflexion that is evident when the knee is both flexed and extended must affect both

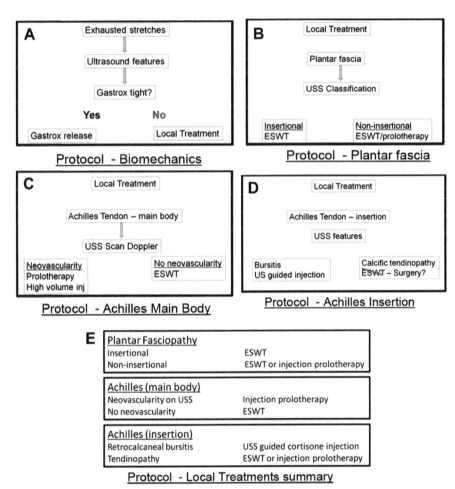

Fig. 7. Summary of treatment protocols. (*A*) Biomechanics. (*B*) Plantar fascia. (*C*) Achilles main body. (*D*) Achilles insertion. (*E*) Local treatments summary. ESWT, extra corporeal shockwave treatment; inj, injection; USS, ultrasound scan.

gastrocnemius and soleus. If the contracture is present with the knee fully extended but improves with knee flexion then the soleus is not contributing to the contracture.

CLINICAL AND EPIDEMIOLOGIC DATA

The best published evidence for the association between plantar fasciitis and contracture of the gastrocnemius is the recent article by Patel and DiGiovanni.[72] They prospectively reviewed 254 patients with plantar fasciitis. The diagnosis was clinical, and the criteria of DiGiovanni and colleagues[30] were used to define contracture of the gastrocnemius-soleus complex or the gastrocnemius. They further stratified the clinical groups into acute and chronic, choosing 9 months as the cutoff.

Eighty-three percent of patients had limited ankle dorsiflexion. Fifty-seven percent had an isolated contracture of the gastrocnemius, 26% had a contracture of the whole gastrocnemius-soleus complex, and 17% had no limitation of dorsiflexion. When patients with acute symptoms were compared with those with more than 9 months of pain the figures were similar. The investigators have shown that limited ankle dorsiflexion is commonly associated with plantar fasciitis.

OPERATIVE TREATMENT

If surgery is considered for the treatment of a calf contracture it is essential that the chosen technique is appropriate to the type of contracture. The Silfverskiöld test[73] allows the surgeon to determine whether the contracture is in both the gastrocnemius and the soleus or confined to the gastrocnemius portion of the triceps surae.

Cadaver studies have shown that the degree by which forefoot pressures increase is similar when force is increased through either the whole triceps or just the gastrocnemius.[71] Surgical release of the Achilles tendon is associated with a risk of weakness caused by overlengthening. There is also a lengthy rehabilitation period. For these reasons, when the Silfverskiöld test confirms that the contracture is confined to the gastrocnemius, release of just this portion of the calf may be preferred.[71]

GASTROCNEMIUS LENGTHENING SURGERY

The pioneering work on gastrocnemius release was by Vulpius and Stoffel,[74] Silfverskiöld,[73] and Strayer.[75] Classification of the anatomic level of the gastrocnemius-soleus complex where the release is performed is helpful in understanding the surgical options (**Fig. 8**).[76]

Silfverskiöld[73] described a procedure whereby the 2 heads of gastrocnemius are released from their origin on the posterior femoral condyles (level 5). There were complications predominantly caused by postoperative knee swelling.

The Bauman procedure requires division of the aponeurosis covering the deep surface of gastrocnemius (level 4).[76] This procedure is performed through a medial incision and places the saphenous nerve and greater saphenous vein at risk.

Strayer[75] described a release at the gastrocnemius insertion onto the tendoachilles (level 3). He allowed the gastrocnemius to retract and reattached the muscle more proximally. Operations at this level place the sural nerve at risk. The sural nerve can be superficial to, deep to, or closely applied to the fascia at the level of a Strayer release.[77] After surgery the patient is immobilized in a cast or boot for a period of at least 2 weeks.[78,79] This immobilization is another disadvantage of a surgical release at this level. The Strayer release has been associated with an overall rate of complications of 6%: 5% of patients complained of poor wound cosmesis, and 3% of patients had nerve damage.

Endoscopic Strayer release has recently been described.[80–83] The sural nerve is still at risk,[83] with neuropraxia reported in 3 of 18 patients in one series.[82] The aponeurosis at this level is a thick structure and there are reports of difficulties using the shaver to release it completely. In a cadaver study half of the specimens had not been fully released.[83]

The Vulpius procedure (level 2) is used for children with spastic diplegia. The external aponeurosis of the gastrocnemius and the underlying superficial aponeurosis of soleus are sectioned transversely just distal to the gastrocnemius muscle belly.[74,84] The Vulpius procedure therefore lengthens both the gastrocnemius and the soleus. Sammarco and colleagues[85] described the effects of a gastrocnemius lengthening at level 2 and found a 5% incidence of paresthesia in the sural nerve distribution and 5% incidence of complaints related to the wound.

Level 1 is the Achilles tendon. Hoke, White, and Paley have each described surgical techniques for lengthening the tendon. Cadaver studies have shown that percutaneous methods are both unreliable[86] and risk damage to adjacent nerves.[87] Open

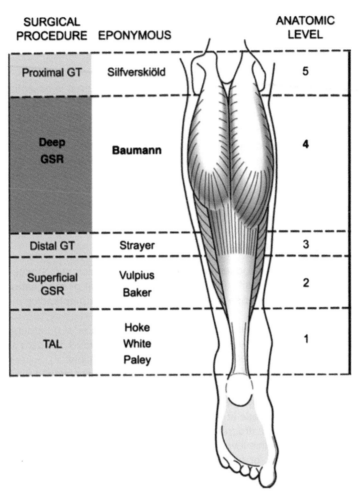

Fig. 8. Other levels of surgical lengthening. (*From* Lamm BM, Paley D, Herzenberg JE. Gastrocnemius soleus recession: a simpler, more limited approach. J Am Podiatr Med Assoc 2005;95:18–25; with permission.)

surgery is therefore recommended.[86] Wound healing and weakness caused by over-lengthening are potentially serious complications.[88]

Level 4 is the ideal level to perform an isolated release of the gastrocnemius. The lengthening is restricted to the tight gastrocnemius aponeurosis. There is no damage to either the insertion or the origin of the muscle, and the risk of neurologic complication is extremely low.

Barouk and colleagues[34] and Kohls-Gatzoulis and Solan,[89] the latter using the technique they learned from L.S. Barouk and P. Barouk, reported a simple and safe gastrocnemius release in level 4 (this is reported in article "Technique, Indications, and Results of Proximal Medial Gastrocnemius Lengthening" in more detail by Dr Pierre Barouk in this issue). When the contracture is pronounced, both heads can be released through a single popliteal crease incision under general anesthesia (GA). Because the medial head has been found to be the source of most of the gastrocnemius tightness, less severe cases can be treated with a proximal release of the aponeurosis of the medial head in isolation. This procedure is safe and can (in adults) be performed under local anesthesia with sedation. Furthermore, patients mobilize immediately after surgery without a protective plaster. The wound heals well with none of the complications seen with the Strayer (**Fig. 9**).[33,89]

RESULTS OF GASTROCNEMIUS LENGTHENING

Short-term reports have shown that ankle dorsiflexion with the knee extended improves by the same amount achieved with the knee flexed.[78] There are no studies to confirm that this correction is maintained over time.

There is limited literature examining whether there is a change in muscle strength with the various lengthening operations described. With the Strayer release there is concern that weakness could occur.[90] Fatty infiltration has been shown on MRI,[91] but little concern about weakness has been noted in surgical series.[30,92]

GASTROCNEMIUS LENGTHENING FOR RECALCITRANT HEEL PAIN

There is very little published literature on this topic. DiGiovanni and colleagues,[30] in a seminal article of 2002, noted plantar fascia and Achilles disorders as conditions that an isolated gastrocnemius contracture would influence. It may be because recalcitrant heel pain is not a priority for orthopedic surgeons that there has been so little attention devoted to the role of gastrocnemius lengthening to treat this group of patients.

Maskil and colleagues[92] recently reported the results of surgical release of the gastrocnemius at the musculotendinous junction. Thirty-eight patients were followed up with good results. This cohort of patients all had foot pain with no structural abnormality. As well as plantar fasciitis (n = 25) there were cases of metatarsalgia and arch

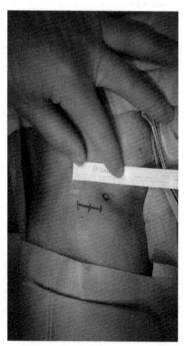

Fig. 9. Posterior view of the left popliteal fossa. Note the central incision.

pain. The investigators do not specify whether the diagnoses were entirely clinical or whether the plantar fasciitis was confirmed with imaging. A note from the journal editor, published alongside the article, notes that the relationship between gastrocnemius contracture and various foot disorders remains intriguing and controversial.

Abassian and colleagues[93] reported the results of proximal medial gastrocnemius release in a cohort of patients with refractory plantar fasciitis. All subjects had failed at least 1 year of nonoperative treatment. Treatment included orthotics, physiotherapy, and in some cases steroid injections. In addition to their previous physiotherapy, all patients underwent at least a further 3-month period of eccentric stretching (as popularized by Alfredson and colleagues[13]) under the supervision of a specialist physiotherapist.

Unlike patients in previous studies all of these patients had radiological as well as clinical diagnosis of plantar fasciitis. Imaging included radioisotope bone scan, MRI, or ultrasonography.

Patients rated the change in the level of their pain on a 5-point Likert scale. They were asked whether they had felt weaker on the released side. Calf power was assessed objectively, by asking the patients to perform 20 consecutive single-stance heel rises on the released side. The power was considered full if this was achieved. Postoperative complaints or complications were also noted. Subjects were also asked whether they would recommend this treatment to a family member.

Seventeen patients (21 heels) were included. The male/female ratio was 3:14 and the average age was 52 years (range, 31–70 years). The duration of heel pain before surgery was from 12 months to 6 years (average, 3.8 years). Fifteen patients (19 heels) had their surgery under local anesthetic infiltration and sedation. The others requested GA.

At an average of 24 months (range, 8–36 months) after surgery, 17 of the 21 heels (81%) reported total or significant pain relief. Note that 10 (58%) noticed this improvement within 1 to 2 weeks of their surgery. The remaining 7 reported a slow but progressive improvement over 3 to 6 months.

Fifteen patients (88%) would recommend this operation to a friend. There were no major complications. One minor wound complication occurred and this resolved without intervention.

PROXIMAL MEDIAL GASTROCNEMIUS RELEASE FOR ACHILLES TENDINOPATHY

The role of gastrocnemius lengthening for the treatment of Achilles pain is even less well researched than the role in plantar fasciopathy. There is a single published case report of Achilles tendinopathy that was treated by Strayer gastrocnemius lengthening,[94] producing a good result.

Gurdezi and colleagues[95] published the results of a small series of patients treated with a proximal release. They were followed for at least 1 year after proximal medial gastrocnemius release (PMGR) for the treatment of refractory Achilles tendinopathy. In this series tendinopathy of the main body of the Achilles (noninsertional tendinopathy) responded more favorably than insertional problems.

This is the only published series of patients to have a PMGR for Achilles tendinopathy. Eleven patients (5 female, 6 male) had 15 PMGRs. Four patients (4 Achilles tendons) required further surgery (1 release of the lateral head, 3 tendon debridements, 1 with supplementary FHL transfer.) Despite these additional procedures, the patient group reported that the gastrocnemius surgery was helpful. Clinical measurements showed the power in the gastrocnemius to be full following release and it was noted that the improvement in ankle dorsiflexion was maintained at 1 year. The investigators concluded that patients with recalcitrant tendinopathy who have tight gastrocnemii can be helped with a PMGR without plaster immobilization. Proximal medial gastrocnemius release is a safe, well-tolerated, and effective procedure, particularly for those patients with noninsertional Achilles tendinopathy who fail an appropriate stretching program.

SUMMARY

Contracture of the gastrocnemius produces subtle alterations to gait and posture. There is a resultant increase in the strain in the Achilles tendon and also the plantar fascia. Patients with recalcitrant heel pain commonly have isolated gastrocnemius contracture that can be shown using the Silfverskiöld test.

Eccentric calf stretching is one of the few interventions that has been proved to be useful in the management of plantar fasciopathy and Achilles tendinopathy. As part of the investigation and management of recalcitrant heel pain any contracture of the gastrocnemius should be identified using the Silfverskiöld's method. If formal eccentric stretching of the gastrocnemius does not result in improvement in the symptoms and the contracture persists, then surgical gastrocnemius lengthening should be considered. PMGR is the preferred technique for most patients because the recovery is rapid, the procedure has a very low morbidity, and it can be performed under local anesthesia with sedation (avoiding the need for full GA in the prone position). If there is extreme contracture then the surgeon must decide whether to release the lateral head of the gastrocnemius proximally at the same time or perform a Strayer procedure instead.

Local treatments for either the Achilles tendon or the plantar fascia should be deferred until any calf contracture has been corrected, which is often by stretching under physiotherapy supervision, but orthopedic surgeons should be aware of the occasional need for gastrocnemius lengthening. The PMGR technique, developed by L.S. Barouk and P. Barouk in France, is an excellent method with extremely good functional results, a low risk of complications, no need for postoperative immobilization, and once mastered is performed under local anesthetic. In time this will become the technique of choice for gastrocnemius lengthening. In our practice the Strayer is reserved for extreme contracture only and in 95% of cases we prefer the Barouk method.

REFERENCES

1. Crawford F. Plantar heel pain and fasciitis. Clin Evid 2003;(10):1431–43.
2. Hennessy MS, Molloy AP, Sturdee SW. Noninsertional Achilles tendinopathy. Foot Ankle Clin 2007;12(4):617–41, vi–vii.
3. Solan M, Davies M. Management of insertional tendinopathy of the Achilles tendon. Foot Ankle Clin 2007;12(4):597–615, vi.
4. Alfredson H, Ohberg L, Zeisig E, et al. Treatment of midportion Achilles tendinosis: similar clinical results with US and CD-guided surgery outside the tendon and sclerosing polidocanol injections. Knee Surg Sports Traumatol Arthrosc 2007;15(12):1504–9.
5. Jarvinen TA, Kannus P, Maffulli N, et al. Achilles tendon disorders: etiology and epidemiology. Foot Ankle Clin 2005;10(2):255–66.
6. Johansson C. Injuries in elite orienteers. Am J Sports Med 1986;14(5):410–5.
7. Kvist M. Achilles tendon injuries in athletes. Sports Med 1994;18(3):173–201.
8. Lysholm J, Wiklander J. Injuries in runners. Am J Sports Med 1987;15(2): 168–71.

9. Murray IR, Murray SA, MacKenzie K, et al. How evidence based is the management of two common sports injuries in a sports injury clinic? Br J Sports Med 2005;39(12):912–6 [discussion: 916].

10. Riddle DL, Schappert SM. Volume of ambulatory care visits and patterns of care for patients diagnosed with plantar fasciitis: a national study of medical doctors. Foot Ankle Int 2004;25(5):303–10.

11. Alfredson H. Chronic midportion Achilles tendinopathy: an update on research and treatment. Clin Sports Med 2003;22(4):727–41.

12. Alfredson H, Cook J. A treatment algorithm for managing Achilles tendinopathy: new treatment options. Br J Sports Med 2007;41(4):211–6.

13. Alfredson H, Pietila T, Jonsson P, et al. Heavy-load eccentric calf muscle training for the treatment of chronic Achilles tendinosis. Am J Sports Med 1998;26(3):360–6.

14. Cullen NP, Singh D. Plantar fasciitis: a review. Br J Hosp Med (Lond) 2006;67(2): 72–6.

15. Fahlstrom M, Jonsson P, Lorentzon R, et al. Chronic Achilles tendon pain treated with eccentric calf-muscle training. Knee Surg Sports Traumatol Arthrosc 2003; 11(5):327–33.

16. Flanigan RM, Nawoczenski DA, Chen L, et al. The influence of foot position on stretching of the plantar fascia. Foot Ankle Int 2007;28(7):815–22.

17. Kingma JJ, de Knikker R, Wittink HM, et al. Eccentric overload training in patients with chronic Achilles tendinopathy: a systematic review. Br J Sports Med 2007;41(6):e3.

18. Knobloch K. Eccentric rehabilitation exercise increases peritendinous type I collagen synthesis in humans with Achilles tendinosis. Scand J Med Sci Sports 2007;17(3):298–9.

19. Maffulli N, Longo UG. How do eccentric exercises work in tendinopathy? Rheumatology (Oxford) 2008;47(10):1444–5.

20. Maffulli N, Longo UG. Conservative management for tendinopathy: is there enough scientific evidence? Rheumatology (Oxford) 2008;47(4):390–1.

21. Maffulli N, Walley G, Sayana MK, et al. Eccentric calf muscle training in athletic patients with Achilles tendinopathy. Disabil Rehabil 2008;30(20–22):1677–84.

22. McLauchlan GJ, Handoll HH. Interventions for treating acute and chronic Achilles tendinitis. Cochrane Database Syst Rev 2001;(2):CD000232.

23. Radford JA, Landorf KB, Buchbinder R, et al. Effectiveness of calf muscle stretching for the short-term treatment of plantar heel pain: a randomised trial. BMC Musculoskelet Disord 2007;8:36.

24. Rompe JD, Furia JP, Maffulli N. Mid-portion Achilles tendinopathy–current options for treatment. Disabil Rehabil 2008;30(20–22):1666–76.

25. Rompe JD, Nafe B, Furia JP, et al. Eccentric loading, shock-wave treatment, or a wait-and-see policy for tendinopathy of the main body of tendo Achillis: a randomized controlled trial. Am J Sports Med 2007;35(3):374–83.

26. Sayana MK, Maffulli N. Eccentric calf muscle training in non-athletic patients with Achilles tendinopathy. J Sci Med Sport 2007;10(1):52–8.

27. Ohberg L, Lorentzon R, Alfredson H. Eccentric training in patients with chronic Achilles tendinosis: normalised tendon structure and decreased thickness at follow up. Br J Sports Med 2004;38(1):8–11 [discussion: 11].

28. DiGiovanni BF, Nawoczenski DA, Lintal ME, et al. Tissue-specific plantar fascia-stretching exercise enhances outcomes in patients with chronic heel pain. A prospective, randomized study. J Bone Joint Surg Am 2003;85-A(7):1270–7.

29. Digiovanni BF, Nawoczenski DA, Malay DP, et al. Plantar fascia-specific stretching exercise improves outcomes in patients with chronic plantar fasciitis. A

prospective clinical trial with two-year follow-up. J Bone Joint Surg Am 2006; 88(8):1775–81.

30. DiGiovanni CW, Kuo R, Tejwani N, et al. Isolated gastrocnemius tightness. J Bone Joint Surg Am 2002;84-A(6):962–70.

31. DiGiovanni CW, Langer P. The role of isolated gastrocnemius and combined Achilles contractures in the flatfoot. Foot Ankle Clin 2007;12(2):363–79, viii.

32. Carlson RE, Fleming LL, Hutton WC. The biomechanical relationship between the tendoachilles, plantar fascia and metatarsophalangeal joint dorsiflexion angle. Foot Ankle Int 2000;21(1):18–25.

33. Barouk LS, Barouk P. Brièveté des gastrocnémiens. Compte rendu du symposium n°3, Journées de Printemps SFMCP-AFCP; 2006. Toulouse (France): Maîtrise Orthopedique; 2006. p. 22–8.

34. Barouk LS, Barouk P, Toulec E. Resultats de la liberation Proximale des Gastrocnemiens. Etude Prospective Symposium « Brieveté des Gastrocnemiens », journées de Printemps SFMCP-AFCP. Toulouse (France): Med Chir Pied; 2006. p. 151–6.

35. Abassian A, Solan MC, Kohl-Gatzoulis J. Proximal medial gastrocnemius release for recalcitrant plantar fasciitis. Windsor (Canada): British foot and ankle society; 2009.

36. Clain MR, Baxter DE. Achilles tendinitis. Foot Ankle 1992;13(8):482–7.

37. Maffulli N, Khan KM, Puddu G. Overuse tendon conditions: time to change a confusing terminology. Arthroscopy 1998;14(8):840–3.

38. Khan KM, Cook JL, Kannus P, et al. Time to abandon the "tendinitis" myth. BMJ 2002;324(7338):626–7.

39. Krishna Sayana M, Maffulli N. Insertional Achilles tendinopathy. Foot Ankle Clin 2005;10(2):309–20.

40. Sharma P, Maffulli N. Understanding and managing Achilles tendinopathy. Br J Hosp Med (Lond) 2006;67(2):64–7.

41. Maffulli N, Cook JL, Khan KM. Re: Recalcitrant patellar tendinosis in elite athletes: surgical treatment in conjunction with aggressive postoperative rehabilitation. Am J Sports Med 2006;34(8):1364 [author reply: 1364–5].

42. Magra M, Maffulli N. Molecular events in tendinopathy: a role for metalloproteases. Foot Ankle Clin 2005;10(2):267–77.

43. Astrom M, Rausing A. Chronic Achilles tendinopathy. A survey of surgical and histopathologic findings. Clin Orthop Relat Res 1995;(316):151–64.

44. Maffulli N, Wong J, Almekinders LC. Types and epidemiology of tendinopathy. Clin Sports Med 2003;22(4):675–92.

45. Paavola M, Orava S, Leppilahti J, et al. Chronic Achilles tendon overuse injury: complications after surgical treatment. An analysis of 432 consecutive patients. Am J Sports Med 2000;28(1):77–82.

46. Fahlstrom M, Lorentzon R, Alfredson H. Painful conditions in the Achilles tendon region: a common problem in middle-aged competitive badminton players. Knee Surg Sports Traumatol Arthrosc 2002;10(1):57–60.

47. Mandelbaum B, Mayerson MS. Disorders of the Achilles tendon and the retrocalcaneal region. In: Myerson MS, editor. Foot and ankle disorders. 1st edition. Philadelphia: WB Saunders; 2000. p. 1367–98.

48. Schepsis AA, Jones H, Haas AL. Achilles tendon disorders in athletes. Am J Sports Med 2002;30(2):287–305.

49. James SL, Bates BT, Osternig LR. Injuries to runners. Am J Sports Med 1978; 6(2):40–50.

50. Silfverskiöld N. Orthopaedische studie über hemiplegia spastica infantilis. Acta Chir Scand 1924;84:393.

51. Bleakney RR, White LM. Imaging of the Achilles tendon. Foot Ankle Clin 2005; 10(2):239–54.
52. Harty J, Soffe K, O'Toole G, et al. The role of hamstring tightness in plantar fasciitis. Foot Ankle Int 2005;26(12):1089–92.
53. Ieong E, Afolayan J, Carne A, et al. Ultrasound scanning for recalcitrant plantar fasciopathy. Basis of a new classification. Skeletal Radiol 2013;42(3):393–8.
54. McMillan AM, Landorf KB, Gilheany MF, et al. Ultrasound guided corticosteroid injection for plantar fasciitis: randomised controlled trial. BMJ 2012;344:e3260.
55. Knobloch K. Eccentric training in Achilles tendinopathy: is it harmful to tendon microcirculation? Br J Sports Med 2007;41(6):e2 [discussion: e2].
56. Knobloch K, Kraemer R, Jagodzinski M, et al. Eccentric training decreases paratendon capillary blood flow and preserves paratendon oxygen saturation in chronic Achilles tendinopathy. J Orthop Sports Phys Ther 2007;37(5):269–76.
57. Knobloch K, Kraemer R, Lichtenberg A, et al. Achilles tendon and paratendon microcirculation in midportion and insertional tendinopathy in athletes. Am J Sports Med 2006;34(1):92–7.
58. Rompe JD. Effectiveness of extracorporeal shock wave therapy in the management of tennis elbow. Am J Sports Med 2005;33(3):461–2 [author reply: 462–3].
59. Rompe JD, Schoellner C, Nafe B. Evaluation of low-energy extracorporeal shock-wave application for treatment of chronic plantar fasciitis. J Bone Joint Surg Am 2002;84-A(3):335–41.
60. Rompe JD. "Extracorporeal shock wave therapy for lateral epicondylitis–a double blind randomized controlled trial" by C.A. Speed et al., J Orthop Res 2002;20:895–8. J Orthop Res 2003;21(5):958–9 [author reply: 961].
61. Speed CA, Nichols D, Wies J, et al. Extracorporeal shock wave therapy for plantar fasciitis. A double blind randomised controlled trial. J Orthop Res 2003;21(5):937–40.
62. Ogden JA. Extracorporeal shock wave therapy for plantar fasciitis: randomised controlled multicentre trial. Br J Sports Med 2004;38(4):382.
63. Seil R, Wilmes P, Nuhrenborger C. Extracorporeal shock wave therapy for tendinopathies. Expert Rev Med Devices 2006;3(4):463–70.
64. Theodore GH, Buch M, Amendola A, et al. Extracorporeal shock wave therapy for the treatment of plantar fasciitis. Foot Ankle Int 2004;25(5):290–7.
65. Trebinjac S, Mujic-Skikic E, Ninkovic M, et al. Extracorporeal shock wave therapy in orthopaedic diseases. Bosn J Basic Med Sci 2005;5(2):27–32.
66. Pettrone FA, McCall BR. Extracorporeal shock wave therapy without local anesthesia for chronic lateral epicondylitis. J Bone Joint Surg Am 2005;87(6):1297–304.
67. Speed CA. Extracorporeal shock-wave therapy in the management of chronic soft-tissue conditions. J Bone Joint Surg Am 2004;86(2):165–71.
68. Gerdesmeyer L, Frey C, Vester J, et al. Radial extracorporeal shock wave therapy is safe and effective in the treatment of chronic recalcitrant plantar fasciitis: results of a confirmatory randomized placebo-controlled multicenter study. Am J Sports Med 2008;36(11):2100–9.
69. Rompe JD, Furia J, Maffulli N. Eccentric loading compared with shock wave treatment for chronic insertional Achilles tendinopathy. A randomized, controlled trial. J Bone Joint Surg Am 2008;90(1):52–61.
70. Rompe JD, Furia J, Maffulli N. Eccentric loading versus eccentric loading plus shock-wave treatment for midportion Achilles tendinopathy: a randomized controlled trial. Am J Sports Med 2009;37(3):463–70.
71. Aronow MS, Diaz-Doran V, Sullivan RJ, et al. The effect of triceps surae contracture force on plantar foot pressure distribution. Foot Ankle Int 2006;27(1):43–52.

72. Patel A, DiGiovanni B. Association between plantar fasciitis and isolated contracture of the gastrocnemius. Foot Ankle Int 2011;32(1):5–8.
73. Silfverskiöld N. Reduction of the uncrossed two-joint muscles of the leg to one joint muscles in spastic conditions. Acta Chir Scand 1924;56:315–30.
74. Vulpius O, Stoffel A. Tenotmie der end schnen der mm. gastrocnemius et soleus mittels rutschenlassens nach vulpius. Orthopadishe Operationslehre. Stuttgart (Germany): Verlag von Ferdinand Enke; 1913.
75. Strayer LM Jr. Recession of the gastrocnemius; an operation to relieve spastic contracture of the calf muscles. J Bone Joint Surg Am 1950;32-A(3):671–6.
76. Herzenberg JE, Lamm BM, Corwin C, et al. Isolated recession of the gastrocnemius muscle: the Baumann procedure. Foot Ankle Int 2007;28(11):1154–9.
77. Pinney SJ, Sangeorzan BJ, Hansen ST Jr. Surgical anatomy of the gastrocnemius recession (Strayer procedure). Foot Ankle Int 2004;25(4):247–50.
78. Pinney SJ, Hansen ST Jr, Sangeorzan BJ. The effect on ankle dorsiflexion of gastrocnemius recession. Foot Ankle Int 2002;23(1):26–9.
79. Rush SM, Ford LA, Hamilton GA. Morbidity associated with high gastrocnemius recession: retrospective review of 126 cases. J Foot Ankle Surg 2006;45(3): 156–60.
80. Barrett SL, Jarvis J. Equinus deformity as a factor in forefoot nerve entrapment: treatment with endoscopic gastrocnemius recession. J Am Podiatr Med Assoc 2005;95(5):464–8.
81. DiDomenico LA, Adams HB, Garchar D. Endoscopic gastrocnemius recession for the treatment of gastrocnemius equinus. J Am Podiatr Med Assoc 2005; 95(4):410–3.
82. Saxena A, Widtfeldt A. Endoscopic gastrocnemius recession: preliminary report on 18 cases. J Foot Ankle Surg 2004;43(5):302–6.
83. Tashjian RZ, Appel AJ, Banerjee R, et al. Endoscopic gastrocnemius recession: evaluation in a cadaver model. Foot Ankle Int 2003;24(8):607–13.
84. Fry NR, Gough M, McNee AE, et al. Changes in the volume and length of the medial gastrocnemius after surgical recession in children with spastic diplegic cerebral palsy. J Pediatr Orthop 2007;27(7):769–74.
85. Sammarco GJ, Bagwe MR, Sammarco VJ, et al. The effects of unilateral gastrocsoleus recession. Foot Ankle Int 2006;27(7):508–11.
86. Hoefnagels EM, Waites MD, Belkoff SM, et al. Percutaneous Achilles tendon lengthening: a cadaver-based study of failure of the triple hemisection technique. Acta Orthop 2007;78(6):808–12.
87. Salamon ML, Pinney SJ, Van Bergeyk A, et al. Surgical anatomy and accuracy of percutaneous Achilles tendon lengthening. Foot Ankle Int 2006;27(6):411–3.
88. Delp SL, Statler K, Carroll NC. Preserving plantar flexion strength after surgical treatment for contracture of the triceps surae: a computer simulation study. J Orthop Res 1995;13(1):96–104.
89. Kohls-Gatzoulis JA, Solan M. Results of proximal medial gastrocnemius release. J Bone Joint Surg Br 2009;91-B(Supp II):361.
90. Mann RA. RE: The effect on ankle dorsiflexion of gastrocsoleus recession, Pinney SJ, et al., Foot Ankle Int. 23(1):26-29, 2002. Foot Ankle Int 2003;24(9):726–7 [author reply: 727–8].
91. Hoffmann A, Mamisch N, Buck FM, et al. Oedema and fatty degeneration of the soleus and gastrocnemius muscles on MR images in patients with Achilles tendon abnormalities. Eur Radiol 2011;21(9):1996–2003.
92. Maskill JD, Bohay DR, Anderson JG. Gastrocnemius recession to treat isolated foot pain. Foot Ankle Int 2010;31(1):19–23.

93. Abbassian A, Kohls-Gatzoulis J, Solan MC. Proximal medial gastrocnemius release in the treatment of recalcitrant plantar fasciitis. Foot Ankle Int 2012; 33(1):14–9.

94. Gentchos CE, Bohay DR, Anderson JG. Gastrocnemius recession as treatment for refractory Achilles tendinopathy: a case report. Foot Ankle Int 2008;29(6): 620–3.

95. Gurdezi S, Kohls-Gatzoulis J, Solan MC. Results of proximal medial gastrocnemius release for Achilles tendinopathy. Foot Ankle Int 2013;34(10):1364–9.

The Use of Ultrasound to Isolate the Gastrocnemius-Soleus Junction Prior to Gastrocnemius Recession

Eugene P. Toomey, MD*, Nicholas R. Seibert, MD

KEYWORDS

- Gastrocnemius recession • Strayer • Ultrasound • Achilles tendon

KEY POINTS

- Gastrocnemius recession has become a popular procedure to release isolated gastrocnemius tightness.
- Using visual anatomic landmarks alone to plan the incision can be deceiving.
- The use of ultrasound preoperatively has been highly reproducible in isolating the gastrocnemius-soleus junction in the authors' practice. This provides confidence for incision placement, a smaller incision, and isolated release of the gastrocnemius fascia while leaving the underlying soleus undisturbed.

INTRODUCTION

Release of the gastrocnemius aponeurosis has become a popular procedure to treat many common pathologies of the foot. Investigators have advocated the procedure for forefoot overload, plantar fasciitis, flatfoot reconstruction, and foot pain related to, or in conjunction with, a tight gastrocnemius.[1–4] A tight gastrocnemius is best defined as an ankle achieving less than 0° of dorsiflexion with a Silverskiöld test when the knee is straight.[5]

Gastrocnemius recession is a much more popular procedure than either open or percutaneous release of the Achilles tendon, because it is unlikely to lead to overlengthening of the Achilles or a calcaneal gait.[6]

The most common way of performing a gastrocnemius recession is through a medial approach to the gastrocnemius fascia just before it becomes confluent with the underlying soleus fascia. The sural nerve and lesser saphenous vein are protected

Disclosures: None.
Orthopedic Physician Associates, Swedish Orthopedic Institute, 601 Broadway, Seattle, WA 98122, USA
* Corresponding author.
E-mail address: e.toomey@proliancesurgeons.com

and the interval between the gastrocnemius fascia and soleus fascia is identified. The gastrocnemius fascia is then cut and the underlying soleus fascia is left undisturbed. The gastrocnemius is then allowed to retract and is either sutured to the underlying soleus muscle or simply left in the lengthened position.[1,4,7]

To achieve a good outcome without weakness or overlengthening, the literature is reasonably clear that only the gastrocnemius fascia should be lengthened and the soleus left alone. If the Silverskiöld test demonstrates contracture of the gastrocnemius and soleus, then it is appropriate to do a lengthening of both muscles with either a Vulpius procedure or Achilles tendon lengthening.

Unfortunately, few calf muscles are the same, and because of these anatomic or cosmetic differences, the incision may be off by several centimeters (**Fig. 1**). An even bigger problem is dividing the fascia and finding underlying soleus muscle rather than fascia and essentially doing a form of Achilles lengthening.[8]

The authors have concluded that some method of predicting the exact location of the gastrocnemius junction is desirable.

PROCEDURE

The authors have begun localizing the junction of the gastrocnemius and soleus with a portable ultrasound machine (SonoSite, Bothell, Washington) and have found that this is a very reproducible method for localizing the gastrocnemius-soleus junction, allowing for accurate incision placement.

The ultrasound evaluation is done with the patient supine and the leg externally rotated. This is done this in a preoperative holding area with the machine used for popliteal nerve blocks.

Conductive gel is placed over the site and the flat wand of the SonoSite machine is placed over the medial head of the gastrocnemius (**Fig. 2**). The wand is then moved distally, until the junction is identified and centered on the screen (**Fig. 3**). The center screen position corresponds to the line on the wand and the skin is then marked for incision placement (**Fig. 4**).

DISCUSSION

Isolated gastrocnemius contracture has been demonstrated to be a component of multiple foot pathologies. It is readily defined by the Silverskiöld test. Many

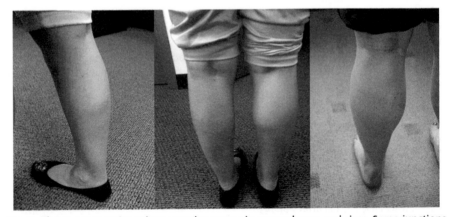

Fig. 1. The gastrocnemius-soleus complex comes in many shapes and sizes. Some junctions are easy to identify and others are not.

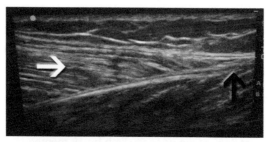

Fig. 2. Ultrasound image demonstrating gastrocnemius muscle belly (*white arrow*) and gastrocnemius-soleus junction (*black arrow*).

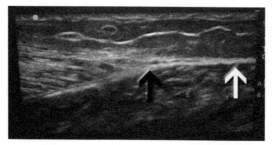

Fig. 3. The wand is moved distally to center the junction (*black arrow*) on the screen. The white arrow indicates the confluence of the 2 muscles and the beginning of the Achilles tendon.

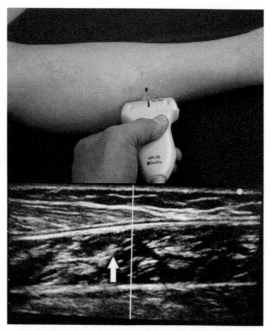

Fig. 4. The centering line on the screen (*lower*) corresponds to the arrow on the wand (*upper*). The site is marked with indelible marker for later incision placement.

investigators have advocated the Strayer procedure, which divides the gastrocnemius fascia from the underlying soleus fascia.[9]

Maskill and colleagues[1] showed an improvement in visual analog scale pain score from 8/10 preoperatively to 2/10 postoperatively; 93% of patients were satisfied with the results. Strength was not measured.

Sammarco and colleagues[10] approached the tendon with a central incision and performed a Vulpius procedure (gastrocnemius-soleus lengthening). Strength was tested with stair climbing in 40 patients; 9 patients had noticeable weakness, and 1 had moderate weakness. Peak torque tested at 6 months was 62.6% of the opposite limb and reached an average of 74% of the opposite limb by 18 months.[11–25]

Rush and colleagues[7] performed a retrospective review of 126 cases of isolated gastrocnemius recession. Total complication rate was 6%. They found all patients could do a single limb heal rise on the operative side at 6 months.

SUMMARY

Gastrocnemius recession is successful at alleviating pain, has low morbidity, and does not lead to overlengthening or significant weakness of the gastrocnemius-soleus complex. The authors have found that the use of ultrasound to isolate the junction of these 2 tendons preoperatively has been useful to do a minimally invasive, true Strayer lengthening.

REFERENCES

1. Maskill JD, Bohay DR, Anderson JG. Gastrocnemius recession to treat isolated foot pain. Foot Ankle Int 2010;31(1):19–23.
2. Pinney SJ, Hanseon ST, Sangeorzan BJ. The effect on ankle dorsiflexion of the gastrocnemius recession. Foot Ankle Int 2002;23(1):26–9.
3. Digiovanni CW, Kuo R, Tejwani N, et al. Isolated gastrocnemius tightness. J Bone Joint Surg Am 2002;84(6):962–70.
4. Abdulmassih S, Phisitkul P, Femino J, et al. Triceps surae contracture: implications for foot and ankle surgery. J Am Acad Orthop Surg 2013;21(7):398–407.
5. Silverskiold N. Reduction of the uncrossed two-joint muscles of the leg to one-joint muscles in spastic conditions. Acta Chir Scand 1924;56:149–59.
6. Chilvers M, Malicky ES, Anderson JG, et al. Heel overload associated with hell cord insufficiency. Foot Ankle Int 2007;28(6):687–9.
7. Rush SM, Ford LA, Hamilton GA. Morbidity associated with high gastrocnemius recession: retrospective review of 126 cases. J Foot Ankle Surg 2006;45(3):156–60.
8. Vulpius OS, Stoffel A. Tenotomie der end schen der mm:Gastrocnemisu et soleus mittels rutschenlassens nach vulpius. In: Orthopadische operationslehre. Stuttgart (Germany): Ferdinand Enke; 1913. p. 29–31.
9. Strayer LM Jr. Recession of the gastrocnemius: an operation to relieve spastic contracture of the calf muscles. J Bone Joint Surg Am 1950;32(3):671–6.
10. Sammarco GJ, Bagwe MR, Sammarco VJ, et al. The effects of unilateral gastrocsoleus recession. Foot Ankle Int 2006;27(7):508–11.
11. Digiovanni CW, Langer P. The role of isolated gastrocnemius and combined Achilles contractures in the hindfoot. Foot Ankle Clin 2007;12(2):363–79.
12. Orendorf MS, Rohr ES, Sangeorzan BJ, et al. An equinus deformity of the ankle accounts for only a small amount of the increased forefoot plantar pressure in patients with diabetes. J Bone Joint Surg Br 2006;88(1):65–8.

13. Cummins EJ, Anson BJ. The structure of the calcaneal tendon (of Achilles) in relation to orthopedic surgery, with additional observations on the plantaris muscle. Surg Gynecol Obstet 1946;83:107–16.
14. O'Brien M. The anatomy of the Achilles tendon. Foot Ankle Clin 2005;10(2): 225–38.
15. Hennessy MS, Molly AP, Sturdee SW. Noninsertional Achilles tendinopathy. Foot Ankle Clin 2007;12(4):617–41.
16. Aronow MS, Diaz-Doran V, Sullivan RJ, et al. The effect of the triceps surae contracture force on plantar foot pressure distribution. Foot Ankle Int 2006; 27(1):43–52.
17. Cheung JT, Zhang M, An KN. Effect of Achilles Tendon loading on plantar fascia tendion in the standing foot. Clin Biomech (Bristol, Avon) 2006;21(2):194–203.
18. Thordarson DB, Schmotzer H, Chon J, et al. Dynamic support of the human longitudinal arch: a biomechanical evaluation. Clin Orthop Relat Res 1995;316: 165–72.
19. Arangio G, Rogman A, Reed JF III. Hindfoot alignment valgus moment arm increases in adult flatfoot with Achilles tendon contracture. Foot Ankle Int 2009; 30(11):1078–82.
20. Downey MS, Banks AS. Gastrocnemius recession in the treatment of nonspastic ankle equinus: a retrospective study. J Am Podiatr Med Assoc 1989;79(4): 159–74.
21. Radford JA, Burns J, Buchbinder R, et al. Does stretching increase ankle dorsiflexion range of motion? A systematic review. Br J Sports Med 2006;40(10): 870–5.
22. Aronow MS. Triceps Surae contractures associated with posterior tibial tendon dysfunction. Tech Orthop 2000;15(3):164–73.
23. Saxena A, Gollwitzer H, Widtfeldt A, et al. Endoscopic gastrocnemius recession as therapy for gastrocnemius equinus. Z Orthop Unfall 2007;145(4):499–504 [in German].
24. Chimera NJ, Castro M, Manal K. Function and strength following gastrocnemius recession for isolated gastrocnemius contracture. Foot Ankle Int 2010;31(5): 377–84.
25. Lamm B, Paley D, Herzenberg J. Gastrocnemisu soleus recession, a simpler more limited approach. J Am Podiatr Med Assoc 2005;95(1):18–25.

Surgical Techniques of Gastrocnemius Lengthening

Raymond Y. Hsu, MD[a], Scott VanValkenburg, MD[b],*,
Altug Tanriover, MD[c], Christopher W. DiGiovanni, MD[b]

KEYWORDS

- Gastrocnemius contracture • Silfverskiold • Baumann • Vulpius • Baker • Strayer

KEY POINTS

- Isolated gastrocnemius contracture is now a well-recognized symptom producer of various foot and ankle pathologies, and its assessment should become a routine part of any patient evaluation.
- Various methods of gastrocnemius recession have been described, and it is paramount the practicing foot and ankle surgeon be familiar with at least 1 technique of surgical release.
- Gastrocnemius recession can be effectively used as sole treatment for remedying primary contracture or in conjunction with other reconstructive procedures as a means of aiding deformity correction and offloading related foot pathology.
- Determining which method to use should be based on surgeon comfort with the particular procedure/anatomy, anticipated patient position, any cosmetic concern, technical considerations (eg, the need for additional reconstructive procedures), and availability of appropriate instrumentation for performing a preferred release.
- Approximately 1 cm of distal Achilles tendon advancement and 10° to 15° of improvement in ankle dorsiflexion can generally be expected after gastrocnemius release in patients without confounding pathology. If further correction is thereafter desired, addition of an Achilles lengthening, soleus fascial release, or posterior ankle capsular release may become necessary.

Conflicts of Interest: None of the authors have any potential conflicts of interest associated with the published material herein.
Funding: None.
[a] Department of Orthopaedic Surgery, Rhode Island Hospital, The Warren Alpert Medical School of Brown University, 593 Eddy Street, Providence, RI 02903, USA; [b] Department of Orthopaedic Surgery, Harvard Medical School, Massachusetts General Hospital, 55 Fruit Street, Boston, MA 02114, USA; [c] Department of Orthopaedic Surgery, Cankaya Hospital, Bulten Street 44, Kavaklıdere, Ankara 06700, Turkey
* Corresponding author.
E-mail address: s.vanvalkenburg22@gmail.com

INTRODUCTION

Surgical release of the entire gastrocnemius-soleus complex has been in use for centuries, and was primarily used to enable plantigrade stance in the face of clubfoot deformity or equinus contracture.[1,2] Initial proposal of isolated gastrocnemius lengthening as a more directed and controlled correction of equinus and related deformity, however, did not occur until the first half of the 20th century. It was over this period that Silfverskiold,[3] Vulpius and Stoffel,[4] and Strayer[1] independently described techniques for treatment of spastic contracture in pediatric neuromuscular disorders. The last 2 decades, in particular, have seen tremendous growth in both a general interest in isolated gastrocnemius contracture and further refinement of various recession procedures to match the demand of expanding applications of gastrocnemius release.

The gastrocnemius-soleus complex is the most powerful dynamic force exerted across the foot and ankle and, thus, always remains a potential contributor to both load-related pathology and deformity. Over the last few decades, release of isolated gastrocnemius contracture has been shown to alleviate symptoms from pathologies associated with abnormal loading.[5-10] More recently, gastrocnemius recession has also received increased attention for its integral role in augmenting the correctability of both planovalgus and cavovarus feet.[11-14]

As derivatives of Silfverskiold's original gastrocnemius technique described in 1924, numerous modifications of isolated gastrocnemius lengthening have evolved over this last century.[3] Despite substantial publication of these individual procedures, however, to our knowledge there have been no reports that directly compare the clinical effectiveness of one form of surgical release to another. This article, therefore, highlights the various mainstream alternatives for direct gastrocnemius lengthening and elucidates the relative strengths and tradeoffs of each as a means of providing balanced perspective in selecting the appropriate procedure for any given patient.

ANATOMIC BASIS

The gastrocnemius-soleus complex, or triceps surae, is the most powerful muscle complex influencing the ankle and subtalar joints. The more superficial gastrocnemius muscle uniquely takes origin from the posterior femoral condyles, while its anterior counterpart, the soleus muscle, originates more inferiorly from the posterior tibia, fibula, and interosseous membrane. Distally, the tendon fibers of these 2 muscles converge to become a confluent Achilles tendon and thereby attach in unison to the calcaneal tuberosity. The anatomic peculiarity of the gastrocnemius in spanning the knee as one of 3 joints across which it exerts force remains paramount to understanding its potential impact on foot and ankle pathology over the course of evolution. Isolated contracture of the gastrocnemius has been well described as an atavistic trait acquired by humans over millennia as a consequence of bipedal gait.[15] In short, the gastrocnemius muscle tendon unit has effectively tightened in humans by virtue of having to stretch out across a straightened knee, ankle, and subtalar joint during upright stance. The biomechanical significance of such leverage forms the basis for the Silfverskiold test, whereby sustained increased dorsiflexion with knee flexion compared with knee extension indicates isolated gastrocnemius contracture.[3]

INDICATIONS

Limited ankle dorsiflexion can exist for many reasons. Although often caused by isolated gastrocnemius contracture and thus typically amenable to gastrocnemius release, any relative equinus must first be differentiated from other causes—such as overt triceps surae tightness, bony impediment, and global arthrofibrosis—before considering the most appropriate intervention. Silfverskiold's original work focused on the difference in strength requirements for dorsiflexing the ankle in knee flexion versus extension as a means of identifying gastrocnemius spasticity.[16] Over the years, however, the relative purpose of this test has changed slightly, in part based on evolved understanding of gastrocnemius pathology. A positive Silfverskiold test is currently defined as greater maximal passive ankle dorsiflexion during knee flexion than during full knee extension while the foot is held in neutral alignment (**Fig. 1**). A 10° difference has been adopted by some as the selective cutoff for determining clinically significant gastrocnemius contracture, and, perhaps not coincidentally, is approximately equivalent to the minimal ankle dorsiflexion requirement for normal gait.[5,17]

Mounting evidence continues to broaden the indications for gastrocnemius recession after identification of a contracture via the Silfverskiold maneuver. Metatarsalgia, plantar fasciitis, Achilles tendinopathy, and diabetic ulcers have all been reported to enjoy significant levels of successful resolution after being treated with gastrocnemius recession.[7–9,18–21] From a biomechanical standpoint, cadaver studies have found that contracture of the triceps surae shifts weight-bearing pressures from hindfoot to forefoot.[22] Gastrocnemius recession is effectively believed to correct for the overload of these symptomatic structures. Additionally, for adult flatfeet and related hindfoot

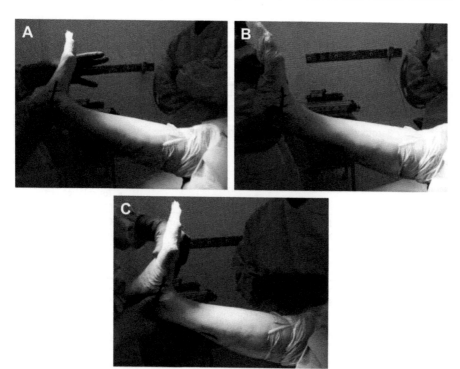

Fig. 1. Examination of ankle. (*A*) Hindfoot eversion and midfoot break can be misinterpreted as ankle pseudodorsiflexion when the foot is not held in neutral alignment through a reduced talonavicular joint. (*B*) Locking the midfoot and hindfoot in neutral shows significant gastrocnemius contracture in the same patient. (*C*) Fifteen degrees of dorsiflexion correction after gastrocnemius release in same patient, again assessed with maintenance of neutral foot alignment.

deformities, gastrocnemius recession can remove one of the major deforming forces that obviates correction of peritalar subluxation and is therefore considered by many to be essential for enabling proper realignment.[11,12,14] DiGiovanni and Langer[11] examined the association between isolated gastrocnemius contracture and the development of flatfoot deformity and highlighted the relationship between gastrocnemius tightness and increased hindfoot valgus.[11] Although commenting that the evidence remains unclear as to which of these pathologies first drives this deformity, the authors show mounting consensus that some form of gastrocnemius contractural release is frequently necessary for proper planovalgus correction.[11]

SURGICAL TECHNIQUES

Although the numerous surgical approaches designed to address gastrocnemius contracture can be classified in accordance with temporal development, they are perhaps best understood by categorizing their anatomic locations along the gastrocnemius complex (**Table 1**). The right technique has yet to be determined for any particular problem, but certainly the best technique for a given circumstance is predicated most on surgeon familiarity and, to a lesser extent, on technical/equipment considerations, perceived patient positioning needs, degree of desired correction, potential complications, and cosmetic concerns.

Table 1 Gastrocnemius recession techniques by anatomic location				
	Author, Year Described	**Released Structure**	**Positioning**	**Other Considerations**
Proximal	Silfverskiold,[3] 1924	Medial and lateral gastrocnemius heads	Prone	• Groin to heel casting for 4–6 wk
	Barouk et al,[23] 2006	Medial gastrocnemius head	Prone	• No postoperative immobilization • Small incision hidden in popliteal fossa • Tourniquet not required
Mid-distal	Baumann and Koch,[27] 1989	Anterior gastrocnemius aponeurosis +/− posterior soleus aponeurosis	Supine	• Controlled serial releases possible
Distal	Vulpius et al/ Baker,[4,59] 1913	Gastrocnemius tendon and posterior soleus aponeurosis	Prone	• Additional soleus release possible
	Strayer et al,[1] 1950	Gastrocnemius tendon	Supine/ prone	• Easiest to incorporate with other foot and ankle procedures • Tourniquet not required
	Saxena,[40] and Trevino and Panchbhavi,[41] 2002	Gastrocnemius tendon	Supine/ prone	• Small incision(s) • Requires endoscopy equipment

Proximal Gastrocnemius Recession Techniques

Traditional medial and lateral gastrocnemius muscle release: the Silfverskiold procedure

In 1924, Silfverskiold became the first to describe complete proximal gastrocnemius recession to correct a degree of spasticity in patients who suffered from neuromuscular disease.[3] His technique was again published in detail by Silver and Simon in 1959.[2] The traditional Silfverskiold procedure was performed under thigh tourniquet control with the patient positioned prone. Initial exposure is gained through an incision made in the popliteal crease (**Fig. 2**). The deep fascia is then opened in line with this skin incision to expose the 2 heads of the gastrocnemius. Care was stressed to identify and define the course of the tibial nerve between these 2 muscular heads. Motor branches emanating directly from the tibial nerve to the proximal gastrocnemius bellies must be identified, and, at least historically, it was advised that half of these branches be purposefully sacrificed to decrease their respective innervation.[2] A curved Kelly clamp would then be placed deep to the proximal end of each head to isolate them from the deeper structures, after which both heads could be sequentially transected with a scalpel from posteriorly to anteriorly. A sponge was described as an ideal tool to then sweep the released heads inferior to the level of the knee joint.

Barouk and colleagues[23] have since described a modification of this original technique, suggesting incision of only the aponeurosis of each head to facilitate reasonable stretch without frank discontinuity of the underlying muscle tissue. Regardless of which approach is taken, caution should be exercised to avoid the popliteal vein immediately deep to the operative field and the peroneal nerve immediately adjacent to the lateral head.

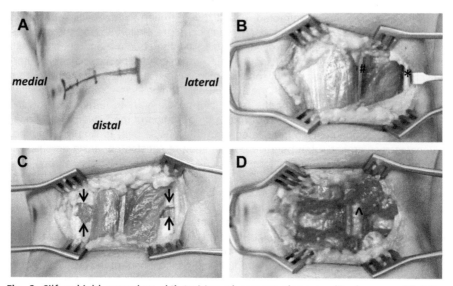

Fig. 2. Silfverskiold procedure. (*A*) Incision placement along popliteal crease. (*B*) After incising fascia, both gastrocnemius heads and the surrounding neurovascular structures are evident. The sural nerve and small saphenous vein (*number sign*) are central, and the peroneal nerve (*asterisk*) is just lateral. (*C*) Barouk describes incising only the aponeuroses (*arrows*).[23] (*D*) Silfverskiold's original procedure involves transecting the complete muscle bellies.[3] Note tibial nerve (*arrowhead*) visible deep to the muscle layer.

Isolated medial gastrocnemius release: a Barouk modification

In recent years, significant interest has emerged with performing proximal release of just the medial gastrocnemius. Advocates of this modification recommend it as a less-invasive, less-risky, and yet perhaps equally effective method of gastrocnemius recession.[8,20,24,25] After experiencing equivalent results with isolated medial recession, Barouk, who originally espoused recessing both heads like Silfverskiold, now favors recessing only the medial head.[25] This approach is purported to offer several advantages over the original procedure: it lessens risk to surrounding neurovascular structures, requires less surgery, and offers a more aesthetically pleasing surgical scar in the popliteal fossa. It should be noted that the medial gastrocnemius head has 2.4 times the cross-sectional area of the lateral head. This lends anatomic credibility to the impression that isolated release of this medial structure alone may provide sufficient correction.[26] The modified technique must still be performed with the patient in a prone position, however, which is not considered optimal for performance of many associated routine foot and ankle procedures. Unlike Silfverskiold's traditional method, however, a tourniquet is not considered necessary for isolated medial release, because it relies on more limited exposure. Infiltration of the subcutaneous tissue using 1% lidocaine with epinephrine apparently provides sufficient temporary hemostasis. It is also advised that the foot be positioned off the end of the table to allow for adequate ankle dorsiflexion during the procedure.

A 2- to 3-cm transverse incision has been specified for adequate exposure, starting 1 cm lateral to the medial dimple of the popliteal crease (**Fig. 3**).[24] This interval is then developed with the short saphenous vein and medial sural cutaneous nerve lying lateral to the plane of dissection, whereas the greater saphenous vein and saphenous nerve rest medial to the exposure. None of these neurovascular structures are routinely encountered, however, and therefore remain at fairly low risk throughout this procedure.[26] The deep fascia should be incised in line with the skin incision, after which the pes anserinus is retracted medially with a deep Langenbeck retractor to expose the medial gastrocnemius head. Hemostats are placed around the aponeurosis of the head proximally and distally to stabilize the structure and enable in situ aponeurotic release between the 2 instruments, which spares the muscle belly.[8] Alternatively, an Adson forceps or small tonsil clamp can be used to extract the head from within the skin incision, after which the aponeurosis can be incised between the 2 tips of the instrument before allowing the remaining muscle body to retract beneath the skin.[24] Regardless, in keeping with Barouk's modification of the Silfverskiold procedure, only the aponeurosis is transected, and the muscle belly is simply stretched. Advocates recommend intraoperative confirmation of satisfactory ankle dorsiflexion to verify acceptable correction before closure.

Whenever any of these popliteal fossa procedures are not performed in isolation, unfortunately, they will generally mandate turning the patient over (supine) to facilitate further foot and ankle reconstructive surgery. When performed alone, however, an added benefit of the proximal release is that it may be performed unilaterally or bilaterally without any postoperative weight-bearing restriction. Two final potential advantages advocated by proponents of the proximal medial release, although not yet definitively proven, include retained strength and concealment of the incisional scar.

Midaspect Gastrocnemius Recession Techniques

The Baumann procedure

In 1989, Baumann and Koch[27,28] became the first to describe an aponeurotic release of the anterior aponeurosis of the central gastrocnemius muscle belly. For this procedure, the patient must be positioned supine with an unsterile tourniquet placed high on

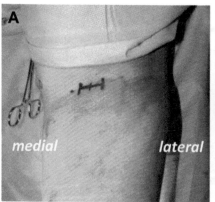
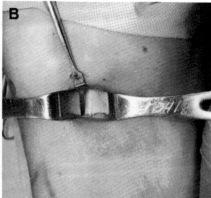

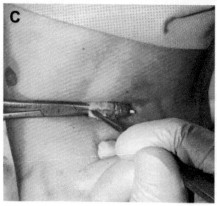

Fig. 3. Isolated proximal medial gastrocnemius release. (*A*) Small 2-cm transverse skin incision made 1 cm lateral to the medial dimple of the popliteal crease, exposing the underlying fascia. (*B*) After incising the fascia, the medial gastrocnemius head is bluntly freed and medial and lateral deep retractors are placed. (*C*) A hemostat is used to elevate the head above the deeper structures, after which the aponeurosis is released.

the patient's thigh. The hip is abducted and externally rotated with the knee flexed in a simulated frog leg position to expose the medial calf. An approximately 8-cm medial longitudinal incision is placed at the junction of the proximal and middle thirds of the leg, 2 finger breaths posterior to the posterior edge of the tibia (**Fig. 4**).[29–31] Blunt dissection is carefully used to avoid damage to the greater saphenous vein and saphenous nerve. The authors describe incising the superficial compartment fascia directly over the gastrocnemius-soleus interval to expose the plane between the 2 muscles. Deep retractors are then placed anteriorly to retract the belly of the soleus and posteriorly to retract the belly of the gastrocnemius. The plantaris tendon is resected. After dorsiflexing the ankle to place tension on the anterior aponeurosis of the gastrocnemius, 2 to 3 sequential parallel transverse incisions are made in the aponeurosis approximately 1 to 2 cm apart. Improvement in dorsiflexion can be checked after each incision to determine if additional incisions are necessary. The soleus aponeurosis can also be lengthened through the same incision when necessary for further correction, although at least 1 cadaver study suggests this may add negligible additional benefit.[29]

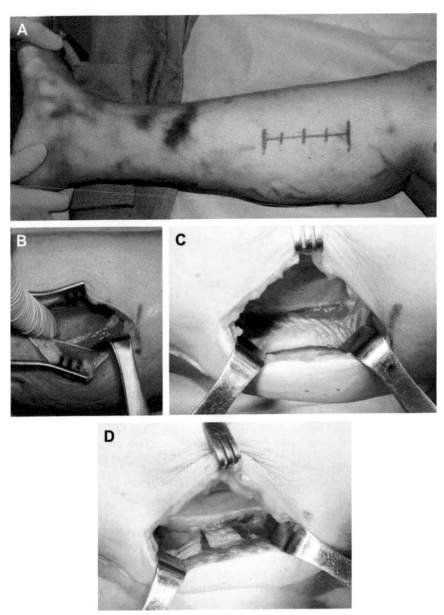

Fig. 4. Baumann procedure. (*A*) An 8-cm longitudinal incision is placed several centimeters behind the posteromedial border of the tibia along the midportion of the proximal gastrocnemius muscle belly (junction of middle and proximal third). (*B*) The fascia is bluntly cleared to avoid damage to the saphenous vein and nerve. Fascia is then incised to define the gastrocnemius–soleus interval by blunt finger dissection. (*C*) Deep retractors expose the anterior aponeurosis of the gastrocnemius. (*D*) Multiple sequential transverse incisions are made in the aponeurosis, sparing the muscle belly to gain release.

Touted advantages of this midcalf intramuscular recession technique are that it allows for a controlled, sequential release and also preserves muscle strength compared with the more distal tendon releases.[29,30] One notable disadvantage, however, is that it requires a larger skin incision in a more proximal and visible area of the calf.

Distal Gastrocnemius Recession Techniques

The original Vulpius and Baker procedures

In 1913, Vulpius and Stoffel[4] were the first to describe a distal gastrocnemius recession, although they originally suggested this procedure in conjunction with release of the soleus aponeurosis. This technique may be most appropriate when the soleus is believed to contribute significantly to the patient's contracture severity.[32,33] A 4-cm longitudinal midline incision is made through skin and fascia at the junction of the middle and distal thirds of the leg (**Fig. 5**). A transverse tenotomy is then created through the terminal tendon of the gastrocnemius and carried deep and through only the aponeurotic fibers of the soleus. Care is taken to specifically spare the soleus muscle belly at this level. In 1956, Baker described a similar technique in which he separated the gastrocnemius tendon as an inverted "U." The resultant distal tongue is then sutured back to the proximal tendon in a lengthened position after release of the deeper soleus aponeurosis.

The Strayer procedure

Strayer[1] published an alternative method of isolated distal gastrocnemius recession in 1950. It should be pointed out, however, that the approach as he initially described differs somewhat from the procedure that today frequently bears his name. A recommended 10- to 12-cm longitudinal midline incision is first centered over the middle of the calf, typically centered at the change in muscle contour posteriorly. This exposure is then carried down through the fascia of the superficial posterior compartment and the gastrocnemius subsequently dissected bluntly off the soleus. The gastrocnemius tendon is then described as being released just distal to its muscle belly and just proximal to its confluence at the Achilles tendon (aponeurosis). To allow greater retraction, Strayer recommended that the proximal tendon be reflected proximally to further dissect the medial and lateral attachments of the muscle body from the surrounding fascia. He also advocated that the proximal tendon then be affixed to the soleus in its new position, at least 1 inch proximal to its original attachment. Care and visual inspection are recommended to avoid injury to the adjacent sural nerve, which can often be found directly posterior to the gastrocnemius aponeurosis.

The modified Strayer procedure (author's preferred technique)

Today's more commonly performed Strayer procedure (or mini open distal gastrocnemius release) is typically executed through a more limited posteromedial incision, which can be accessed with the patient either supine or prone, and without any requirement for a tourniquet, as the proper anatomic plane is essentially bloodless (**Fig. 6**).[13,33,34] An assistant (or padded Mayo stand) supports the heel and knee with the leg elevated, the hip externally rotated, the knee slightly flexed, and the ankle dorsiflexed. This position keeps the gastrocnemius tendon under reasonable tension to facilitate release and also allows for easy, unimpeded access to the medial calf. A 3-cm posteromedial incision is recommended, centered over the junction of the gastrocnemius-soleus complex. The level can reliably be found where the calf contour gently transitions from the convexity of the proximal gastrocnemius muscle belly to the rapid taper of the Achilles confluence more distally. On average, this junction is 2 cm distal to the skin indentation marking the distal extent of the gastrocnemius muscle.[34]

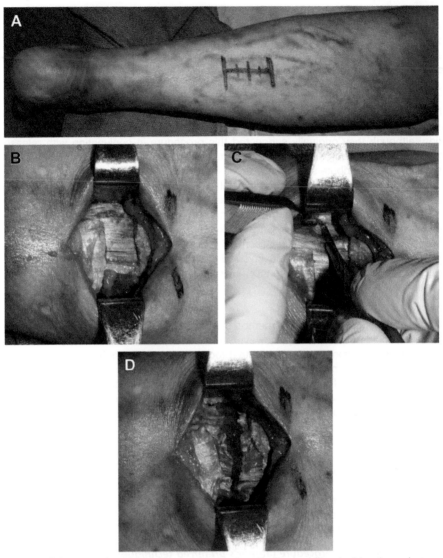

Fig. 5. Vulpius procedure. (*A*) A 4-cm posterior longitudinal midline incision is made two-thirds of the way down the leg (at the junction of the middle and distal third of the gastroc-nemius muscle). (*B*) After incising fascia, the gastrocnemius tendon is cut at its distal extent, exposing the underlying soleus. (*C, D*) The soleus aponeurosis is then similarly incised, with care taken to spare its muscle belly.

Alternatively, if bony surface anatomy is more prominent than muscle contour, this junction can be identified halfway between the ends of the fibula.[35] When in doubt, it is advocated that a smaller incision first be centered over the presumed location. This initial incision can then be lengthened 1 to 2 cm in the appropriate proximal or distal direction once the superficial posterior compartment is opened to identify the exact aponeurotic location.

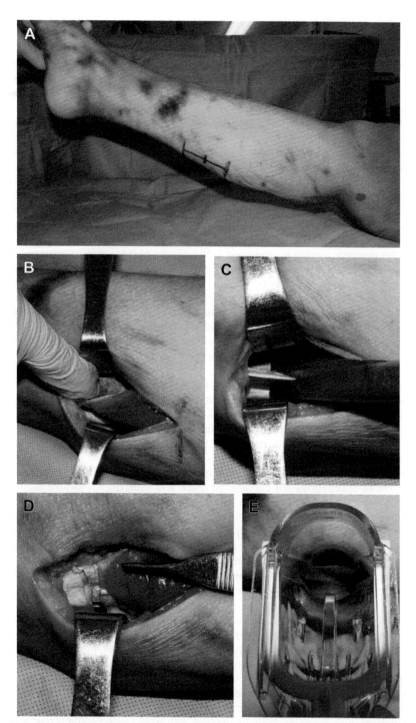

Fig. 6. Strayer procedure (*A*) A 2- to 3-cm posteromedial longitudinal incision is made along the distal contour of the gastrocnemius muscle. (*B*) Blunt dissection over the fascia protects the saphenous nerve and vein. After incising fascia, the intervals in front of and behind the gastrocnemius tendon are bluntly defined to avoid the sural nerve. (*C, D*) With deep retractors in place, the gastrocnemius tendon is transected under direct visualization. (*E*) Use of a speculum in lieu of these deep retractors has also been described.

Blunt dissection to the level of the superficial compartment fascia helps avoid injury to the greater saphenous vein and saphenous nerve. After incising the fascia in line with the skin incision and extending this initial fascial release both proximally and distally with a gloved finger, the gastrocnemius tendon can be readily identified. The sural nerve is typically deep to the fascia at this level, close to midline, and within the substance of surrounding adipose tissue. In some cases, it can even be found directly adherent to the posterior surface of the gastrocnemius tendon. A Freer elevator is recommended to dissect any superficial tissues off the posterior aspect of the gastrocnemius tendon as a means of developing a clear plane for inserting a deep right-angled retractor to protect this structure (even if it is not directly visualized). A finger can then be used to separate and reflect the soleus anteriorly, after which the posteriorly located gastrocnemius tendon is thereby isolated and easily transected sharply from medial to lateral using a curved Mayo scissor. This should be performed under constant visualization, and, when the plantaris tendon is visualized in the course of dissection, it is advised that this structure be released as well. Suturing of the reflected proximal gastrocnemius muscle, as described originally by Strayer,[1] is considered optional. Desired improvement in dorsiflexion is confirmed before closure, and, if still inadequate, the senior author recommends proceeding with either soleus fascial release or tendo-Achilles lengthening depending on the degree of further correction required.

Several other authors have described using a speculum, either vaginal or nasal, to improve visualization, decrease risk to the sural nerve, and limit the size of the incision.[7,36–38] The speculum can be placed parallel to the incision, retracting soleus anteriorly and sural nerve posteriorly while isolating the gastrocnemius tendon between the instrument's blades.[37,38] Some have described placing both blades of the speculum in the interval between the gastrocnemius and soleus, turning the speculum 90°, and cutting down on the gastrocnemius.[7,36] This method also provides adequate visualization but is arguably less protective of the sural nerve along the far side of the exposure.

The Strayer procedure and its aforementioned modifications offer several advantages. These approaches are considered quick and safe, do not require tourniquet use, and, perhaps most importantly, do not necessitate any special positioning or repositioning when performed in conjunction with other procedures. Potential disadvantages, which must be particularly considered in younger women and discussed preoperatively, include scar visibility and the small degree of differential calf atrophy and contour change noted after release. In the senior author's experience, however, increased medial transposition of the skin incision can minimize the most common cause of postoperative dissatisfaction (an unsightly scar).

Endoscopic distal gastrocnemius recession

Since its earliest descriptions, endoscopic gastrocnemius recession (EGR) has garnered attention as a means for avoiding the potential morbidity of an open procedure, although few studies have been published on the results of EGR.[39–41] Although the procedure holds promise, open gastrocnemius release seems to still remain today's gold standard.[42] There is no doubt that these endoscopic procedures result in improved cosmetic acceptability and perhaps even faster postoperative recovery. Their performance, however, appears to come with an increased surgical risk, steeper learning curve, additional operating time for set up and (at least initially) performance, and adjunct operating room equipment—all of which must be taken into account when considering what is most appropriate for any given patient.

EGR is generally performed with the patient supine, although it can be performed with the patient prone if the patient requires such positioning. The technique generally benefits from the use of a thigh tourniquet to ensure adequate visualization and muscle excursion, although this is not considered mandatory. Similar to an open Strayer procedure, the contour of the calf should be used to estimate the location of the musculotendinous junction of the gastrocnemius. Carl and Barrett[43] more precisely described an endoscopic zone, in which the recession can be carried out safely. They have found this to be an average length of 3.6 cm, centered 16.4 cm proximal to the insertion of the Achilles tendon. They concluded that the ideal point to introduce the surgical endoscopic equipment was 15 to 17 cm from the superior tuberosity of the calcaneus with the foot in a neutral position. Before initiating the portals, it is recommended to mark out the landmarks of the most distal point of the medial gastrocnemius, the insertion of the Achilles tendon on the calcaneus, and the path of the sural nerve from the ankle to the calf muscle groove (**Fig. 7**).[44]

A longitudinal 1-cm skin incision is first made posteromedially within the previously described zone.[39] Dissection is then carried bluntly down to the compartmental fascia, which is subsequently opened in line with the skin incision. The free end of the aponeurosis is then identified using a fascial elevator, and a plane is developed between the gastrocnemius tendon and the fascia in both a medial and lateral direction. This elevator is subsequently replaced with an endoscopic cannula using a blunt obturator. The cannula should be advanced until it tents the lateral skin to define an ideal location of the 1-cm lateral incision, which can then be made. The medial and lateral edges of the gastrocnemius aponeurosis are then retracted using hemostats through these respective incisions. This is recommended to facilitate complete endoscopic release

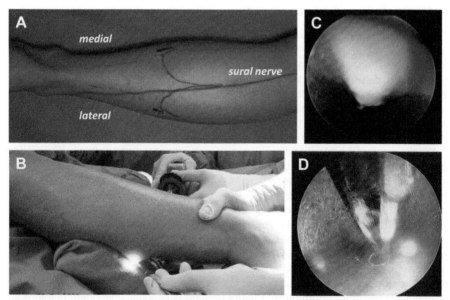

Fig. 7. Endoscopic gastrocnemius recession. (*A*) The medial and approximate lateral incisions are marked based on surface landmarks. (*B*) After blunt dissection, the endoscope is inserted medially. If a hook knife is to be used for release, a lateral portal is first made by tenting the skin for location. This is not necessary if an endoscope-mounted blade is being used. The gastrocnemius tendon is initially visualized anteriorly (*C*), and the soleus muscle then becomes visible after gastrocnemius recession (*D*). ([B] *From* Saxena A, DiGiovanni CW. Endoscopic gastrocnemius recession. In: Scuderi GR, Tria AJ, editors. Minimally invasive surgery in orthopedics: foot and ankle handbook. New York: Springer; 2012. p. 9–16.)

and counteract the naturally biplanar contour of the gastrocnemius muscle. After proper positioning is confirmed, the trocar is replaced with a 4.0-mm 30° endoscope to first visualize the gastrocnemius anteriorly and then to inspect the fascia, adipose tissue, and perhaps sural nerve posteriorly. Before any aponeurotic transection, this anatomic plane should be examined in its entirety from medial to lateral as a means of determining where the sural nerve might be at any risk during the course of recession. With the endoscope docked medially, a hook knife is then inserted through the lateral portal incision. Although the ankle is held in dorsiflexion and gentle traction placed on the medial and lateral hemostats to keep the gastrocnemius tendon edges under tension, the entire aponeurosis is cut from medial to lateral in a direction which proceeds away from the endoscope. The endoscope and knife are then exchanged in position to release any remaining tendon from lateral to medial. Small dissecting scissors can also be used to release the extreme medial and lateral edges of the tendon, if necessary.

Yeap and colleagues[45] described a modification of the above technique using a straight arthroscopic punch to cut across the tendon while visualizing from the opposite portal. This may be a good alternative if equipment options are limited, because this device is invariably part of any basic arthroscopy set. Techniques with more specialized equipment have also been described. Trevino and colleagues[46] first published a single portal technique using a carpal tunnel release endoscope system, and multiple companies have since marketed dedicated EGR systems with endoscope-mounted blades.[47,48]

POSTOPERATIVE CARE

The postoperative care recommended after performance of the original Silfverskiold and Strayer procedures for spastic contracture included groin-to-heel casting with the knee extended and the ankle in neutral for 4 to 6 weeks.[1,2] For the population of patients with cerebral palsy, some have even advocated casting the ankle in hyperdorsiflexion, although the duration of long-leg casting can be shortened if these patients are able to maintain knee extension independently.[49] Today, as a result of changing indications, which include treatment for nonneurogenic isolated contracture and deformity, the postoperative care has also significantly changed.

For the general adult population, gastrocnemius lengthening is often performed in conjunction with other reconstructive foot and ankle procedures. In most cases, therefore, postoperative immobilization and weight-bearing restrictions will be primarily dictated by these additional procedures. When recession is performed in isolation, however, there are some minor protocol differences in postoperative rehabilitation that are predicated on surgical level. When the distal procedures (Vulpius, Baker, or Strayer) are performed in isolation, most investigators advocate an initial postsurgical splint for the first 1 to 2 weeks, followed by a removable walking boot to maintain ankle neutrality for 2 to 6 weeks thereafter.[18,50–53] After the first 2 weeks postoperatively, these boots are often advocated predominantly for nighttime use—to minimize any potential for recurrent contracture. Weight bearing is typically advanced as tolerated after suture removal. Stretching exercises are also permitted to tolerance after the first postoperative visit. These patients are typically weaned into regular shoe wear once they can fully bear weight without an assistive device.

Exceptions to this general protocol exist for the less-invasive techniques. After endoscopic recession, some advocate for immediate range of motion, whereas others have maintained more conservative care with a removable walking boot for 4 weeks.[45,54] Proximal medial gastrocnemius recession may mandate the least amount of restriction postoperatively, as several investigators have described success with no immobilization or weight-bearing limitations of any kind.[8,20,24]

OUTCOMES

Objectively controlled outcome assessment after these various gastrocnemius lengthening methods, particularly for the earlier described techniques, unfortunately remain limited.[1–4,28] Furthermore, heterogeneous patient populations and potentially confounding differences caused by the effects of concomitant procedures make generalizations or any comparison between these procedures extremely difficult.[30,32,54–56] Although certain patient populations could be considered reasonably similar, there has also been no standardization of measurement parameters used for determining correction (absolute dorsiflexion, correction obtained/maintained, and clinical outcome) nor of acceptable timing of the evaluation relative to the index procedure.[10,31,50] Moreover, some of the arguably most valuable results have been subjective assessments by experienced observers, but this level V evidence does not lend itself well to scientific comparison.

Maximal ankle dorsiflexion during full knee extension remains the most consistently tested outcome parameter. Because this is not only the most frequently and easily documented preoperative indication of contracture but also the most common postoperative measure of correction, perhaps its use is appropriate. Unfortunately, however, although this parameter may represent an extremely useful and obtainable clinical measure, it has yet to be proven a scientifically reproducible or validated one. In contradistinction, direct measurement of muscle tendon unit lengthening in cadaver studies is known to be a more precise measurement, but it obviously becomes less meaningful and entirely impractical in the clinical setting.[57] An equally accurate but more reproducible assessment tool for the clinical setting would be most welcome.

Arguably related to its early development and the many iterations of its technique that have evolved since, no detailed range-of-motion outcome studies of the original Silfverskiold procedure are currently available. A minimum result of 10° of dorsiflexion with the knee extended, however, can be inferred from Silver and Simon's 1959 publication.[2] More recently, however, Barouk and colleagues[23] have reported on a large series of 185 proximal gastrocnemius releases for equinus contracture. Preoperatively, all ankles in the series had less than neutral passive dorsiflexion with the knee extended, and more than 76% were found to be more than 15° shy of neutral. In the postoperative setting, three-quarters of these had at least passive dorsiflexion to neutral with the knee in extension. Similar degrees of correction of dorsiflexion have also been reported for isolated proximal medial gastrocnemius releases.[24] In a comparison of 15 patients who underwent isolated medial release on one side and contralateral combined medial and lateral releases on the other, Barouk and Barouk[25] found equivalent ankle dorsiflexion between groups during knee extension at 6-months of follow up, providing strong support for isolated medial release.

More detailed results are available for the Baumann, Vulpius, Strayer, and endoscopic recession procedures, although few, if any, definitive comparative conclusions can be drawn (**Table 2**). What can be reasonably stated, however, is that despite wide variation in study populations, methods of assessment, and length of follow-up, in general all of these procedures demonstrate an ability to impart roughly 10° to 15° of improvement in passive ankle dorsiflexion during full knee extension (**Fig. 8**).

Table 2
Range of motion improvements by procedure

	Study, Year Pub.	Primary Indication	Change in Max Dorsiflexion (deg)	Preop DF (deg)	Postop DF (deg)	Concomitant Procedures	Length of Follow-up (mean)	No. Patients
Baumann	Herzenberg et al,[29] 2007[a]	N/A	8/14[b]	1	9/15[b]	N/A	N/A	15
	Saraph et al,[30] 2000	Cerebral palsy	28.8	-16.9	11.9	Multilevel tendon releases	24 mo	22 (28 limbs)
	Svehlik et al,[31] 2012	Cerebral palsy	15.5	-6.4	9.1	Multilevel tendon releases	10 y	18 (21 limbs)
Vulpius	Yngve et al,[58] 1996	Cerebral palsy	6	-3	3	Multilevel tendon releases	12 mo	22
	Takahashi and Shrestha,[32] 2002	Hemiplegia (CVA)	10	1.5	11.5	FHL/FDL lengthenings	N/A	140
	Park et al,[56] 2012	Clubfeet (residual/relapsed)	15.2	-0.7	14.5	Posterior tibialis aponeurotic lengthening	24 mo	17 (22 limbs)
	Sammarco et al,[55] 2006	Post. tibial def., total ankle arthroplasty, posttraumatic deformity	18.8	-3.5	15.3	Multiple reconstruction procedures	25.4 mo	40
Strayer	Pinney et al,[50] 2002	Isolated contracture	18.2	5.1	23.3	None	Immediate	20 (26 limbs)
	Chimera et al,[51] 2012	Isolated contracture	14	-1	13	None	3 mo	6
	Duthon et al,[10] 2011	Achilles tendinopathy	13	-6	7	None	12 mo	14 (17 limbs)
Endoscopic recession	Tashjian et al,[39] 2003[a]	N/A	22	-12	10	N/A	N/A	15
	Saxena and Widtfeldt,[54] 2004	Mixed deformity	14.9	-8.7	6.2	Multiple reconstructive procedures	3 mo	15
			12.3		3.6		6 mo	
	Rabat,[44] 2012	Mixed deformity	8.5	3.5	12	Multiple reconstructive procedures	6-36 mo	42

Abbreviations: CVA, cerebrovascular accident; DF, dorsiflexion; FDL, flexor digitorum longus; FHL, flexor hallucis longus; N/A, not applicable.
[a] Cadaver study.
[b] 1 recession/2 recessions.

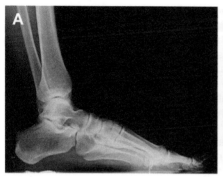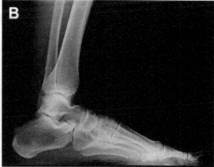

Fig. 8. Radiographic results of the modified Strayer procedure. Lateral weight-bearing radiographs of a 35-year-old man with gastrocnemius contracture refractory to aggressive physical therapy. Radiographs are taken with the patient in maximum dorsiflexion (*A*) preoperatively and (*B*) 6 weeks postoperatively after a modified Strayer procedure.

COMPLICATIONS

Reports of complication after proximal gastrocnemius recession techniques are scarce, but this nonetheless warrants some discussion in terms of guiding technique selection. Silfverskiold noted that the major complication he encountered in his patients after complete release of both gastrocnemius heads was postoperative knee swelling.[3] Advocates of isolated proximal medial gastrocnemius release purport that the decreased amount of dissection required for the procedure generally avoids such risk, although this has not been proven in a study. Reported complications for the isolated medial release do, however, include large calf hematomas (up to approximately 20% of patients in one series), one deep venous thrombosis and one hypertrophic scar (in one patient from another series of 12 patients), and one case of persistent drainage for 2 weeks in a third series of 17 patients.[8,20,24]

The major perioperative risks and side effects reported after open distal gastrocnemius recession have been sural nerve injury, weakness, and poor cosmesis; although, again, few large series exist. In a series of 126 modified Strayer procedures published by Rush and colleagues,[53] 4% complained of dissatisfaction with the incisional scar, 3% of patients experienced superficial wound dehiscence or infection, 2% had sural nerve irritation, and there were no complaints of weakness. In contrast, Maskill and colleagues,[18] published another series of 29 Strayer procedures with no wound complications, sural nerve irritation, weakness, or dissatisfaction with scar, although these subjective measures were not queried specifically. Sammarco and colleagues,[55] in a series of 40 Vulpius procedures frequently performed in concordance with other reconstructions, found sural nerve irritation in 5% and subjective weakness in 25%, but made no mention of any dissatisfaction with cosmesis. From these studies, it appeared that overall careful dissection, gentle retraction, and atraumatic closure minimizes wound and sural nerve issues.

Ever since its initial description, a primary concern of EGR has been possible increased risk to the sural nerve.[39] In a clinical series of 18 procedures, Saxena and Widtfeldt[54] reported 3 (18%) cases of sural nerve irritation. In contrast, Trevino and colleagues[46] in a series of 31 procedures reported no sural nerve problems. They did note, though, two cases of incisional placement at the wrong level requiring second incisions, one superficial wound infection, and one conversion to an open recession.[44] Rabat similarly found no sural nerve injuries amongst his series of 42 patients, but did remark that during his entire experience with over 200 procedures, he had documented one transection of the sural nerve, one case of severe dysesthesia, and 2 cases of temporary dysesthesia which recovered promptly.[44] Overall, while endoscopic recession may pose a higher risk of injury to the sural nerve as compared to open techniques, it does represent a reasonable option if the scar associated with an open recession is unacceptable.

Weakness and atrophy are also often stated as unavoidable complications of distal gastrocnemius recession. Actual data on these sequelae, however, remain inconclusive. Although Sammarco and colleagues[55] found that plantarflexion of operative legs was weaker than the contralateral nonoperative leg even beyond 18 months, preoperative strength was not available for comparison, and these findings were not statistically significant. Chimera and colleagues[51] examined patients with isolated gastrocnemius contracture 3 months after Strayer recession and similarly found that postoperative plantar flexion was weaker than that of controls. However, they also found that there was increased strength in isokinetic plantar flexion and no decrease in isometric plantar flexion compared with preoperative measurements. Duthon and colleagues[10] examined patients 1 year after the Strayer procedure for Achilles tendinopathy and found plantarflexion strength to be equal to that of the contralateral leg. It therefore seems that postoperative weakness still exists as a potential concern after gastrocnemius recession, although concrete objective data corroborating any validity of this complication are limited.

Even less attention and outcomes data have been published regarding atrophy after distal recession. One recent small series showed no change compared with the contralateral leg at 35 months of follow up.[9] In the senior author's experience, at least a slight degree of comparative atrophy always seems to exist in these patients well into their postoperative course, although this is often measured to be on the order of millimeters, and any clinical or functional consequence of this finding remains unknown.

SUMMARY

Gastrocnemius tightness has been implicated in numerous common pathologic conditions of the foot and ankle. When such isolated contracture is appropriately identified with use of the Silfverskiold maneuver, gastrocnemius lengthening can be expected to aid both the degree of equinus and the severity of any related symptomatic pathology. Many different techniques to recess the gastrocnemius along the length of its muscle–tendon unit have been described, and several continue to be used and modified with regularity today. Selection of the ideal technique for a specific clinical scenario is dictated by surgeon experience, technical and equipment considerations, cosmetic expectations, and the existence of any potential concurrent procedures that might influence positioning or tourniquet placement. In properly selected patients, however, both proximal and distal releases have been found to provide substantial correction of ankle dorsiflexion with relatively low risk—although no good direct clinical comparisons currently exist in the literature to demonstrate superiority of one technique over another. Although nerve injury and postoperative weakness have traditionally been the most voiced concerns after release, complication rates remain relatively rare. As evidence in support of the beneficial effects of gastrocnemius release on various types of foot and ankle pathology continue to mount, it seems clear that at least some form of this procedure needs to become an integral part of every foot and ankle surgeon's technical armamentarium.

REFERENCES

1. Strayer LM Jr. Recession of the gastrocnemius; an operation to relieve spastic contracture of the calf muscles. J Bone Joint Surg Am 1950;32-A(3):671–6.
2. Silver CM, Simon SD. Gastrocnemius-muscle recession (Silfverskiold operation) for spastic equinus deformity in cerebral palsy. J Bone Joint Surg Am 1959; 41-A:1021–8.
3. Silfverskiold N. Reduction of the uncrossed two-joints muscles of the leg to one-joint muscles in spastic conditions. Acta Chir Scand 1924;56:315–30.
4. Vulpius O, Stoffel A. Tenotomie der end schnen der mm. gastrocnemius el soleus mittels rutschenlassens nach vulpius. Stuttgart (Germany): Ferdinand Enke; 1913.
5. DiGiovanni CW, Kuo R, Tejwani N, et al. Isolated gastrocnemius tightness. J Bone Joint Surg Am 2002;84-A(6):962–70.
6. Patel A, DiGiovanni B. Association between plantar fasciitis and isolated contracture of the gastrocnemius. Foot Ankle Int 2011;32(1):5–8.
7. Greenhagen RM, Johnson AR, Peterson MC, et al. Gastrocnemius recession as an alternative to tendoAchillis lengthening for relief of forefoot pressure in a patient with peripheral neuropathy: a case report and description of a technical modification. J Foot Ankle Surg 2010;49(2):159.e9–13.
8. Gurdezi S, Kohls-Gatzoulis J, Solan MC. Results of proximal medial gastrocnemius release for achilles tendinopathy. Foot Ankle Int 2013;34:1364–9.
9. Kiewiet NJ, Holthusen SM, Bohay DR, et al. Gastrocnemius recession for chronic noninsertional Achilles tendinopathy. Foot Ankle Int 2013;34(4): 481–5.
10. Duthon VB, Lubbeke A, Duc SR, et al. Noninsertional Achilles tendinopathy treated with gastrocnemius lengthening. Foot Ankle Int 2011;32(4):375–9.
11. DiGiovanni CW, Langer P. The role of isolated gastrocnemius and combined Achilles contractures in the flatfoot. Foot Ankle Clin 2007;12(2):363–79, viii.
12. Kou JX, Balasubramaniam M, Kippe M, et al. Functional results of posterior tibial tendon reconstruction, calcaneal osteotomy, and gastrocnemius recession. Foot Ankle Int 2012;33(7):602–11.
13. Chen L, Greisberg J. Achilles lengthening procedures. Foot Ankle Clin 2009; 14(4):627–37.
14. Sammarco VJ, Magur EG, Sammarco GJ, et al. Arthrodesis of the subtalar and talonavicular joints for correction of symptomatic hindfoot malalignment. Foot Ankle Int 2006;27(9):661–6.
15. Morton DJ. The human foot: its evolution, physiology and functional disorders. New York: Columbia University Press; 1935.
16. Singh D. Nils Silfverskiold (1888-1957) and gastrocnemius contracture. Foot Ankle Surg 2013;19(2):135–8.
17. Kadaba MP, Ramakrishnan HK, Wootten ME. Measurement of lower extremity kinematics during level walking. J Orthop Res 1990;8(3):383–92.
18. Maskill JD, Bohay DR, Anderson JG. Gastrocnemius recession to treat isolated foot pain. Foot Ankle Int 2010;31(1):19–23.
19. DiGiovanni BF, Moore AM, Zlotnicki JP, et al. Preferred management of recalcitrant plantar fasciitis among orthopaedic foot and ankle surgeons. Foot Ankle Int 2012;33(6):507–12.
20. Abbassian A, Kohls-Gatzoulis J, Solan MC. Proximal medial gastrocnemius release in the treatment of recalcitrant plantar fasciitis. Foot Ankle Int 2012; 33(1):14–9.

21. Laborde JM. Midfoot ulcers treated with gastrocnemius-soleus recession. Foot Ankle Int 2009;30(9):842–6.
22. Aronow MS, Diaz-Doran V, Sullivan RJ, et al. The effect of triceps surae contracture force on plantar foot pressure distribution. Foot Ankle Int 2006;27(1):43–52.
23. Barouk LS, Toullec E, Barouk P. Resultat de la liberation proximale des gastrocnemiens. Etude Prospective. Symposium "Brievete des Gastrocnemiens". Medecine Et Chirurgie Du Pied 2006;22:151.
24. De los Santos-Real R, Morales-Munoz P, Payo J, et al. Gastrocnemius proximal release with minimal incision: a modified technique. Foot Ankle Int 2012;33(9): 750–4.
25. Barouk P, Barouk LS. Comparaison de deux types de liberation proximale des gastrocnemiens: mediale et laterale versus liberation mediale. Symposium "Brievete des Gastrocnemiens". Medecine Et Chirurgie Du Pied 2006;22:156.
26. Hamilton PD, Brown M, Ferguson N, et al. Surgical anatomy of the proximal release of the gastrocnemius: a cadaveric study. Foot Ankle Int 2009;30(12):1202–6.
27. Baumann JU, Koch HG. Ventrale aponeurotische Verläängerung des Musculus gastrocnemius. Operative Orthopädie und Traumatologie 1989;1:254–8.
28. Baumann JU, Koch HG. Lengthening of the anterior aponeurosis of musculus gastrocnemius through multiple incisions. Orthoped Traumatol 1992;1(4):278–82.
29. Herzenberg JE, Lamm BM, Corwin C, et al. Isolated recession of the gastrocnemius muscle: the Baumann procedure. Foot Ankle Int 2007;28(11):1154–9.
30. Saraph V, Zwick EB, Uitz C, et al. The Baumann procedure for fixed contracture of the gastrosoleus in cerebral palsy. Evaluation of function of the ankle after multilevel surgery. J Bone Joint Surg Br 2000;82(4):535–40.
31. Svehlik M, Kraus T, Steinwender G, et al. The Baumann procedure to correct equinus gait in children with diplegic cerebral palsy: long-term results. J Bone Joint Surg Br 2012;94(8):1143–7.
32. Takahashi S, Shrestha A. The vulpius procedure for correction of equinus deformity in patients with hemiplegia. J Bone Joint Surg Br 2002;84(7):978–80.
33. Barske HL, DiGiovanni BF, Douglass M, et al. Current concepts review: isolated gastrocnemius contracture and gastrocnemius recession. Foot Ankle Int 2012; 33(10):915–21.
34. Pinney SJ, Sangeorzan BJ, Hansen ST Jr. Surgical anatomy of the gastrocnemius recession (Strayer procedure). Foot Ankle Int 2004;25(4):247–50.
35. Tashjian RZ, Appel AJ, Banerjee R, et al. Anatomic study of the gastrocnemius-soleus junction and its relationship to the sural nerve. Foot Ankle Int 2003;24(6): 473–6.
36. Tellisi N, Elliott AJ. Gastrocnemius apneourosis recession: a modified technique. Foot Ankle Int 2008;29(12):1232–4.
37. Roberts MM, Hansen ST. Technique tip: using a vaginal speculum for gastrocnemius recession. Operat Tech Orthop 2004;14(1):11–2.
38. Roche AJ, Calder JD. User-friendly instrument for modified Strayer procedure: technical tip. Foot Ankle Int 2012;33(12):1159–60.
39. Tashjian RZ, Appel AJ, Banerjee R, et al. Endoscopic gastrocnemius recession: evaluation in a cadaver model. Foot Ankle Int 2003;24(8):607–13.
40. Saxena A. Endoscopic gastrocnemius tenotomy. J Foot Ankle Surg 2002;41(1):57–8.
41. Trevino SG, Panchbhavi VK. Technique of endoscopic gastrocnemius recession: a cadaver study. Foot Ankle Surg 2002;8(1):45–7.
42. Saxena A, DiGiovanni CW. Endoscopic gastrocnemius recession. In: Scuderi GR, Tria AJ, editors. Minimally invasive surgery in orthopedics: foot and ankle handbook. New York: Springer; 2012. p. 9–16.

43. Carl T, Barrett SL. Cadaveric assessment of the gastrocnemius aponeurosis to assist in the pre-operative planning for two portal endoscopic gastrocnemius recession (EGR). Foot 2005;15:137–40.
44. Rabat E. Endoscopic gastrocnemius recession. In: Barouk LS, Barouk P, editors. Gastrocnemius tightness: from anatomy to treatment. Paris: Sauramps Medical; 2012. p. 351–73.
45. Yeap EJ, Shamsul SA, Chong KW, et al. Simple two-portal technique for endoscopic gastrocnemius recession: clinical tip. Foot Ankle Int 2011;32(8):830–3.
46. Trevino S, Gibbs M, Panchbhavi V. Evaluation of results of endoscopic gastrocnemius recession. Foot Ankle Int 2005;26(5):359–64.
47. Schroeder SM. Uniportal endoscopic gastrocnemius recession for treatment of gastrocnemius equinus with a dedicated EGR system with retractable blade. J Foot Ankle Surg 2012;51(6):714–9.
48. Roukis TS, Schweinberger MH. Complications associated with uni-portal endoscopic gastrocnemius recession in a diabetic patient population: an observational case series. J Foot Ankle Surg 2010;49(1):68–70.
49. Craig JJ, van Vuren J. The importance of gastrocnemius recession in the correction of equinus deformity in cerebral palsy. J Bone Joint Surg Br 1976;58(1):84–7.
50. Pinney SJ, Hansen ST Jr, Sangeorzan BJ. The effect on ankle dorsiflexion of gastrocnemius recession. Foot Ankle Int 2002;23(1):26–9.
51. Chimera NJ, Castro M, Davis I, et al. The effect of isolated gastrocnemius contracture and gastrocnemius recession on lower extremity kinematics and kinetics during stance. Clin Biomech (Bristol, Avon) 2012;27(9):917–23.
52. Laborde JM. Neuropathic plantar forefoot ulcers treated with tendon lengthenings. Foot Ankle Int 2008;29(4):378–84.
53. Rush SM, Ford LA, Hamilton GA. Morbidity associated with high gastrocnemius recession: retrospective review of 126 cases. J Foot Ankle Surg 2006;45(3):156–60.
54. Saxena A, Widtfeldt A. Endoscopic gastrocnemius recession: preliminary report on 18 cases. J Foot Ankle Surg 2004;43(5):302–6.
55. Sammarco GJ, Bagwe MR, Sammarco VJ, et al. The effects of unilateral gastrocsoleus recession. Foot Ankle Int 2006;27(7):508–11.
56. Park SS, Lee HS, Han SH, et al. Gastrocsoleus fascial release for correction of equinus deformity in residual or relapsed clubfoot. Foot Ankle Int 2012;33(12):1075–8.
57. Firth GB, McMullan M, Chin T, et al. Lengthening of the gastrocnemius-soleus complex: an anatomical and biomechanical study in human cadavers. J Bone Joint Surg Am 2013;95(16):1489–96.
58. Yngve DA, Chambers C. Vulpius and Z-lengthening. J Pediatr Orthop 1996;16(6):759–64.
59. Baker LD. A rational approach to the surgical needs of the cerebral palsy patient. J Bone Joint Surg Am 1956;38-A(2):313–23.

Gastrocnemius Recession

John G. Anderson, MD[a],*, Donald R. Bohay, MD[b],
Erik B. Eller, MD[c], Bryan L. Witt, DO[d]

KEYWORDS

- Gastrocnemius recession • Gastrocnemius equinus • Foot and ankle conditions
- Flat foot • Arch collapse

KEY POINTS

- The Grand Rapids Arch Collapse classifications create a novel and simple system for categorizing and correlating numerous common foot and ankle conditions related to a failing arch.
- Gastrocnemius equinus diagnosis plays a crucial role in the pathology of arch collapse.
- A contracture of the gastrocnemius muscle is increasingly recognized as the cause of a multitude of foot and ankle conditions.
- Therapeutic treatments should focus on stretching, splinting, and other therapeutic modalities for this muscle once a contracture is identified. If conservative therapy fails, a gastrocnemius recession can successfully relieve refractory foot pain with an acceptable complication profile.

BACKGROUND

Orthopedic foot and ankle surgeons commonly identify gastrocnemius contractures as the cause of multiple pathologic foot and ankle conditions. DiGiovanni and colleagues[1] identified an 88% incidence of gastrocnemius contractures (characterized by <10° dorsiflexion) in patients with symptomatic foot pain as opposed to only 44% in asymptomatic controls. Another common diagnosis for the condition, equinus contracture, describes the vertical orientation of the tibiotalar joint similar to that seen in horse anatomy. This orientation, although advantageous for quadrupedal motion, is problematic with human bipedal motion. During bipedal motion, passive dorsiflexion with an extended knee is important, especially during the second rocker phase of gait. With a tight gastrocnemius muscle, the heel elevates from the ground, prematurely transferring more weight for a prolonged period to the forefoot. This

Disclosure: None.
[a] Spectrum Health Department of Orthopaedics, Orthopaedic Associates of Michigan, PC, 1111 Leffingwell Avenue NE, Grand Rapids, MI 49525, USA; [b] Orthopaedic Associates of Michigan, PC, 1111 Leffingwell Avenue NE, Grand Rapids, MI 49525, USA; [c] The CORE Institute, 26750 Providence Parkway suite 200, Novi, MI 48374, USA; [d] Suncoast Orthopedics, 13211 Walsingham Road, Largo, FL 33774, USA
* Corresponding author.
E-mail address: John.Anderson@oamichigan.com

Foot Ankle Clin N Am 19 (2014) 767–786
http://dx.doi.org/10.1016/j.fcl.2014.09.001
1083-7515/14/$ – see front matter © 2014 Elsevier Inc. All rights reserved.

foot.theclinics.com

transmission occurs through the Achilles tendon, then to the plantar fascia, and ultimately to the forefoot. Thus, the increased stress through the Achilles tendon elevates the load on the plantar fascia.[2] The consequence of this overload is tension of the soft tissue of the posterior calf and plantar aspect of the foot, leading to insertional and noninsertional Achilles tendinopathy, plantar fasciitis, neuromas, metatarsalgia, and progressive arch collapse.[3]

An isolated gastrocnemius contracture is measured and differentiated from a gastrocnemius/soleus contracture using the Silfverskiold test. This assessment is performed by measuring dorsiflexion of the foot with the knee flexed and then extended. A gastrocnemius contracture is identified when dorsiflexion is less than 10° with the knee extended. During the terminal phase of stance, 10° of passive dorsiflexion with the knee extended is required for tibial advancement.[4] A lesser amount of dorsiflexion can potentially alter gait and lead to foot and ankle dysfunction.

ANATOMY

The gastrocnemius muscle lies in the superficial, posterior compartment of the calf, along with the soleus and plantaris muscles. The muscle is a component of what is known as the triceps surae. It contributes two muscle bellies and one tendon to this complex, whereas the soleus muscle contributes one head and one tendon. The 2 tendons merge at the distal two-thirds of the calf, about 6 to 9 cm from the point of calcaneal insertion, to become the Achilles tendon. The calcaneal insertion is 1.2 to 2.5 cm wide and roughly 5 to 6 mm thick, depending on the individual's size.[5,6] Before the tendons merge, they glide independently of one other. The muscle belly of the soleus continues much more distal along the tibia than the gastrocnemius muscle fibers. The fibers of the Achilles tendon rotate 90° to insert into the posterior aspect of the calcaneus. The medial and lateral heads of the gastrocnemius muscle are the only components that cross the knee joint; therefore, they can be isolated with the Silfverskiold test. They insert into the medial and lateral femoral condyles, respectively. The sural nerve is a terminal branch of the peroneal nerve and lies close to the gastrocnemius fascia. In an anatomic study by Pinney and colleagues,[7] the sural nerve was superficial to the fascia in 42.5% of the extremities and deep to the fascia in 57.5% of the calves. This nerve provides sensation to the lateral aspect of the leg and, if damaged, can bring about numbness and a painful neuroma. It is imperative that the sural nerve is identified and protected during gastrocnemius release.

ARCH COLLAPSE

The Grand Rapids Arch Collapse Classification (GRACC) (**Table 1**) was designed to highlight the progressive collapse of the arch, noted with tensile failure of the plantar soft tissues and compression failure of the dorsal midfoot joints (**Fig. 1**A). **Fig. 1** demonstrates what happens clinically as the arch collapses. This progressive collapse typically occurs over several years. In this classification, type I is a precollapse condition associated with pain in the posterior or plantar foot. Initially, an isolated gastrocnemius contracture, or Grand Rapids type I deformity, leads to midfoot and forefoot overload of the structures maintaining the arch of the foot. This pathologic contracture can initiate Achilles tendinopathy, plantar fasciitis, metatarsalgia, and arch pain without radiographic abnormality. With persistent gastrocnemius contracture, the arch begins to collapse with forefoot deformity denoting a Grand Rapids type II. This continued overload creates hypermobility in the first tarsometatarsal (TMT) joint and first ray elevation. This hypermobility can bring about further forefoot deformities including hallux valgus. Furthermore, the unstable first tarsometatarsal joint leads to

Table 1
The Grand Rapids Arch Collapse Classification (GRACC)

Classification	Affected Part of the Foot	Presenting Pathology	Biomechanics
Type 1	Gastrocnemius (Precollapse, no foot deformity)	• Gastrocnemius equinus • Plantar fasciitis • Metatarsalgia • Achilles tendon pain	• Weakened support of the arches • Tensile failure of posterior and plantar soft tissues
Type 2	Forefoot	• Hypermobile first ray • Hallux valgus • Lesser toe deformity • Metatarsalgia • Metatarsal stress fracture	• Medial column incompetence with weight bearing transfer to lesser rays

Type 3	Midfoot	• Midfoot arthritis:
		  ○ Second and third TMT Arthritis
		  ○ Medial navicular arthritis
			• Transverse arch collapse

Type 4	Hindfoot	• Hindfoot valgus • Peritalar subluxation • Posterior tibial tendon (PTT) pathology • Lateral hindfoot/subtalar arthritis • Sinus tarsi impingement	• Medial arch collapse with spring ligament attenuation and hindfoot valgus
Type 5	Ankle	• Valgus ankle arthritis	• Deltoid ligament attenuation

an overload of the lesser metatarsals, causing metatarsalgia, intractable plantar keratoses, metatarsophalangeal joint synovitis, and hammer toe deformities.

Less commonly, dorsiflexion/compression stress at the lesser tarsometatarsal joints leads to midfoot arthritis rather than the forefoot failing at the metatarsophalangeal joints. A Grand Rapids type III deformity characterizes such a midfoot deformity. The typical pattern of arthritis involves the second and third TMT joints and progresses to the medial naviculocuneiform joint in more advanced midfoot deformity.

As the arch continues to collapse, further elevation of the first ray can produce spring ligament attenuation leading to lateral or dorsolateral peritalar subluxation and subsequent hindfoot valgus deformity. This hindfoot valgus pathology is the defining characteristic of the Grand Rapids type IV deformity.

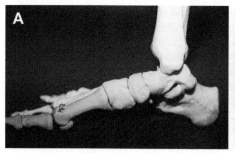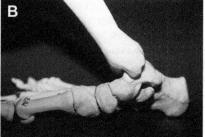

Fig. 1. (*A, B*) Clinical example of how the foot fails. Note compression failure dorsally and tension failure plantarly. (*Courtesy of* Orthopaedic Associates of Michigan, PC.)

Finally, with continued valgus malalignment of the hindfoot, in concert with the attenuation of the deltoid ligament, valgus deformity and degenerative joint changes of the tibiotalar joint are the primary traits of a Grand Rapids type V deformity, the final stage of arch collapse.

Gastrocnemius lengthening is an important component of correcting all stages of arch collapse. In the beginning phase of arch collapse, gastrocnemius stretching exercises, night splinting, and therapeutic modalities are the foundation of treatment. If conservative measures fail, surgical lengthening of the gastrocnemius muscle proves to be successful at alleviating the pain and pathology of Achilles tendinosis, plantar fasciitis, and metatarsalgia.[3] In the later phases of arch collapse, a gastrocnemius recession is not only important to alleviate the overload of the midfoot and forefoot but is also vital to protect the midfoot and forefoot reconstructive procedures.

OUTCOMES

The benefits of performing a gastrocnemius recession or an Achilles tendon lengthening in diabetics have been established for some time. Mueller and colleagues[8] followed up with patients who had diabetes and neuropathic ulcers treated with either total contact casting or tendoachilles lengthening (TAL) and found a 75% lower incidence of ulcer recurrence at 7 months and 52% lower incidence at 2 years in those patients who underwent TAL. The gastrocnemius recession has had similar success rates as demonstrated by Laborde[9] who performed a Vulpius procedure in combination with selected lengthening of peroneal tendons and healed 19 of 20 neuropathic ulcers with only 3 reported recurrences.

Grand Rapids Type I Outcomes

The type I deformity is an isolated gastrocnemius equinus contracture, causing the overload of the structures that support the arch of the foot. In this stage of collapse, radiographs are normal (**Fig. 2**). Gastrocnemius recession can be performed in isolation or as a part of a larger foot correction. As part of a more complicated correction, patient strength was found to reach 82% of unaffected side at 18 months.[10] When performed for isolated Achilles tendinopathy, strength between the 2 legs was equal at 1 year according to observations by Duthon and colleagues.[11] In isolation, gastrocnemius release has been used to successfully treat isolated foot pain associated with or without Grand Rapids type I deformities. Maskill and colleagues[3] reviewed their experience with isolated gastrocnemius recession for isolated foot pain and noted marked improvement in all groups at an average follow-up of 19.5 months. Of their 29 patients, 25 had plantar fasciitis, 6 had metatarsalgia, and 3 had arch pain. All patients had failed a course of conservative treatment measures. The subgroup with plantar fascia had significantly improved Visual Analog Scale (VAS) scores from 8.1 preoperatively to 1.9 postoperatively. The metatarsalgia subgroup also improved significantly from 7.5 to 2.2 per the VAS. Too few patients were in the arch pain group to achieve statistical significance, but VAS improvement from 9.3 to 3.3 was noted comparatively.

Duthon and colleagues[11] followed up with 14 patients prospectively who had chronic noninsertional Achilles tendinopathy for greater than 1 year. Using a primarily clinical diagnosis, all patients were found to have a gastrocnemius contracture and underwent an isolated Strayer procedure for correction. At 1 year of follow-up, American Orthopaedic Foot & Ankle Society (AOFAS), Foot Function Index, and SF-12 scores had significantly improved, and strength was equal. Nine patients

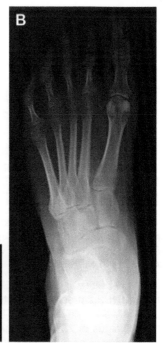

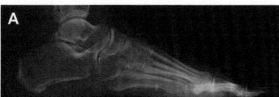

Fig. 2. (*A, B*) Grand Rapids type I deformity. Radiographically there is no abnormality. This patient presented with intractable plantar fasciitis with a gastrocnemius equinous contracture. She underwent an isolated gastrocnemius recession. (*Courtesy of* Orthopaedic Associates of Michigan, PC.)

reported no pain, and 5 reported mild/occasional pain at last follow-up. At the 1- to 2-year follow-up 13 of 14 patients indicated that they would undergo the procedure again. Range of motion significantly increased from −6° preoperatively to 7° postoperatively.

Grand Rapids Type II Outcomes

Once forefoot deformity occurs with associated symptoms (hallux valgus, metatarsalgia, and hammertoes) (**Fig. 3**), a specific course of action addresses these problems. Based on the GRAC classification, the source of a gastrocnemius contracture with forefoot deformity is related to an unstable/hypermobile first TMT joint. Thus, in addition to the gastrocnemius recession, the first TMT joint needs to be stabilized by means of a first TMT arthrodesis. Any hallux valgus deformity is addressed using a modified McBride realignment. The hammering of the toes is managed with a modified Girdlestone-Taylor procedure if the interphalangeal joint is flexible or proximal interphalangeal resection or arthrodesis if the interphalangeal joint is rigid. If the metatarsophalangeal joint is subluxated or dislocated, or in the event there are intractable plantar keratoses under the metatarsal heads, a metatarsal shortening osteotomy is performed (**Fig. 4**). Habbu and colleagues[12] reviewed their experience with this algorithm and reported good results. In a review of 374 patients (412 feet) treated with this methodology, they found a first TMT union rate of 96% and a lesser metatarsal shortening osteotomy union rate of 98%. Of the 292 patients available for phone interview after an average of 52.4 months, 88% were satisfied with their results. The mean VAS improved

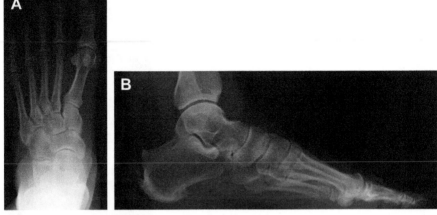

Fig. 3. (*A, B*) Grand Rapids type II deformity. Gastrocnemius contracture, hallux valgus with clinical first TMT hypermobility, and second metatarsal overload. (*Courtesy of* Orthopaedic Associates of Michigan, PC.)

from 6.6 ± 2.2 preoperatively to 2.5 ± 2.5 postoperatively. The most common complications were delayed wound healing in 4.9%, first TMT nonunion in 3.8%, recurrent hallux valgus in 2.7%, and metatarsal osteotomy nonunion in 2.2% of participants. Less common complications that were observed include hallux varus, metatarsal overload, deep infection, and toe gangrene. One patient required a below-the-knee amputation for chronic infection.

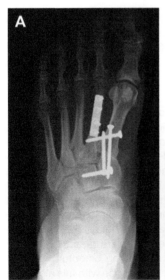
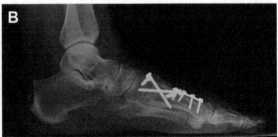

Fig. 4. (*A, B*) Grand Rapids type II correction. This was treated with a gastrocnemius recession, first TMT arthrodesis with a modified McBride, 1-2 intermetatarsal and 1-2 intercuneiform arthrodesis, and a second metatarsal shortening osteotomy. (*Courtesy of* Orthopaedic Associates of Michigan, PC.)

The surgical technique is consistent. The gastrocnemius recession is performed at the musculotendinous junction, and the fascia is not repaired. The first TMT fusion is completed using crossed 3.5-mm screws. More recently, the authors have routinely fused the first intermetatarsal and first intercuneiform joints as well. A modified Mcbride is performed using the standard technique with adductor hallucis, lateral capsule, and transverse metatarsal ligament release with medial capsular plication. The lesser metatarsal osteotomies are performed with a segmental shortening technique using dorsal $\frac{1}{4}$ tubular plate fixation.[13,14] Hammertoes are addressed with the modified Girdlestone-Taylor procedure (transferring the flexor longus to the extensor longus following a metatarsophalangeal capsulotomy and extensor tenotomy and releasing the flexor brevis).

Grand Rapids Type III Outcomes

The Grand Rapids type III deformity is defined by midfoot pathology—typically radiographically evident arthritis (**Fig. 5**). This is the result of a compression failure of the dorsum of the midfoot, following the development of first TMT hypermobility that leads first to second TMT dorsal compression, then third TMT dorsal compression, and finally medial navicular-cuneiform compression, depending on the degree of intercuneiform incompetence. With an ineffectual medial column, the lesser metatarsals are obliged to bear more weight. Conservative treatment consists of injections, carbon fiber insoles with a rocker bottom shoe, and activity modification. Failure of conservative measures leads to operative correction of this problem by fusing the affected joints. By definition, the medial column is unstable and a first TMT arthrodesis is required for stabilization. After this, involved lesser TMT (second and third) joints need to be dealt with accordingly (**Fig. 6**). Nemec and colleagues[15] reviewed their results of midfoot fusions in 96 patients with 104 feet. The average VAS score improved from 6.9 ± 1.7 preoperatively to 2.3 ± 2.4 postoperatively. The AOFAS score improved

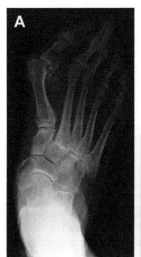
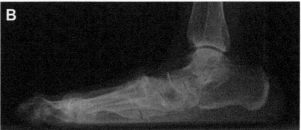

Fig. 5. (A, B) Grand Rapids type III deformity. This patient has a gastrocnemius contracture, first TMT hypermobility clinically and exhibited by the significant hallux valgus radiographically. Note the severe arthritis of the second and third TMT joints from the compressive failure, but no involvement of the first navicular cuneiform joint. (*Courtesy of* Orthopaedic Associates of Michigan, PC.)

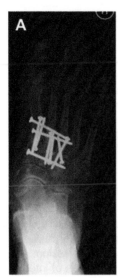
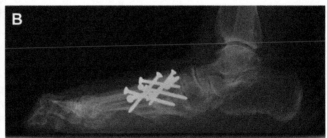

Fig. 6. (*A, B*) Grand Rapids type III correction. This deformity was corrected with a gastroc-nemius recession, first TMT arthrodesis with a modified McBride, 1-2 intermetatarsal and 1-2 intercuneiform arthrodesis, and second and third TMT arthrodesis to treat the midfoot pain/instability. (*Courtesy of* Orthopaedic Associates of Michigan, PC.)

from a preoperative mean of 32 to 79 at last follow-up. The fusion rate was reported as 92% with a major complication rate of 4% (3 deep infections and 1 complex regional pain diagnosis). Twenty-five percent of the feet required removal of hardware.

Grand Rapids Type IV Outcomes

The Grand Rapids type II deformity (forefoot deformity) can progress into the type IV deformity (hindfoot deformity) with spring ligament attenuation and progressive triceps surae contracture (**Fig. 7**). The type IV deformity is a pes planovalgus deformity and can be either flexible or rigid. Conservative management includes orthotics, bracing, anti-inflammatories, and activity modification. When these interventions fail to alleviate pain, surgical intervention is warranted. The flexible deformity is treated with gastrocnemius recession, medial column stabilization (accomplished through first TMT joint arthrodesis), a medializing calcaneal osteotomy, PTT debridement with a flexor digitorum longus (FDL) tendon transfer to navicular, and with or without lateral column lengthening depending on degree of deformity/talar head uncovering (**Fig. 8**). Pomeroy and Manoli[17] demonstrated very good outcomes with the double calcaneal osteotomy and FDL tendon transfer in patients with Johnson type II deformities. In one review, they showed an improvement in AOFAS scores from 51.4 preoperatively to 82.8 postoperatively after 17.5 months of follow-up with radiographic maintenance of correction. In another study, they found a postoperative AOFAS ankle-hindfoot score of 90 with no calcaneal nonunions reported. One patient in this study went on to require fusion for subsequent calcaneocuboid arthritis that developed in 14% of their patients.[16,17]

A rigid deformity often requires arthrodesis—traditionally a triple arthrodesis. However, alternatives to a triple arthrodesis include isolated talonavicular arthrodesis or a double arthrodesis (talonavicular and calcaneocuboid). The talonavicular arthrodesis is reserved for those with a rigid deformity but maintains motion at the subtalar joint

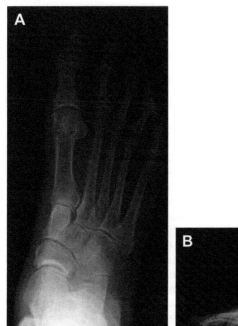
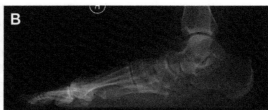

Fig. 7. (*A, B*) Grand Rapids type IV deformity. This patient has a gastrocnemius contracture, first TMT hypermobility with significant uncovering of the talar head. This was a flexible deformity clinically. (*Courtesy of* Orthopaedic Associates of Michigan, PC.)

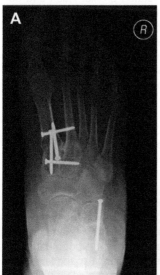
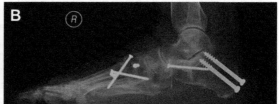

Fig. 8. (*A, B*) Grand Rapids type IV correction. This deformity was treated with a gastrocnemius recession, first TMT arthrodesis, 1-2 intermetatarsal and 1-2 intercuneiform arthrodesis to restore the medial column integrity, a medializing calcaneal osteotomy with a lateral column lengthening, and an FDL to navicular tendon transfer. (*Courtesy of* Orthopaedic Associates of Michigan, PC.)

with no noted arthrosis. This arthrodesis does not correct midtarsal instability or excessive hindfoot valgus. An adjunct calcaneus osteotomy may be required to remedy these conditions. The double arthrodesis is reserved for those patients with rigid deformity originating in the transverse tarsal joint and a passively correctable hindfoot.

Mann and Bearman[18] retrospectively evaluated their results with the double arthrodesis and found a patient satisfaction rate of 83%. Four talonavicular nonunions occurred, and progressive adjacent joint arthrosis was commonly reported. Although there are several ways to treat this deformity, there is widespread consensus that the triceps surae muscle complex is a considerable component of the deformity.

Type V Deformity

The last stage of arch collapse terminates with ankle joint involvement. Once the arch has collapsed, the valgus stress at the ankle leads to deltoid incompetence and lateral ankle joint wear (**Fig. 9**). Under these circumstances, a staged approach is often applied. The problem that is more symptomatic is addressed first. The foot deformity is addressed as discussed previously (**Fig. 10**) and then the ankle can undergo either an arthroplasty (**Fig. 11**) or an arthrodesis (**Figs. 12–18**) depending on the patient suitability factors. At this time, the benefit of ankle arthroplasty is, in theory, improved gait mechanics and preservation of ancillary joints. The benefit of ankle arthrodesis is its longevity. Currently, the reported survivability of ankle arthroplasty is 70% to 90% at 10 years.[19] The arthrodesis has similar functional and satisfaction outcomes; however, the risk of progressive adjacent joint arthritis is 96% at 20 years.[20–23] Paramount to the understanding of how a type V arch collapse occurs is the realization that treatment of the ankle deformity will require either a TAL or a gastrocnemius recession to restore proper talar declination relative to the longitudinal axis of the tibia, regardless of whether an ankle fusion or total ankle arthroplasty is the chosen treatment.

Gastrocnemius recession has an acceptable complication profile. Rush and colleagues[24] performed a retrospective review of 126 patients that underwent an open gastrocnemius recession (Strayer technique) with a mean follow-up of 19 months (range, 6–50 months). Postsurgical complications were identified in 6% (9 of 126) patients: 6 (4%) had scar problems, 2 (1.33%) had wound dehiscence, 2 (1.33%) had infection, 3 (2%) had nerve problems, and 1 (0.67%) had a complex regional pain syndrome. None of the patients complained of either a limp or gait disturbance, and no persistent decrease in muscle strength was noted.

Techniques

Several surgical techniques can increase ankle dorsiflexion, thus, correcting an equinus deformity. These different surgical procedures are determined by the level at which the resection takes place and what portion of the muscle is being resected. The more proximal the resection, the more stable the lengthening but the lesser degree of correction. The more distal the resection, the less stable the release (ie, a prolonged period of immobilization); however, a greater degree of dorsiflexion is achieved. The original description of the gastrocnemius recession technique was that of Silverskiold, in which a transverse incision is made in the popliteal fossa, and both heads of the gastrocnemius muscle are released just distal to the knee joint. More distally, the Baumann technique involves transecting the gastrocnemius muscle aponeurosis proximal to the myotendinous junction. The Strayer procedure is performed at the level of the gastrocnemius musculotendinous junction and is an isolated release of the gastrocnemius tendon. The most distal procedures are the Achilles tendon lengthening techniques, including the Hoke procedure, which involves 3 hemisections of the Achilles tendon (2 medial and 1 lateral hemisection).

Silfverskiold Procedure

The patient is placed in the prone position on a well-padded operating table. A tourniquet is placed about the affected thigh. The lower extremity is sterilely prepped and draped in the usual fashion. An Esmarch bandage is used to exsanguinate the lower extremity, and the tourniquet is inflated to 300 mm Hg. A transverse incision is made through skin, subcutaneous tissue, and deep fascia using a #15 blade scalpel in the popliteal crease. The tibial nerve is identified, and the motor branches

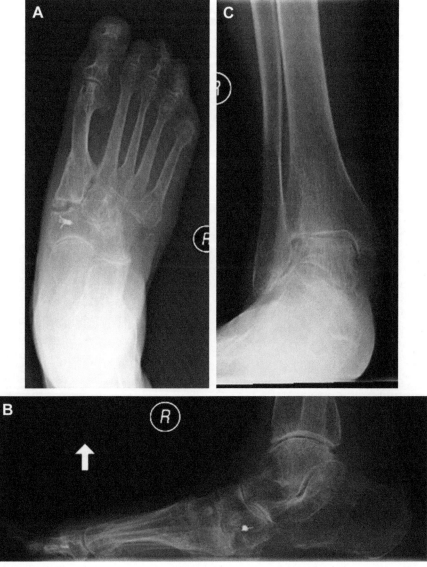

Fig. 9. Grand Rapids type V. Note that this is essentially a Grand Rapids type IV deformity of the foot (*A, B*) that has now caused valgus ankle arthritis (*C*). (*Courtesy of* Orthopaedic Associates of Michigan, PC.)

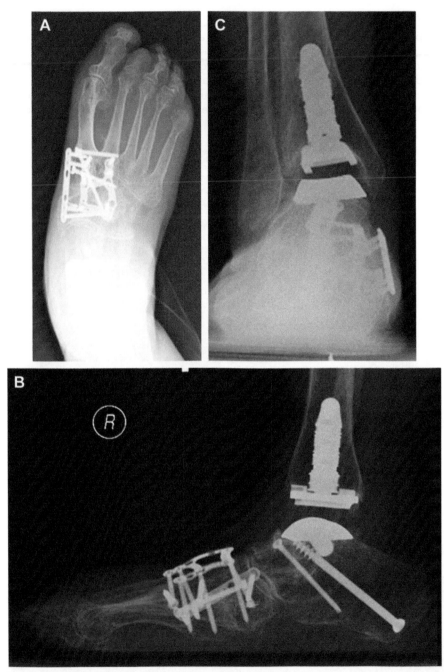

Fig. 10. (*A–C*) Grand Rapids type V correction. The first step is to address the foot deformity. Note this is a Grand Rapids IV foot correction with a TAL, first TMT arthrodesis, a second TMT arthrodesis, 1-2 intermetatarsal and 1-2 intercuneiform, and naviculocuneiform arthrodesis to restore the medial column integrity; a subtalar arthrodesis was performed to correct the hindfoot position. The valgus ankle arthritis is treated with a total ankle arthroplasty. (*Courtesy of* Orthopaedic Associates of Michigan, PC.)

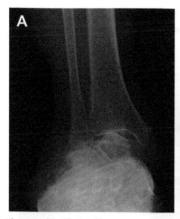
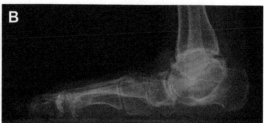

Fig. 11. (*A, B*) Another example of a Grand Rapids type VI deformity denoted by the valgus ankle arthritis. (*Courtesy of* Orthopaedic Associates of Michigan, PC.)

to the gastrocnemius muscle are isolated. One to 2 branches are observed both medially and laterally innervating the medial and lateral heads of the gastrocnemius muscle. The motor branches to the medial and lateral head of the gastrocnemius muscles are transected with a #15 blade scalpel. The medial and lateral heads of the gastrocnemius muscle are isolated and transected using a #15 blade scalpel from the posterior aspect of the femoral condyles. After the transection is complete, there should be a noticeable increase of ankle dorsiflexion compared with the patient's preoperative dorsiflexion measurement. The wound is then copiously irrigated with sterile normal saline solution. The deep fascia of the lower leg is reapproximated using 2-0 Monocryl suture in a simple interrupted fashion. The subcuticular layer of skin is closed using 2-0 Monocryl suture in a running subcuticular fashion. Finally, skin closure is completed using 3-0 nylon suture. Then the tourniquet is deflated, and a soft sterile dressing is applied over the wound. The patient is placed into a walking boot and allowed to weight bear as tolerated. Approximately 6 weeks

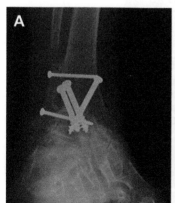
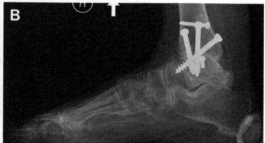

Fig. 12. (*A, B*) Grand Rapids type V deformity (see **Fig. 11**). The ankle arthritis was addressed first through ankle arthrodesis. Note the correction of the foot deformity by simply correcting the ankle position. (*Courtesy of* Orthopaedic Associates of Michigan, PC.)

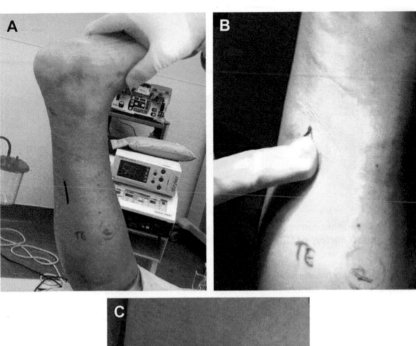

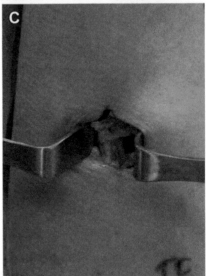

Fig. 13. (A–C) The incision is performed at the musculotendinous junction of the gastrocnemius in the distal two-thirds of the calf. A finger is used to get down bluntly to the fascia. The fascia is incised longitudinally and then the gastrocnemius tendon is resected under direct visualization while protecting the sural nerve. (*Courtesy of* Orthopaedic Associates of Michigan, PC.)

after surgery, the patient is allowed to transition into a supportive shoe as pain and swelling permits.

Baumann Procedure

The patient is placed in the supine position on a well-padded operating table. A tourniquet is placed around the affected thigh. The lower extremity is sterilely prepped and

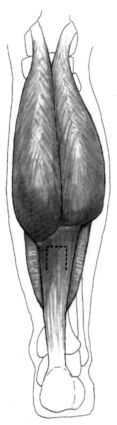

Fig. 14. Example of Hoke excision technique for gastrocnemius recession. (*Courtesy of* Lindsey A. Behrend, BS; with permission.)

draped in the usual fashion. An Esmarch bandage is used to exsanguinate the lower extremity, and the tourniquet is inflated to 300 mm Hg. With the knee extended on the operating table, a 4- to 8-cm longitudinal incision is made with a #15 blade scalpel at the level of the midcalf along the medial aspect of the lower leg, in line with the medial malleolus. The subcutaneous tissue is bluntly dissected with use of tenotomy scissors. The saphenous nerve and vein are identified and both are retracted using soft tissue retractors. A rent is then made in the superficial fascia of the lower leg using tenotomy scissors, and extended proximally and distally in line with the skin incision. A plane between the gastrocnemius and soleus muscle is created with blunt finger dissection from medial to lateral. The plantaris tendon is identified and sharply transected with a #15 scalpel. With the knee extended and the foot dorsiflexed, a #15 blade scalpel is used to carefully cut the posterior surface of the gastrocnemius fascia from medial to lateral without disrupting the muscle fibers of the gastrocnemius muscle. The intramuscular septum between the medial and lateral heads of the gastrocnemius muscle is identified. Using a #15 blade scalpel, the septum is incised longitudinally along the septum. After the transection is completed, there should be a noticeable increase of the patient's ankle dorsiflexion compared with preoperative measurements. The wound is then copiously irrigated using sterile normal saline solution. The superficial fascia of the lower leg is reapproximated using 2-0 Monocryl suture in a simple

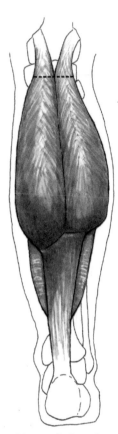

Fig. 15. Example of Silfverskiold excision technique for gastrocnemius recession. (*Courtesy of* Lindsey A. Behrend, BS; with permission.)

interrupted fashion. The subcuticular layer of skin is closed using 2-0 Monocryl suture in a running subcuticular fashion. Finally, skin closure is achieved using Steri-strips. The tourniquet is deflated, and a soft sterile dressing is applied over the wound. The patient is placed into a walking boot and allowed to weight bear as tolerated. Approximately 6 weeks after surgery, the patient is allowed to transition into a supportive shoe as pain and swelling permit.

Strayer Procedure

The patient is placed in the supine position on a well-padded operating table. A tourniquet is placed about the affected thigh. The lower extremity is prepped and draped in customary sterile fashion. An Esmarch bandage is used to exsanguinate the lower extremity, and the tourniquet is inflated to 300 mm Hg. With the knee extended on the operating table, the surgical assistant holds the ankle in dorsiflexion. A 2- to 3-cm incision is made using a #15 blade scalpel through skin at the level of the musculotendinous junction of the gastrocnemius in line with the posterior border of the medial malleolus. Tenotomy scissors are used to bluntly dissect down through the subcutaneous tissue to the superficial fascia of the lower leg. Soft tissue retractors are used retract the subcutaneous tissue out of the operative site. Tenotomy scissors are then used to make a rent into the superficial fascia of the lower leg then extended

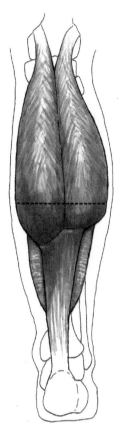

Fig. 16. Example of Baumann excision technique for gastrocnemius recession. (*Courtesy of Lindsey A. Behrend, BS; with permission.*)

both proximally and distally in line with the skin incision. The superficial fascia of the lower leg is bluntly dissected from the gastrocnemius musculotendinous junction. A ribbon retractor is applied to retract the superficial fascia of the lower leg from the gastrocnemius tendon, thus, protecting the sural nerve. A #15 scalpel is placed along the ribbon retractor, and the blade is rotated 90° toward the gastrocnemius tendon, transecting the medial portion of the tendon at the musculoskeletal junction. The ribbon retractor is removed and blunt finger retraction is used to separate the superficial fascia of the lower leg from the gastrocnemius tendon. At this point, tenotomy scissors are used to complete the transection from medial to lateral across the gastrocnemius tendon at the musculotendinous junction. After the transection is complete, there should be a noticeable increase of ankle dorsiflexion compared with the preoperative motion. The wound is then copiously irrigated with sterile normal saline solution. The superficial fascia of the lower leg is reapproximated using 2-0 Monocryl suture in a simple interrupted fashion. The subcuticular layer of skin is closed using 2-0 Monocryl suture in a running subcuticular fashion. Finally, Steri-strips are applied. The tourniquet is deflated, and a soft sterile dressing is applied over the wound. The patient is placed into a walking boot and allowed to weight bear as tolerated. Approximately 6 weeks after surgery, the patient is allowed to transition into a well-supportive shoe as pain and swelling allow.

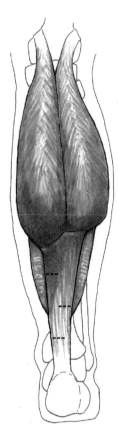

Fig. 17. Example of Z-lengthening excision technique for gastrocnemius recession. (*Courtesy of* Lindsey A. Behrend, BS; with permission.)

Hoke (Tendoachilles Lengthening) Procedure

The patient is placed in the supine position on a well-padded operating table with the affected lower extremity sterilely prepared and draped. The surgical assistant lifts the lower extremity off the operating table, maintaining knee extension and ankle dorsiflexion throughout the procedure. The surgeon starts distally over the midsubstance of the Achilles tendon. A longitudinal stab incision, using a #15 blade scalpel, is made along the midportion of the Achilles tendon through skin, subcutaneous tissue, and the Achilles tendon. Here, the scalpel blade is turned 90° in a medial direction performing a partial medial tenotomy of the Achilles tendon. Another stab incision is made approximately 1 to 2 cm proximal to the previous partial Achilles tenotomy through skin, subcutaneous tissue, and Achilles tendon. The scalpel blade is rotated 90° laterally, performing a partial lateral tenotomy of the Achilles tendon. Finally, another stab incision is made approximately 1 to 2 cm proximal to the previously lateral tenotomy. Once again, the scalpel is placed through skin, subcutaneous tissue, and Achilles tendon. The scalpel blade is then rotated 90° medially performing a partial medial tenotomy. An increase of dorsiflexion after the third and final partial tenotomy should be visualized by the surgeon. The patient is placed into a walking boot for approximately 6 weeks and is allowed to weight bear as tolerated in the walking boot. Six weeks after surgery, the patient can be transitioned into a well supportive shoe as pain and swelling are tolerated.

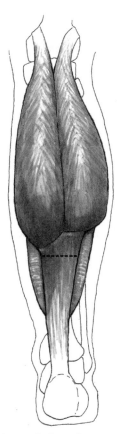

Fig. 18. Example of Strayer excision technique for gastrocnemius recession. (*Courtesy of* Lindsey A. Behrend, BS; with permission.)

SUMMARY

The GRACC create a novel and simple system for categorizing and correlating numerous common foot and ankle conditions related to a failing arch. As noted previously, the algorithm for treating these conditions is exceptionally replicable, and that has excellent outcomes. Gastrocnemius equinus diagnosis plays a crucial role in the pathology of arch collapse.

A contracture of the gastrocnemius muscle is increasingly recognized as the cause of several foot and ankle conditions. Therapy should focus on stretching, splinting, and other modalities for this muscle once a contracture is identified. If conservative therapy fails, a gastrocnemius recession can successfully relieve refractory foot pain with an acceptable complication profile. The authors have expanded their indications for gastrocnemius recession to include arch pain without radiographic abnormality, calcaneus apophysitis, plantar fasciitis/fibromas, Achilles tendonosis, early-onset diabetic Charcot arthropathy, and neuropathic forefoot ulcers. The authors would like to gratefully acknowledge the assistance of Michelle A. Padley, BS, CRC and Lindsey A. Behrend, BS with the completion of this article.

REFERENCES

1. DiGiovanni CW, Kuo R, Tejwani N, et al. Isolated gastrocnemius tightness. J Bone Joint Surg Am 2002;84-A:962–70.

2. Cheung JT, Zhang M, An K. Effect of Achilles tendon loading on plantar fascia tension in the standing foot. Clin Biomech (Bristol Avon) 2006;21:194–203.
3. Maskill JD, Bohay DR, Anderson JG. Gastrocnemius recession to treat isolated foot pain. Foot Ankle Int 2010;31(1):19–23.
4. Root M, Orien W, Weed J. Normal and abnormal function of the foot, vol. 2. Los Angeles (CA): Clinical Biomechanics Corporation; 1977.
5. Abdulmassih S, Phisitkul P, Femino JE, et al. Triceps surae contracture: implications for foot and ankle surgery. J Am Acad Orthop Surg 2013;21(7):398–407.
6. Bohay DR, Anderson JG. Stage IV posterior tibial tendon insufficiency: the tilted ankle. Foot Ankle Clin 2003;8:619–36.
7. Pinney SJ, Sangeorzan BJ, Hansen ST. Surgical anatomy of the gastrocnemius recession (Strayer procedure). Foot Ankle Int 2004;25(4):247–50.
8. Mueller MJ, Sinacore DR, Hastings MK, et al. Effects of achilles tendon lengthening on neuropathic plantar ulcers: a randomized clinical trial. J Bone Joint Surg Am 2003;85(8):1436–45.
9. Laborde JM. Midfoot ulcers treated with gastrocnemius-soleus recession. Foot Ankle Int 2009;30(9):842–6.
10. Sammarco GJ, Mahesh RB, Sammarco VJ, et al. The Effects of Unilateral Gast-11 Recession. Foot & Ankle International 2006;7:508–11.
11. Duthon VB, Lubbeke A, Duc Sylvain SR, et al. Noninsertional Achilles tendinopathy treated with gastrocnemius lengthening. Foot Ankle Int 2011;32(4):375–9.
12. Habbu R, Holthusen SM, Anderson JG, et al. Operative correction of arch collapse with forefoot deformity: a retrospective analysis of outcomes. Foot Ankle Int 2011;32(8):764–72.
13. Galluch DB, Bohay DR, Anderson JG. Midshaft metatarsal segmental osteotomy with open reduction and internal fixation. Foot Ankle Int 2007;28(2):169–74.
14. Gentchos CE, Anderson JG, Bohay DR. Management of the rigid arthritic flatfoot in the adults: alternatives to triple arthrodesis. Foot Ankle Clin N Am 2012;17:323–35.
15. Nemec SA, Habbu RA, Anderson JG, et al. Outcomes following midfoot arthrodesis for primary arthritis. Foot Ankle Int 2011;32(4):355–61.
16. Moseir-LaClair S, Pomeroy G, Manoli A. Intermediate follow-up on the double osteotomy and tendon transfer procedure for stage II posterior tibial tendon insufficiency. Foot Ankle Int 2001;22(4):283–91.
17. Pomeroy GC, Manoli A. A new operative approach for flatfoot secondary to posterior tibial tendon insufficiency: a preliminary report. Foot Ankle INt 1997;18(4):206–12.
18. Mann RA, Beaman DN. Double arthrodesis in the adult. Clin Orthop Rel Res 1999;(365):74–80.
19. Easley ME, Adams SB, Hembree C, et al. Current concepts review:results of total ankle arthroplasty. J Bone Joint Surg Am 2011;93:1455–68.
20. Haddad SL, Coetzee JC, Estok R, et al. Intermediate and long-term outcomes of total ankle arthroplasty and ankle arthrodesis. J Bone Joint Surg Am 2007;89(9):1899–905.
21. Herzenberg JE, Lamm BM, Corwin C, et al. Isolated recession of the gastrocnemius muscle: the Baumann procedurel. Foot Ankle Int 2007;28(11):1154–9.
22. Sheridan BD, Robinson DE, Hubble MJ, et al. Ankl arthrodesis and its relationship to ipsilateral arthritis of the hind and mid-foot. J Bone Joint Surg Br 2006;88-B:206–7.
23. Silver C, Simon S. Gastrocnemius-muscle recession (Silverskiold operation) for spastic equinus deformity in cerebral palsy. J Bone Joint Surg Am 1959;41(6):1021–8.
24. Rush SM, Ford LA, Hamilton GA. Morbidity associated with high gastrocnemius recession: retrospective review of 126 cases. J Foot Ankle Surg 2006;45(3):156–60.

Endoscopic Gastrocnemius Release

Joshua N. Tennant, MD, MPH[a],*, Annunziato Amendola, MD[b], Phinit Phisitkul, MD[b]

KEYWORDS

- Endoscopic gastrocnemius release • Ankle equinus contracture
- Modified strayer

KEY POINTS

- The starting point is medially 2 cm distal to the inferior extent of the visible medial gastrocnemius muscle belly, at a distance approximately 1 cm anterior to the palpable medial edge of the gastrocnemius tendon.
- The cannula/trochar placement should be easily palpable, depending on the density of subcutaneous tissue, on the posterior (superficial) surface of the gastrocnemius tendon, using proprioceptive twisting and oscillating motions to define the surgical plane, with the location of the sural nerve considered while making the lateral portal.
- Confirmation of plane identifies clearly the gastrocnemius tendon and that the sural nerve is not visible before using the retrograde knife.

INTRODUCTION

Endoscopic gastrocnemius recession (EGR) is a reliable option for surgical management of ankle equinus contracture. In the authors' experience and in other authors' findings, adequate release is obtainable with improved cosmesis and decreased wound-healing concerns with smaller percutaneous incisions. The amount of tendon released, the ability to carefully perform a thorough gastrocnemius recession with or without the release of the soleal fascia, and the identification of the proper tissue plane for the cannula to avoid injury to the sural nerve are all important considerations for the procedure.

The initial description of EGR appeared in 2002 in peer-reviewed orthopedic literature by Tashjian and colleagues[1] in a cadaveric study with 15 specimens. A 2-portal technique was used with an endoscopic carpal tunnel system slotted cannula and

Disclosures: None.
[a] Department of Orthopaedics, University of North Carolina School of Medicine, 3144 Bioinformatics Building, CB# 7055, Chapel Hill, NC 27599, USA; [b] Department of Orthopaedic Surgery and Rehabilitation, University of Iowa Hospitals and Clinics, 200 Hawkins Drive, 0102X JPP, Iowa City, IA 52242-1088, USA
* Corresponding author.
E-mail address: josh_tennant@med.unc.edu

trochar, and a 30° 4.0-mm arthroscope, and a retrograde knife. The authors noted complete resection (100%) of the gastrocnemius aponeurosis after a modification of the 2-portal technique for the final 8 specimens. Mean dorsiflexion improvement was 20°. One specimen had an identifiable sural nerve injury on postoperative dissection; only 33% of the specimens had a sural nerve that was identifiable intraoperatively. Medial and lateral incision lengths averaged 18 mm and 17 mm, respectively.

An understanding of the surgical anatomy, particularly that of the sural nerve, is critical to the success of EGR. The location of the sural nerve has been described in 2 anatomic studies of note. Immediately preceding their work noted above, Tashjian and colleagues[2] performed a cadaveric study identifying the location of the traversing sural nerve at the gastrocnemius-soleus junction to be an average of 12 mm medial to the lateral border of the gastrocnemius aponeurosis, on the lateral aspect—20% of the width across—of the posterior leg at this level.[2] Pinney and colleagues[3] studied the location of the sural nerve in 40 consecutive Strayer gastrocnemius recessions, noting that the sural nerve was superficial to the superficial posterior compartment fascia in 42.5% of cases, deep to the fascia in 57.5% of cases, and directly applied to the gastrocnemius tendon in 12.5% of cases. During EGR, the proper placement of the cannula from the medial portal and identification of the proper surgical plane depends on this key anatomic knowledge of the sural nerve.

Using an endoscopic technique, options for surgical release include open correlates of the previously described isolated Strayer gastrocnemius recession,[4] or a modified Strayer including both the gastrocnemius aponeurosis and the fascia of the soleus.[5] The choice and specificity of the lengthening procedure is guided by the surgical indications for the patient. Portal sites must be carefully chosen to be able to release the gastrocnemius aponeurosis at the proper level and to avoid overlengthening. The importance of the level of release for both stability and ability to correct contracture has been theorized in computer modeling[6] and further substantiated in recent cadaveric biomechanical testing.[7]

SURGICAL TECHNIQUE

The patient is positioned in the supine position with a small bump under the operative hip. The patient should be placed toward the end of the table so that the distal part of the heel is slightly exposed beyond the end of the table. If associated procedures are to be performed that necessitate prone positioning, the following technique is easily modified by rotating the instrumentation. The ankle dorsiflexion with the knee bent and extended and the subtalar joint in reduced position is measured preoperatively under anesthesia. A thigh tourniquet is placed. The lower extremity is prepared and draped in a sterile fashion, with drapes positioned at least above the level of the visible gastrocnemius musculature. The extremity is elevated and the thigh tourniquet is raised for the procedure to allow for maximal visibility.

The medial portal is selected 2 cm distal to the inferior extent of the visible medial gastrocnemius muscle belly, at a distance approximately 1 cm anterior to the palpable medial edge of the gastrocnemius tendon (**Fig. 1**). This location is approximately located at 50% of the distance between the proximal tip of the head and the distal tip of the lateral malleolus.[2] A 5-mm stab incision is made, and a curved hemostat is used to spread through subcutaneous fat and the crural fascia. Passage of the slotted cannula and trochar (ECTRA II, Smith & Nephew, Andover, MA, USA) is performed carefully in the plane just posterior to gastrocnemius tendon and superficial to the crural fascia. Gentle twisting and fine side-to-side windshield-wiping motions help to define the proper plane of the gastrocnemius tendon as the cannula and

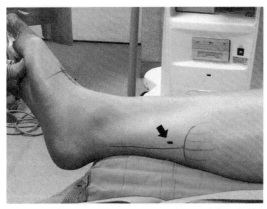

Fig. 1. Intraoperative markings of the right leg indicate medial gastrocnemius muscle bellies, gastrocnemius aponeurosis, and the medial portal (*arrow*).

trochar advance from medial to lateral. Keeping the ankle in slight dorsiflexion will facilitate the identification of the correct plane because the gastrocnemius tendon is under some tension. Care should be made to stay as close to the gastrocnemius tendon as possible while advancing the trocar laterally to keep the sural nerve and saphenous vein on the posterior aspect of it. The nerve is usually palpable subcutaneously in the posterior aspect of the cannula at the junction of middle and lateral thirds of the soft tissue tunnel. As the trochar tip becomes subcutaneous at the lateral calf, the skin is tented by the blunt tip, and a second 5-mm incision is made to allow both cannula ends to rest outside the leg (**Fig. 2**). The trochar is removed, and 1 or 2 cotton-tipped applicators are passed through the cannula for cleaning.

The 4.0-mm arthroscope with a 30° lens is placed into the medial side of the cannula, with the lens facing anteriorly toward the slot and the gastrocnemius tendon. The white tendon should be clearly visible, with no subcutaneous fat, nerve, or other tissue visible within the slot or the trocar must be reinserted. An arthroscopic probe can be used to palpate the tendon and make sure there are no other structures trapped in this plane (**Fig. 3**).

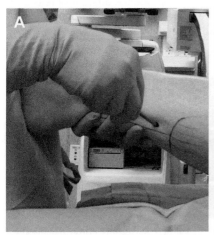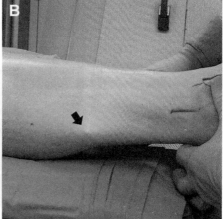

Fig. 2. (*A*) A trocar is inserted from the medial portal into a plane dorsal to the gastrocnemius aponeurosis. (*B*) The lateral portal is located using inside-out technique (*arrow*).

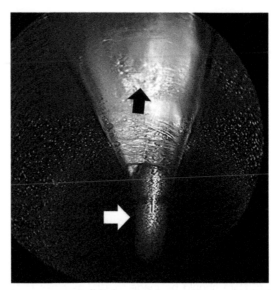

Fig. 3. Gastrocnemius aponeurosis (*black arrow*) is visualized and palpated with an arthroscopic probe (*white arrow*) through a slotted cannula.

The retrograde knife is inserted in the cannula and the tendons of the gastrocnemius and soleus are incised under endoscopic visualization. A standard straight surgical punch has also been described as an alternative to the retrograde knife, which in its current form is a disposable item with slightly more expense.[8] The knife is controlled by keeping the thumb of the hand holding the knife on the cannula end while pulling the knife to maximize proprioceptive control. The patient's foot is held against the surgeon's lower chest and the ankle is dorsiflexed to tighten the tendon to facilitate the release. The scope and knife may be switched from one side to the other. Underlying soleus muscle fibers will be visualized while the aponeurosis is released (**Fig. 4**). Dorsiflexion can be measured intraoperatively to determine the amount of release to be performed. When adequate release has been performed, the 2 wounds are irrigated and closed with a single simple skin suture on each side.

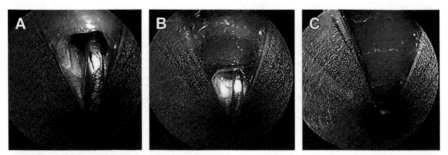

Fig. 4. The gastrocnemius aponeurosis is released by using a retrograde knife. The diagrams demonstrate an initial cut (*A*), the exposure of the underlying soleus muscle as the release progresses (*B*), and the final appearance after a complete release (*C*).

Table 1
Review of endoscopic gastrocnemius release clinical literature

Authors/Year	Technique	No. of Patients (Limbs)	Range of Motion Improvement	Strength	Functional Outcome	Complications
Trevino et al,[9] 2005	Endoscopic, single portal	28 (31)	Subjective increase at time of release, otherwise not measured	Not reported	Modified Molander and Olerud score, statistically significant (P<.05) improvement in pain, swelling, stiffness, and overall average score	• No sural nerve injury nor Achilles tendon injury • 1 infection (3.2%) • 2 initial incisions were put in the wrong place, requiring a second incision (6.5%) • 1 procedure converted to an open release (3.2%)
Grady & Kelly,[10] 2010	Endoscopic, 2 portals	23 (40)	15 + 4°	Not reported	Not reported	No sural nerve injuries
Schroeder,[12] 2012	Endoscopic, 1 portal	53 (60)	15.7 ± 1.8° (12–19°)	Not specifically measured; 1 case (1.7%) of focal triceps surae weakness that resolved after 4 wk of physical therapy	93% good or excellent subject patient scar cosmesis assessment; no other outcome scoring	1 patient (1.7%) had persistent sural nerve paresthesias at 4 mo
DiDomenico et al,[13] 2005	Endoscopic, 2 portals	28 (31)	18° (11–32°)	Not reported	Not reported	1 hematoma; 3 complaints of subjective weakness; 1 persistent pain that "resolved with elevation and administration of pain medication"
Roukis & Schweinberger,[14] 2010	Endoscopic, 1 portal	18 (23)	Not reported	Not reported	Not reported	No nerve injuries. 3 conversions to an open procedure; 3 wound-healing problems; 3 undercorrections
Yeap et al,[8] 2011	Endoscopic, 2 portals	7 (9)	11.1° (6–18°)	Not reported	Not reported	No sural nerve injuries
Saxena & Widtfeldt,[11] 2004	Endoscopic, 1 or 2 portals	15 (18)	12.6°	Able to do single-leg heel raise at 13.0 + 6.0 wk postoperatively	Not reported	3 sural nerve injuries (16.5%) (lateral foot dysesthesias)

Postoperative protocol is typically dictated by concomitant procedures. With an isolated EGR, patients are asked to be weight-bearing to tolerance in a walking boot with crutches for assistance.

RESULTS

Clinical study of EGR has been completed in a limited series of patients. Trevino and colleagues[9] reported on a series of 28 patients (31 procedures) who underwent EGR through a single portal with the use of an endoscopic carpal tunnel release system. No sural nerve injury or Achilles tendon injury was noted postoperatively. One infection (3.2%) occurred; 2 initial incisions were put in the wrong place, requiring a second incision (6.5%), and one procedure was aborted and converted to an open release (3.2%). Statistically significant clinical improvement was noted on a modified Molander and Olerud outcome score. A series of 23 pediatric patients (40 procedures) without significant neurologic pathologic abnormality and diagnosed with ankle equinus contracture was treated with EGR by a 2-portal technique. Ankle dorsiflexion was improved by a mean of 15° (SD + 4°). No outcome measures were reported, nor whether the patients' presenting symptoms were changed. No sensory deficit from nerve injury was found postoperatively at 2 weeks, 6 months, and 2 years for all patients.[10] Other smaller series exist both with[11] and without[8] reports of sural nerve injury. Results of clinical studies are summarized in **Table 1**.

One of the senior authors (P.P.) has performed endoscopic gastrocnemius recession since 2009 on a total of 320 patients (344 legs). Most of the procedures were done concomitantly with other indicated procedures. The preoperative ankle dorsiflexion was improved from $-0.82 \pm 5.36°$ (range, $-50–10$) to $14.65 \pm 6.66°$ (range, $0–30$) intraoperatively and $10.89 \pm 6.24°$ (range, $-10–30$) at final follow-up, average follow-up 17.96 ± 8.88 months (range, 6–53 months). Dorsiflexion was always determined with the knee in full extension and the subtalar joint in neutral alignment, while providing a moderate dorsiflexion force to the forefoot until an endpoint is reached. The visual analogue scale scores for pain improved from 7.33 ± 2.19 (range, 0–10) to 3.38 ± 2.73 (range, 0–10) after the procedure. There were 10 of 320 patients (3.13%) with postoperative sural nerve symptoms. Eleven of 320 patients (3.44%) had subjective complaints of ankle weakness.

FUTURE DIRECTIONS

The surgical technique for endoscopic gastrocnemius recession is relatively simple but requires some experience in arthroscopy. The instrumentation currently used is adopted from the endoscopic carpal tunnel release and may not entirely match with a procedure in the lower limbs. Improvement in surgical equipment may allow shortening of the learning curve while increasing safety of the procedure. The sural nerve should always be protected, and surgeons should be aware of potential variations of the nerve. Finally, a more refined and standardized postoperative protocol may allow early mobilization and return to activities, while avoiding plantarflexion weakness.

SUMMARY

In summary, EGR is a relatively new surgical option for the treatment of ankle equinus contracture. Although limited clinical studies exist to date, growing experience shows the benefit of cosmesis and wound healing, with the equivalent ability to release the gastrocnemius aponeurosis and soleal fascia. Injury to the sural nerve may be avoided by the knowledge of surgical anatomy and meticulous surgical technique. Further

> **Box 1**
> **Surgical instrumentation**
>
> 4.0-mm arthroscope with 30° lens
>
> Slotted cannula with trochar
>
> Retrograde knife
>
> Cotton tip cleaners
>
> Curved hemostat
>
> Scalpel

clinical study and development of improved instrumentation are indicated for the EGR technique (**Box 1**).

REFERENCES

1. Tashjian RZ, Appel AJ, Banerjee R, et al. Endoscopic gastrocnemius recession: evaluation in a cadaver model. Foot Ankle Int 2003;24(8):607–13.
2. Tashjian RZ, Appel AJ, Banerjee R, et al. Anatomic study of the gastrocnemius-soleus junction and its relationship to the sural nerve. Foot Ankle Int 2003; 24(6):473–6.
3. Pinney SJ, Sangeorzan BJ, Hansen ST Jr. Surgical anatomy of the gastrocnemius recession (Strayer procedure). Foot Ankle Int 2004;25(4):247–50.
4. Strayer LM Jr. Recession of the gastrocnemius; an operation to relieve spastic contracture of the calf muscles. J Bone Joint Surg Am 1950;32A(3):671–6.
5. Vuillermin C, Rodda J, Rutz E, et al. Severe crouch gait in spastic diplegia can be prevented: a population-based study. J Bone Joint Surg Am 2011;93(12):1670–5.
6. Delp SL, Statler K, Carroll NC. Preserving plantar flexion strength after surgical treatment for contracture of the triceps surae: a computer simulation study. J Orthop Res 1995;13(1):96–104.
7. Firth GB, McMullan M, Chin T, et al. Lengthening of the gastrocnemius-soleus complex: an anatomical and biomechanical study in human cadavers. J Bone Joint Surg Am 2013;95(16):1489–96.
8. Yeap EJ, Shamsul SA, Chong KW, et al. Simple two-portal technique for endoscopic gastrocnemius recession: clinical tip. Foot Ankle Int 2011;32(8):830–3.
9. Trevino S, Gibbs M, Panchbhavi V. Evaluation of results of endoscopic gastrocnemius recession. Foot Ankle Int 2005;26(5):359–64.
10. Grady JF, Kelly C. Endoscopic gastrocnemius recession for treating equinus in pediatric patients. Clin Orthop Relat Res 2010;468(4):1033–8.
11. Saxena A, Widtfeldt A. Endoscopic gastrocnemius recession: preliminary report on 18 cases. J Bone Joint Surg Am 2004;43(5):302–6.
12. Schroeder SM. Uniportal endoscopic gastrocnemius recession for treatment of gastrocnemius equinus with a dedicated EGR system with retractable blade. J Foot Ankle Surg 2012;51(6):714–9.
13. DiDomenico LA, Adams HB, Garchar D. Endoscopic gastrocnemius recession for the treatment of gastrocnemius equinus. J Am Podiatr Med Assoc 2005; 95(4):410–3.
14. Roukis TS, Schweinberger MH. Complications associated with uni-portal endoscopic gastrocnemius recession in a diabetic patient population: an observational case series. J Foot Ankle Surg 2010;49(1):68–70.

Technique, Indications, and Results of Proximal Medial Gastrocnemius Lengthening

 CrossMark

Pierre Barouk, MD

KEYWORDS

- Gastrocnemius • Equinus • Hallux valgus • Metatarsalgia
- Proximal gastrocnemius release

KEY POINTS

- Gastrocnemius proximal lengthening was first performed to correct spasticity in children, and was adapted for the patient with no neuromuscular condition in the late 1990s.
- Since that time, the proximal gastrocnemius release has become less invasive and has evolved to include only the fascia overlying the medial head of the gastrocnemius muscle.
- The indications for performing this procedure are a clinically demonstrable gastrocnemius contracture that influences a variety of clinical conditions in the forefoot, hindfoot, and ankle.
- Proximal gastrocnemius release is a safe and easy procedure that can be performed bilaterally simultaneously, and does not require immobilization of the ankle after surgery.
- Proximal gastrocnemius release can be performed either as an isolated procedure, or in conjunction with additional foot or ankle surgeries.

INTRODUCTION

When equinus is caused only by tightness of the gastrocnemius, lengthening only the gastrocnemius is logical. This procedure can be performed at 3 levels: proximal, intermediate, and distal. The distal open techniques are described in the article "Surgical Techniques of Gastrocnemius Lengthening" by Dr. DiGiovanni and colleagues in this issue. The intermediate-level technique was described by Bauman,[1–4] but is one with which the authors have no experience, and it involves a section of the anterior aponeurosis of the gastrocnemius.

Silfverskiold[5] was the first to describe proximal gastrocnemius lengthening in 1923 in cases of cerebral palsy. He cut the medial and lateral gastrocnemius at their insertion on the femoral condyle (**Fig. 1**). According to Gage,[6] spasticity first affects the

Disclosures: None.
Foot Surgery Center at the Sport's Clinic, 2 Rue Georges Nègrevergne, Merignac 33700, France
E-mail address: pierre.barouk@wanadoo.fr

Foot Ankle Clin N Am 19 (2014) 795–806
http://dx.doi.org/10.1016/j.fcl.2014.08.012
1083-7515/14/$ – see front matter © 2014 Elsevier Inc. All rights reserved.

foot.theclinics.com

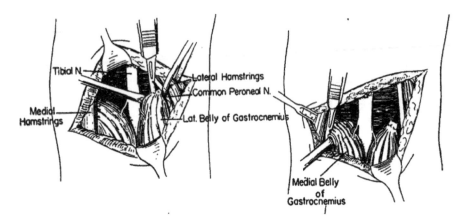

Fig. 1. Silfverskiold's technique. Lat, lateral; N, nerve. (*From* Silfverskiold N. Reduction of the uncrossed two-joints muscles of the leg to one-joint muscles in spastic conditions. Acta Chir Scand 1923;56:315–30.)

biarticular muscles, and the technique for this indication is still used and provides good results.[7]

The authors' technique of proximal release of the fascia of the medial gastrocnemius is derived from experience with the Silfverskiold's method. This procedure began with the work of Barouk[7] in 1970, when the original technique of Silfverskiold was used in cerebral palsy cases. From 1997 to 2005, the authors performed section of only the white fibers (aponeurosis), but of both the medial and lateral gastrocnemius (**Fig. 2**) in patients with static problems (as opposed to dynamic associated with neuromuscular conditions such as spasticity) mainly related to the forefoot.[8]

From 2005 to present, the authors have sectioned only the aponeurosis of the medial gastrocnemius (**Fig. 3**) for reasons that are explained later.

Indications for Proximal Gastrocnemius Release

In the authors' practice, indications for the procedure are based on the presence of gastrocnemius tightness (a positive Silfverskiold sign), particularly when this tightness has influenced the problem for which the patient has sought help. Additional symptoms will be relieved by the proximal release, including the presence of lumbar pain cramps in the calf, calf tension, or difficulty walking in bare feet or flat shoes.[9,10,11]

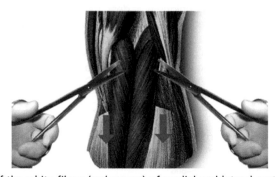

Fig. 2. Section of the white fibers (*red arrows*) of medial and lateral gastrocnemius. (*From* Barouk LS. Forefoot reconstruction. New York: Springer-Verlag; 2003; with permission.)

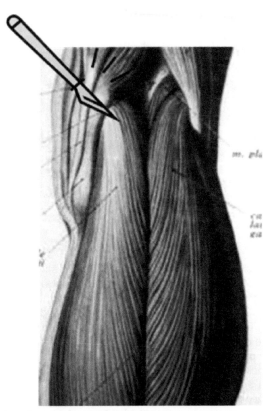

Fig. 3. Section of the white fibers of the medial gastrocnemius. (*From* Barouk LS. Forefoot reconstruction. New York: Springer-Verlag; 2003; with permission.)

Surgical Technique

General anesthesia can be used, but the authors' choice is peripheral local or regional anesthesia using a sciatic nerve block with a subgluteal lateral approach, guided with ultrasound. The choice of local anesthetic agent depends on the duration of the stay of the patient. The authors use either mepivacaine, 15 mg/mL for ambulatory patients, or a mix of mepivacaine, 20 mg/mL and ropivacaine, 7.5 mg/mL for hospitalized patients. The volume injected is approximately 20 mL.

This block is, however, ineffective for cutaneous anesthesia, particularly the posterior cutaneous nerve of the thigh, and is therefore supplemented with local anesthesia just above the popliteal fossa (lidocaine, 20 mg/mL with adrenalin) just before the incision.

Preparation

Surgery is performed in the prone position, with a pillow under the ankles to relax the gastrocnemius. The authors have used a supine position, but this requires additional retraction and a larger incision, with more traction on the soft tissues, and they do not commonly perform the procedure in the supine position. No need exists for a tourniquet. Having 2 kinds of retractors available is preferable: 1 narrow for the superficial layers and 1 broader for the deep layer.

The incision is made in the flexion crease, 1 cm lateral to the medial fovea. It is approximately 3 cm in length (**Fig. 4**). At this level, no vascular or nervous structures

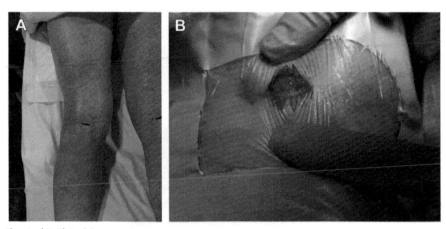

Fig. 4. (A, B) Incision.

can be damaged, as is well described by the anatomic study of Hamilton and colleagues.[12] The subcutaneous fat is retracted and the authors look for the posterior fascia of the leg, which is opened in the axis of the leg. The authors find, just underneath, the medial gastrocnemius covered by a thin aponeurosis and marked by a fat layer of variable thickness. The tendon is on the medial side, extending anteriorly (**Fig. 5**). All the white fibers are cut with scissors (**Fig. 6**). The authors use a finger to check that no more tension is present in the muscle while they move the ankle into dorsiflexion.

Indications for including the lateral head are limited, but this may be considered in some cases when a medial section alone is insufficient. The authors divided both heads systematically for several years. To do this, the incision is extended laterally. The authors then locate the muscle with the finger, lateral to the popliteal artery. The posterior fascia of the leg is opened carefully because the sural communicating branch of the common peroneal nerve is at risk, and this now places the authors on the muscle. The white fibers are in fact a narrow aponeurotic band, slightly lateral (**Fig. 7**). Here again, one must be careful of the common peroneal nerve, which is close and must be seen before the white fibers are sectioned.

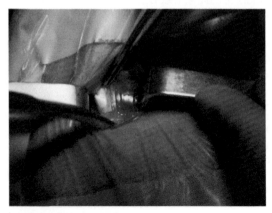

Fig. 5. Medial tendon, lateral aponeurosis.

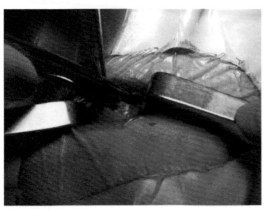

Fig. 6. Tendinous fibers already cut, and aponeurotic ones in progress.

Hemostasis is checked and the authors close subcutaneous tissue and skin with an intradermal suture. Use of a drain is not necessary.

Postoperatively, no immobilization is recommended. Walking is allowed as soon as the local anesthesia has worn off. A rehabilitation program is begun by the physiotherapist, and consists of passive dorsiflexion of the ankle with the knee in extension (**Fig. 8**). The authors recommend walking in a shoe without a heel to keep the ankle in dorsiflexion.

The authors reviewed a series of 354 proximal gastrocnemius releases—274 medial and lateral and 80 only medial—at 2 years' follow-up. In 354 interventions they noted:

- Four cases of moderate pain of the calf, resolved at 1 year, except one with persistent unexplained popliteal pain
- One case of deep vein thrombosis (this patient was operated on for correction of hallux valgus simultaneously)
- One case of lateral tension of the calf in a patient who had medial release only

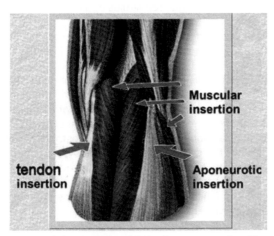

Fig. 7. Proximal insertion of the medial and lateral gastrocnemius. (*From* Barouk LS. Forefoot reconstruction. New York: Springer-Verlag; 2003; with permission.)

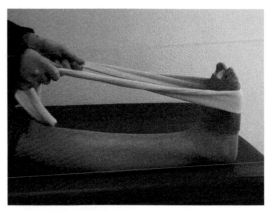

Fig. 8. Patient-directed rehabilitation.

- Two cases of transient lateral dysesthesia (in the case of lateral and medial release)
- Ten cases of keloid scar, each time when lateral and medial gastrocnemius were elongated, which tends to be associated with greater scarring
- Ten cases of weakness (subjective evaluation by the patient) in 7 cases of medial and lateral lengthening; in these 10 cases, 1 was really symptomatic (excessive lengthening with too much dorsiflexion of the ankle that restricted the patient in sports activities)

Since this study, the authors have performed medial gastrocnemius release in 368 patients, among whom they observed:

- Four hematomas: 2 that spontaneously regressed and 2 that had to be drained; the authors believe that this coincided with the use of a new antithrombosis prophylaxis agent that they have since discontinued
- Two deep vein thrombosis (both patients underwent simultaneous hallux valgus correction)
- No dysesthesia, no keloid scar, and no weakness

With section of only the medial gastrocnemius aponeurosis, complications are rare and of no significance.

Whether the release was performed to include the medial head only or both heads, ankle dorsiflexion with the knee extended was improved in all the cases of the series described.

However, estimation of the results depends on the manner in which the gastrocnemius is examined. The authors test for an equinus contracture with the subtalar joint reduced to slight varus and then with moderate strength to dorsiflex the ankle. If one is going to compare these results, the maneuver must be able to be reproduced from one patient to another, and preoperatively and postoperatively.

Preoperatively, 69% of the patients had an equinus contracture of –15°, with the ankle in dorsiflexion and the knee extended, and this decreased to 4% postoperatively. A contracture between 0° and –15° was seen in 22% of the patients, and 19% postoperatively. The ankle dorsiflexion test with the knee extended increased from 9% to 77% postoperatively.

In a blinded series of 30 patients, no differences were seen in the amount of improvement of ankle dorsiflexion with the medial alone compared with the medial and lateral (**Table 1**).

Table 1 Ankle dorsiflexion, knee extended					
>1°		Between 0° and −15°		<−15°	
Preoperatively	Postoperatively	Preoperatively	Postoperatively	Preoperatively	Postoperatively
9%	77%	22%	19%	69%	4%

The influence of gastrocnemius release on the forefoot is difficult to assess because simultaneous forefoot surgery is often performed. Nevertheless, the proximal release can be sufficient to avoid surgery on the foot in some of these cases, such as for correction of ankle instability, Achilles tendinopathy, plantar fasciitis, metatarsalgia, and hallux rigidus. If local surgery to the foot or ankle is required anyway, the authors believe that proximal gastrocnemius release can decrease the potential for recurrence or even ensure a good result, but they cannot prove it statistically.

DISCUSSION

Few reports exist on the proximal gastrocnemius release.[13–18] One series was presented at the French foot meeting in Toulouse in 2006,[13,14] the ones of Solan and colleagues[15,16] in England, and De los Santos and colleagues.[17,18] In fact, few surgeons routinely use the proximal release. The most popular way to lengthen the gastrocnemius is the Strayer procedure.[19]

The authors' technique is efficient: Silfverskiold's sign disappears and ankle dorsiflexion with the knee extended normalizes in 79% of cases. The 19% of cases with postoperative moderate equinus (from −1° to −15°) correspond in fact to the patients who present preoperatively with a larger equinus contracture of more than −15°. These contractures are improved, even if a degree of equinus persists. Similar results were reported by Colombier,[14] who noted a 95% improvement in ankle dorsiflexion with the knee extended.

The amount of improvement is probably less than that obtained with distal lengthening (Strayer procedure) which is 18°.[20] Rabat,[21] with the endoscopic section, obtained an average of 12° of dorsiflexion. Nevertheless, distal lengthening, whatever the technique, involves the gastrocnemius tendon and less or more of the soleus aponeurosis.

Bilaterality

Another advantage of proximal gastrocnemius release is that it can be performed bilaterally. This aspect is important, because shortening of the gastrocnemius generally occurs bilaterally, and it is also logical when considering patient complaints of lumbar pain, cramps, and difficulty walking without a heel, because these are bilateral complaints. It would be useless to permit to a woman to walk with a flat shoe on just one foot.

Five Reasons to Lengthen Just the Medial Gastrocnemius

1. The medial head of gastrocnemius is a strong tendon, whereas the lateral side has a thin aponeurosis. Hamilton and colleagues[12] showed that the tendinous fibers of the medial gastrocnemius are 2.4 times thicker than the lateral.
2. Tennis leg always occurs on the medial side because of a preponderance of tension.[22]
3. Fewer complications occur, especially lateral dysesthesia, scarring, and postoperative pain (**Fig. 9**), if the lateral is not lengthened.

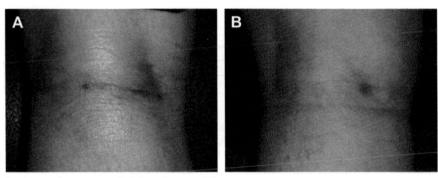

Fig. 9. Results at 1 month (*A*) and 1 year (*B*).

4. It is a minimally invasive surgery and the operating time is very short.
5. Finally, the medial gastrocnemius lengthening is as efficient as the medial and lateral (shown in the authors' comparative series).[13]

Reasons to Prefer Proximal Versus Distal Lengthening

1. Distal section involves the gastrocnemius tendon and often the aponeurosis of the soleus, because the junction between these 2 structures is wide and cannot be found every time. Therefore, the distal section is not always a pure gastrocnemius lengthening.
2. Distal section leads to an interruption of the muscle continuity that can provoke weakness.[20] However, this strength decrease has not been found in recent series.[23,24]
3. Distal section allows the septum dividing the soleus (**Fig. 10**) to break secondarily. This problem and the one mentioned just previously provide the rationale for postoperative immobilization. In their original description, Vulpius and Stoffel[25] recommend its section. Endoscopically, Rabat recommends it also if it is seen, but not if it represents an additional technical difficulty.[21]
4. Bilateral lengthening is difficult in cases of distal section.
5. The scar of distal section is less aesthetic than the proximal one; therefore, the authors prefer an endoscopic section over an open one.
6. The complications caused by a distal section are not negligible.[26,27]

However, indications still exist for distal lengthening, such as when immobilization is required because of the foot surgery (eg, rear foot osteotomy); to avoid having to shift

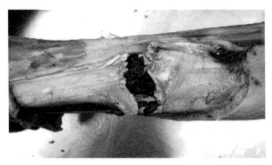

Fig. 10. The soleus septum.

the patient from the prone to the supine position between the gastrocnemius lengthening and the foot surgery; and when the contracture involves both the gastrocnemius and the soleus. In these cases, a distal section is more powerful. The authors believe an endoscopic section is efficient, safe, and noninvasive.

Final Points

Proximal medial gastrocnemius lengthening is technically easy and fast, with simple postoperative care and immediate ambulation, and requires no immobilization. Complications are rare, self-limiting, and without consequences like loss of strength, pain, and scar problems. Except for one patient who experienced a loss of strength, the authors have not noted any cases of weakness. One patient with overcorrection complained of weakness, but most of the patients were not involved in high-level sports.

These results lead the authors to frequently recommend this procedure for cases of gastrocnemius tightening in patients with foot abnormalities, especially if direct or indirect signs are associated.

CHRONOLOGY

Gastrocnemius lengthening must be performed before the foot surgery for several reasons:

1. To decrease the need for the surgery. For example, for a hallux valgus with metatarsalgia, caused mainly by the gastrocnemius tightness, making lesser metatarsal osteotomies will not be necessary because correction of the hallux valgus and gastrocnemius lengthening will be sufficient.

A

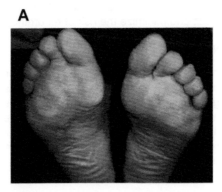

B

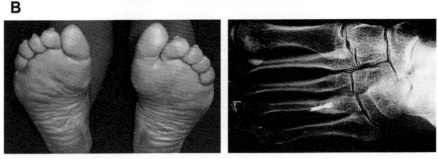

Fig. 11. (*A*) Bilateral metatarsalgia before intervention. (*B*) Results at 6 months after (*right*) medial gastrocnemius lengthening and isolated M4 elevation (Barouk Rippstein Toullec osteotomy) and (*left*) only medial gastrocnemius lengthening.

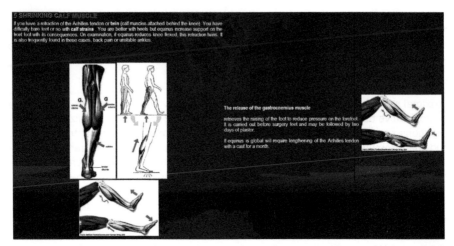

Fig. 12. An information brochure and the Web site http://s407977265.onlinehome.fr/lsb/brievete_des_jumeaux.htm are useful resources to complement the oral explanations. (*Adapted from* Barouk LS. Forefoot reconstruction. New York: Springer-Verlag; 2003. Available at: http://s407977265.onlinehome.fr/lsb/eng_pb_hallux_valgus.htm.)

2. To avoid the need for the surgery. For example, for metatarsalgia,[28] in which the gastrocnemius lengthening favorably replaces multiple metatarsal osteotomies (which do not cure the associated signs), the authors propose performing gastrocnemius lengthening first and then reevaluating the patient. Addressing the cause rather than the consequences is always more logical. **Fig. 11** illustrates these advantages.
3. To ensure a good result and minimize the risk of recurrence.

PATIENT INFORMATION

This surgery requires that the patient be educated about the abnormality, and have an understanding of what will be done behind the knee and why it is necessary. The presence of direct signs (eg, cramps, tension in the calf) or indirect signs (eg, lumbar pain, difficulty walking without a heel, instability) will help guide the decision. An information brochure (**Fig. 12**) and the Web site www.barouk-ls-p.com are useful resources to complement the oral explanations. The patient will then be able to accept and understand this operation and why it occurs away from the foot.

SUMMARY

Proximal medial gastrocnemius release is a simple, effective, and particularly logical procedure that helps patients with foot abnormalities and gastrocnemius tightness.

The gastrocnemius tightness needs to be recognized and then carefully explained to the patient so that they understand its contribution to the abnormality and the associated conditions.

In more than 12 years, the authors have performed greater than 1000 proximal gastrocnemius releases. The reliability of the results and the near-absence of complications lead them to continue using this procedure.

REFERENCES

1. Bauman JU, Koch HG. Ventral aponeurotische verlängerung des musculus gastrocnemius. Oper Orthop Traumatol 1989;1:254–8.

2. Saraph V, Zwick EB, Uitz C, et al. The Baumann procedure for fixed contracture of the gastrosoleus in cerebral palsy. Evaluation of function of the ankle after multi-level surgery. J Bone Joint Surg Br 2000;82(4):535–40.

3. Herzenberg JE, Lamm BM, Corwin C, et al. Isolated recession of the gastrocnemius muscle: the Bauman procedure. Foot Ankle Int 2007;28(11):1154–9.

4. Tellisi N, Elliot AJ. Gastrocnemius recession: a modified technique. Foot Ankle Int 2008;29(12):1232–4.

5. Silfverskiold N. Reduction of the uncrossed two-joints muscles of the leg to one-joint muscles in spastic conditions. Acta Chir Scand 1923;56:315–30.

6. Gage JR. Gait analysis. An essential tool in the treatment of cerebral palsy. Clin Orthop Relat Res 1993;(288):126–34.

7. Barouk LS. Les brièvetés musculaires postérieures du pied de l'infirme moteur cérébral (IMC). Rev Chir Orth 1984;70(Suppl 2):163–6.

8. Barouk LS. Forefoot reconstruction. New York: Springer; 2003. p. 151–61.

9. Barouk P. Signes directs. In: Baudet B, Baudet P, Bonnel F, et al, editors. Brièveté des gastrocnémiens: de l'anatomie au traitement. Montpellier (France): Sauramps; 2012. p. 219–23.

10. Barouk P. Lombalgies. In: Baudet B, Baudet P, Bonnel F, et al, editors. Brièveté des gastrocnémiens: de l'anatomie au traitement. Montpellier (France): Sauramps; 2012. p. 225–6.

11. Barouk P. L'instabilité des membres inférieurs. In: Baudet B, Baudet P, Bonnel F, et al, editors. Brièveté des gastrocnémiens : de l'anatomie au traitement. Montpellier (France): Sauramps; 2012. p. 227–30.

12. Hamilton PD, Brown M, Ferguson N, et al. Surgical anatomy of the proximal release of the gastrocnemius: a cadaveric study. Foot Ankle Int 2009;30(12):1202–6.

13. Barouk LS, Barouk P, Toulec E. Resulltats de la liberation Proximale des Gastro-cnemiens. Etude Prospective Symposium « Brieveté des Gastrocnemiens »,jour-nées de Printemps SFMCP-AFCP. Toulouse. Med Chir Pied 2006;22:151–6.

14. Colombier JA. Liberation Proximale Pure dans la prise en charge thérapeutique des Gastrocnemiens. Courts Symposium « Brieveté des Gastrocnemiens »,jour-nées de Printemps SFMCP-AFCP, Toulouse, 2006. Med Chir Pied 2006;22:156–7.

15. Abassian A, Kohl-Katsoulis J, Solan MC. Proximal medial release of the gastroc-nemius in the treatment of recalcitrant plantar fasciitis. Foot Ankle Int 2012;33(1):14–9.

16. Gurdezi S, Kohls-Gatzoulis JA, Solan M. Results of proximal medial gastrocne-mius release for tendinopathy. Foot Ankle Int 2013;34(10):1364–9.

17. De los Santos-Real R, Morales-Muñoz P, Payo Rodriguez J, et al. Liberación prox-imal del gemelo medial por mínima incisión. Medial Gastrocnemius release with minimal incisión. Rev Pie y Tobillo 2011;XXV(1):37–41.

18. De Los Santos R. La liberation proximale du gastrocnémien medial. Experience madrilène. In: Baudet B, Baudet P, Bonnel F, et al, editors. Brièveté des gastro-cnémiens: de l'anatomie au traitement. Montpellier (France): Sauramps; 2012. p. 389–97.

19. Strayer LM. Gastrocnemius recession. J Bone Joint Surg Am 1958;40A(5):1019–30.

20. Pinney SJ, Hansen ST Jr, Sangeorzan BJ. The effect on ankle dorsiflexion of gas-trocsoleus recession. Foot Ankle Int 2002;23(1):26–9.

21. Rabat E. Allogement endoscopique du gastrocnémien. In: Baudet B, Baudet P, Bonnel F, et al, editors. Brièveté des gastrocnémiens: de l'anatomie au traitement. Montpellier (France): Sauramps; 2012. p. 351–73.

22. Baudet B. Tennis leg. In: Baudet B, Baudet P, Bonnel F, et al, editors. Brièveté des gastrocnémiens: de l'anatomie au traitement. Montpellier (France): Sauramps; 2012. p. 321–7.

23. Mann RA. RE: The effect on ankle dorsiflexion of gastrocsoleus recession, Pinney SJ, et al., Foot Ankle Int. 23(1):26-29, 2002. Foot Ankle Int 2003;24(9):726–7 [author reply: 727–8].

24. Maskill JD, Bohay DR, Anderson JG. Gastrocnemius recession to treat isolated foot pain. Foot Ankle Int 2010;31(1):19–23.

25. Vulpius O, Stoffel A. Orthopädische operationslehre. Stuttgart (Germany): Verlag von Ferdinand Enke; 1924.

26. Rush SM, Ford LA, Hamilton GA. Morbidity associated with high gastrocnemius recession: retrospective review of 126 cases. J Foot Ankle Surg 2006;45(3): 156–60.

27. Rodineau J. Stratégie thérapeutique médicale dans les rétractions des triceps suraux. In: Baudet B, Baudet P, Bonnel F, et al, editors. Brièveté des gastrocnémiens: de l'anatomie au traitement. Montpellier (France): Sauramps; 2012. p. 329–38.

28. Colombier JA. Brièveté des gastrocnémiens dans les métatarsalgies. In: Baudet B, Baudet P, Bonnel F, et al, editors. Brièveté des gastrocnémiens: de l'anatomie au traitement. Montpellier (France): Sauramps; 2012. p. 285–94.

The Effect of Gastrocnemius Tightness on the Pathogenesis of Juvenile Hallux Valgus: A Preliminary Study

CrossMark

Louis Samuel Barouk, MD

KEYWORDS

- Hallux valgus causes • Juvenile hallux valgus causes
- Hallux valgus and Gastrocnemius tightness • Plantar aponeurosis
- Windlass mechanism

KEY POINTS

- Hallux valgus is the most frequent consequence of gastrocnemius tightness in the foot. This condition is particularly evident in juvenile hallux valgus.
- There are anatomic and biomechanical links between the gastrocnemius muscles and the hallux: Achilles tendon, calcaneum, plantar aponeurosis, plantar plate, and sesamoids. Gastrocnemius tightness exerts a deforming force on the hallux.
- Clinical consequences for clinicians are that it is essential to evaluate the gastrocnemius tightness in any case of juvenile hallux valgus, then to consider correcting this tightness each time it is required: this not only serves to secure the results of the bunionectomy but also to avoid, diminish, or at least to ensure the success of surgery of the lesser rays in cases of metatarsalgia.

INTRODUCTION

Isolated gastrocnemius tightness is equinus of the ankle that is present with the knee extended but that disappears when the knee is flexed.[1] The technique for assessment (Silverskiold test)[2] should be performed with only light pressure (average 1 kg[3]) applied to the forefoot (**Fig. 1**A, B).[4]

The consequences of this tightness on the foot and ankle have been well documented, particularly for Achilles tendinopathy,[5–10] plantar fasciitis,[11–16] and generally for hindfoot disorders.[17] However, there are fewer studies of the effects of the gastrocnemius on the forefoot, particularly the association with hallux valgus deformity.[18–21]

DiGiovanni and colleagues[22] and Barouk and Barouk[23] reported the clinical consequences of gastrocnemius tightness on the foot and ankle. Drakos and DiGiovanni[21] studied a series of 34 patients all with foot problems, and these formed the experimental

The Author has nothing to disclose.

39, chemin de la Roche, Yvrac 33370, France

E-mail address: samuel.barouk@wanadoo.fr

Foot Ankle Clin N Am 19 (2014) 807–822

http://dx.doi.org/10.1016/j.fcl.2014.08.005

foot.theclinics.com

1083-7515/14/$ – see front matter © 2014 Elsevier Inc. All rights reserved.

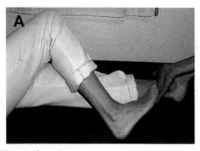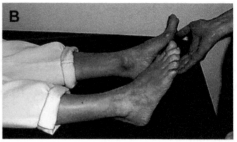

Fig. 1. (A, B) Equinus caused by gastrocnemius tightness: note the light plantar pressure applied.

cohort. The control group included 34 age-matched patients who had no foot and ankle symptoms. In the experimental group they observed an almost 3-fold higher prevalence of isolated gastrocnemius contracture. In this patient group, 13 (38%) had hallux valgus deformity and 7 (19%) had metatarsalgia.

Barouk and Barouk[23] presented a series of 107 patients with gastrocnemius tightness in 182 lower limbs. Of these 182 cases, they observed 128 instances of hallux valgus (77%). Most of the hallux valgus deformities were of the juvenile type (71% juvenile, 29% acquired).

These two studies show that hallux valgus, in particular juvenile hallux valgus, is the most frequent consequence of the gastrocnemius tightness on the foot. We chose to further study the effect of gastrocnemius tightness on juvenile hallux valgus.

There is an anatomic connection between the gastrocnemius and the hallux; namely the plantar aponeurosis and the plantar plate. This article presents the strong association of gastrocnemius tightness with hallux valgus in relation to these anatomic structures.

ANATOMY

The concept that the triceps sural and the Achilles tendon continue distally as the plantar aponeurosis is not widely appreciated by clinicians, but has nevertheless been established by many investigators. Of particular note are the works of Sarrafian[24] and Snow and colleagues.[11] There is an obvious functional biomechanical link, with the posterior calcaneus affording attachment to both the Achilles tendon and the plantar fascia, as shown by Arandes and Viladot[25] in 1954 (**Fig. 2**).

The Plantar Aponeurosis

The plantar aponeurosis or fascia has 3 components.[24,26,27] The lateral component is reserved to the fifth ray. The central component begins proximally from a common origin, on the calcaneum, and then divides into 4 bands reaching each of the 4 medial rays, including the first ray, which is the focus of this article. The medial band is notably separate and diverges from the 3 central bands, making the sheath of the abductor muscle. It does not insert on the calcaneum, so does not belong to the Achilles tendon complex (**Fig. 3**A, B).

Golano[27] and Bonnel[26] showed that each band divides distally in 3 slips, 1 superficial and 2 deep septae orientated sagittally. These slips are located around the flexor tendons (**Fig. 4**A, B).

Distal insertion

All the sagittal septae insert distally onto the corresponding plantar plate. In the first ray, the plantar plate incorporates the sesamoid bones. In addition, the plantar plate inserts onto the base of the proximal phalanx.

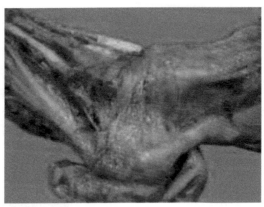

Fig. 2. The Achilles system is anatomically in continuity distally with the plantar aponeu-rosis. (*Courtesy of* J. Pascual Huerta, MD, Universidad Europea de Madrid, Madrid, Spain.)

In conclusion, the anatomic links between the hallux and the gastrocnemius are, from proximal to distal, the junction with the soleus muscle, the Achilles tendon, the calcaneus, the plantar aponeurosis, and the plantar plate (inlaid by the sesamoids) inserting into the plantar aspect of the proximal phalanx.

PATHOGENESIS OF HALLUX VALGUS DEFORMITY IN RELATION TO GASTROCNEMIUS TIGHTNESS

The biomechanical link between the Achilles tendon complex and the hallux is the plantar aponeurosis.

It is well established that tightness of the gastrocnemius continues distally with plantar aponeurosis tightness.[11,25] Pascal Huerta[29] and Maceira and Orejana[30] pub-lished a complete literature review on this subject.

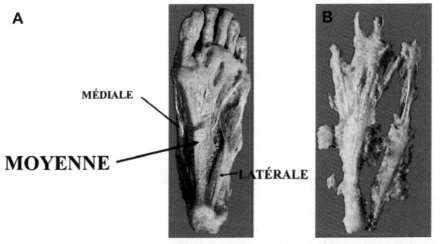

Fig. 3. (*A*, *B*) Plantar aponeurosis, superficial and proximal bands. The plantar aponeurosis includes a lateral component and a medial component, which is the fascia of the abductor muscle. The central band (moyenne), which is the most important, divides distally in 1 band for each ray; the band for the first ray is separated from the 3 central bands, and deviates medially. (*Courtesy of* F. Bonnel, MD, Toulouse, France.)

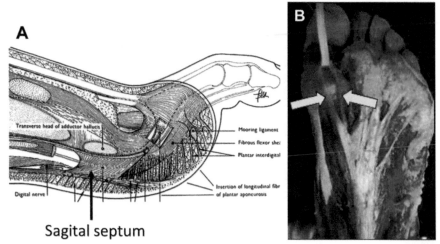

Sagital septum

Fig. 4. (*A*, *B*) Distal part of plantar aponeurosis: deep sagittal septum on the first ray. The distal sagittal septum of the plantar aponeurosis goes deeply along the long flexor tendon (*yellow arrows*) toward the plantar plate, inlaid with sesamoids, and then it attaches on the plantar aspect of the proximal phalanx. ([*A*] *From* Bojsen-Moller F, Flagstad KE. Plantar aponeurosis and internal architecture of the ball of the foot. J Anat 1976;121(Pt 3):599–611; and [*B*] *Courtesy of* F. Bonnel and F. Molinier, MD, Toulouse, France.)

Gastrocnemius tightness is evident at the beginning of the midstance phase of the gait cycle, when the knee and the hip joints are extended. This tightness was shown by Cazeau and Stiglitz,[31] who conducted a dynamic and electromyogram study showing that the maximum tightness of the gastrocnemius occurs in zone C, with a peak on the X point.

The relation to hallux valgus depends on the attachment of the plantar aponeurosis to the plantar plate and the sesamoids. The medial part of the central portion of the plantar aponeurosis has an oblique orientation, becoming more medial as it passes distally. Thus tightness of the plantar fascia contributes to increased valgus deforming force at the metatarsophalangeal (MTP) joint (MTPJ) (**Fig. 5**A–C).

Diebold[32] observed during bunion surgery that the abductor tendon is displaced plantarly and laterally. This displacement results in increasing the imbalance forces, thus increasing the valgus of the toe.

When there is already hallux valgus, all the muscles and tendons crossing the MTPJ contribute to increase the valgus of the toe. This condition is seen in the long flexor tendon, which acts like a bow string, and also in the medial band of the central component of plantar aponeurosis and all the intrinsic muscles, including the abductor hallucis, which moves plantarly and laterally (**Fig. 6**A, B).

Role of Reduced Dorsiflexion of the Metatarsophalangeal Joint

In hallux limitus

Kirby and Roukis[33] studied the effect of plantar aponeurosis tightness on the first MTP dorsiflexion and noted stiffness of the joint. Several investigators, particularly Kowalski and colleagues[34] and Maceira and Orejana,[30] observed decreasing dorsiflexion of the MTPJ, at least when weight bearing. The distal plantar aponeurosis is inserted on the plantar aspect of base of the proximal phalanx. This loss of flexion disappears when the plantar aponeurosis is relaxed; for example, when the ankle is in plantar flexion, as shown with the windlass mechanism (**Fig. 7**A).

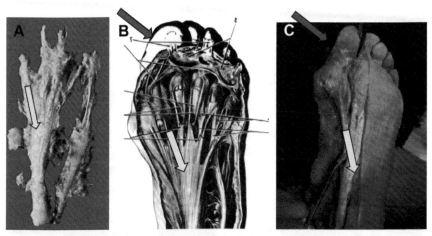

Fig. 5. The medial part of the central band of plantar aponeurosis, including the deep distal septum, when it is tightened by the gastrocnemius, contributes to increasing valgus of the hallux (*yellow arrows*, then *red arrows*). ([*A, C*] *Courtesy of* F. Bonnel, MD, Toulouse, France; and [*B*] *From* Henkel A. Die aponeurosis plantaris. Arch Anat Anat Ab Arch Anat Physiol. 1913;113.)

There is a relationship between the plantar aponeurosis and an equinus posture, such that an equinus position of the foot is involved in the windlass mechanism. The author observed that dorsiflexion of the first metatarso phalangeal joint (1st MTPJ) can be restored when the knee is flexed and the gastrocnemius is relaxed (Barouk test) (see **Fig. 7**B). The only muscle in which tension changes when the knee is flexed is the gastrocnemius. Thus it seems that tightness of the gastrocnemius increases the windlass mechanism through tension of the plantar aponeurosis.

Dorsal flexion of the interphalangeal joint
The distal phalanx is not involved in the insertion of the plantar plate, so a dorsiflexion of the interphalangeal joint (IPJ) may be seen. Kowalski and colleagues[34] Maceira[30] described the spoonlike appearance of the great toe, caused by the associated dorsal flexion of the IPJ. It is caused by the elevation of the first metatarsal, the plantar flexion of the MP1 and dorsiflexion of the IPJ, and is the result of chronic overload of the IPJ and gradual stretching out of the plantar IP ligaments and the flexor hallucis longus (FHL) attachment (**Fig. 8**A, B).

In juvenile hallux valgus
This reduced dorsiflexion of the MTPJ has also been observed by other investigators, including Kowalski and colleagues,[34] Barouk and Colleagues[18] and Diebold.[32] The loss of movement is compensated for in many cases by dorsiflexion of the IPJ. Nevertheless, it was also noted that the extra pressure at the IPJ, producing a characteristic callosity, is not plantar but is located on the medioplantar aspect because the deformity is not only in a sagittal plane but is combined with valgus deviation and axial rotation. This deformity is the familiar pronation of the toe (**Fig. 9**A–C).

A significant difference is observed in MTPJ dorsiflexion when the forefoot is compressed laterally, by the examiner, to manually correct the intermetatarsal (IM) angle (see **Fig. 9**). This diminished dorsiflexion is also caused by tightening of the plantar aponeurosis, but also by an abnormal distal metatarsal articular angle (DMAA) when a congruent joint is present.

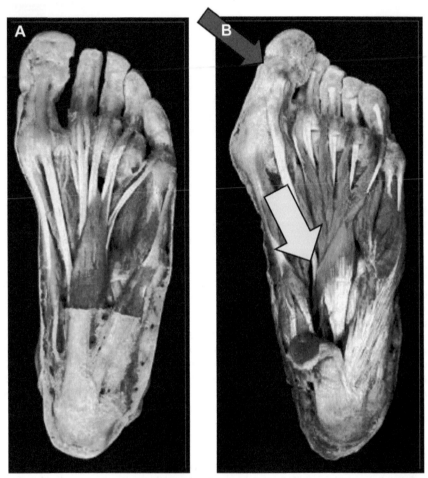

Fig. 6. (*A*) Case without no already hallux valgus: almost any tension of the muscles and tendons cannot result in a valgus of the toe. (*B*) Case with a previous hallux: all the muscles and tendons crossing the first MTPJ (*yellow arrow*) increase the valgus of the toe (*red arrow*). Not only the flexor longus, working like a bow string, but also the medial band of the central component of plantar aponeurosis and all the intrinsic muscles.

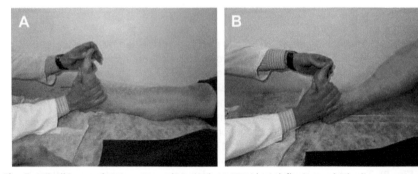

Fig. 7. Windlass mechanism. Barouk test: the MTPJ dorsal flexion, which disappears when the plantar aponeurosis is tightened (*A*), is restored when the gastrocnemius is relaxed (*B*, knee flexed). (*Courtesy of* E. Maceira, MD, Madrid, Spain.)

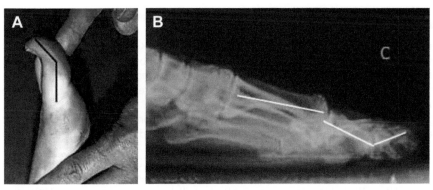

Fig. 8. (*A*) Hyperextension of the IPJ associated with hallux rigidus. (*B*) Corresponding radiograph, standing lateral view. (*Courtesy of* E. Maceira, MD, Madrid, Spain.)

Summary
The loss of MTP dorsiflexion caused by equinus from gastrocnemius tightness is a major contributory factor in the cause of valgus of the toe, because the foot, and particularly the great toe, is forced into valgus as weight passes to the forefoot so early in the stance phase of gait.

The 2 components of the forces acting on the hallux (plantarly and in a valgus direction) combine to exacerbate or create hallux valgus deformity. These forces depend on the intrinsic muscles but also on gastrocnemius tightness, through the plantar aponeurosis. This effect is called the lateral oblique windlass, emphasizing how the windlass effect can include a valgus component acting on the 1st MTPJ.

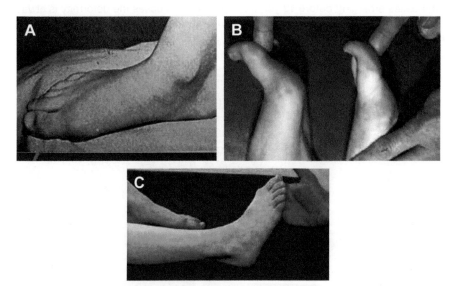

Fig. 9. Typical juvenile hallux valgus, with decreased dorsiflexion of the 1st MTPJ. (*A*) Callus on the medioplantar part of the IPJ (*red arrow*). (*B*) Loss of MTP dorsal flexion observed when the examiner attempts to reduce the intermetatarsal (IM) angle. This condition may be caused by tightening of the plantar aponeurosis. (*C*) Equinus caused by gastrocnemius tightness.

Problems Associated with the Planovalgus Foot

Gastrocnemius tightness is present in most of cases planovalgus foot deformity, and this has been noted by many investigators, particularly Kowalski,[34] De los Santos,[35] and Rabat.[9] The overall foot shape then serves to exacerbate the valgus forces acting on the great toe. Several investigators have observed that pes planus is associated with juvenile hallux valgus. Scranton and Zuckerman[36] reported a 41% incidence of this association, and Trott[37] reported a 25% incidence.

Therefore, because of its well-documented association with pes planovalgus foot posture, gastrocnemius tightness should be considered to be a cause of juvenile hallux valgus.

In contrast, in cavus foot, and especially varus foot, the tightness of the plantar aponeurosis, resulting for instance in a triceps contracture, does not result in hallux valgus: it is particularly obvious in cerebral palsy with hemiplegia, as noted by Holstein.[28]

Spastic Paraplegia in Children

Barouk[38] observed a high rate of hallux valgus in paraplegic children. The dual problems of forefoot overload and valgus foot posture combine to produce hallux valgus (**Fig. 10**). This situation is observed in early static juvenile hallux valgus, in which the same dual constraints are present, albeit to a much lesser extent. Furthermore, Barouk[38] observed that in children with spasticity there is demonstrable isolated gastrocnemius tightness before full triceps contracture develops.

RELATIONSHIP BETWEEN GASTROCNEMIUS TIGHTNESS AND JUVENILE HALLUX VALGUS

It is difficult to determine the age at which gastrocnemius tightness is first evident. By contrast, the emergence of hallux valgus is well studied.[36–42] It can be very early, in some cases emerging before 12 years of age. In these cases the deformity is always pronounced,[18] with a round metatarsal head, an increased DMAA, loss of plantar sesamoid crest, and a long first metatarsal.

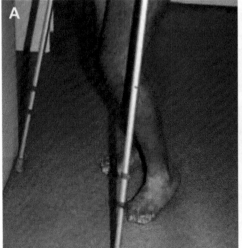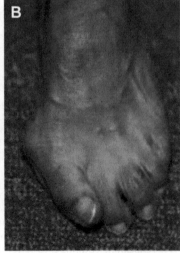

Fig. 10. (A, B) Constraints on the forefoot in a diplegic child. Note the triad of hallux, pes planovalgus, and triceps contracture.

Development of gastrocnemius tightness seems to occur at the same age, but there are no published statistical studies on this topic. Nevertheless, clinical assessment of patients less than 12 years of age with hallux valgus frequently reveals associated gastrocnemius contracture (**Fig. 11**).

We studied the prevalence of hallux valgus in a series of 182 cases with gastrocnemius tightness. Of the 182 cases, we observed 128 with hallux valgus (77%), with 71% of these having a juvenile pattern and 29% an acquired deformity. As has already been noted by DiGiovanni and colleagues[22] and Drakos and DiGiovanni,[21] the most frequent clinical problem associated with gastrocnemius tightness is therefore hallux valgus. This condition is more common than the other associated disorders, namely metatarsalgia, plantar fasciitis, and Achilles tendinopathy.

A weakness of this study is that the prevalence of gastrocnemius tightness in the population of juvenile hallux valgus is not known. However, a study is in progress, and early results show that there is often gastrocnemius tightness in children younger than 12 years presenting with hallux valgus.

Discussion

Gastrocnemius shortness is not the only cause of hallux valgus. In considering the cause, clinicians should try to distinguish between factors that increase the deformity and those that may be its cause.

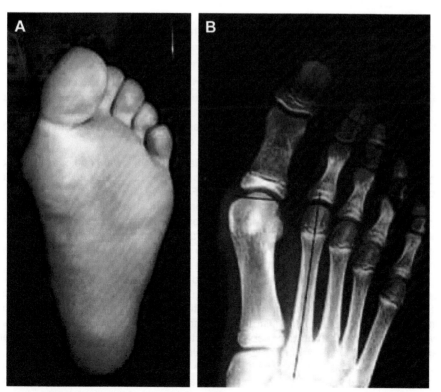

Fig. 11. Associated equinus and juvenile hallux valgus. (*A*) Six-year-old child (same foot) with triangular foot caused by equinus. (*B*) Typical radiograph of juvenile hallux valgus with a normal IM angle, increased DMAA, and a long first metatarsal.

Elements Increasing the Deformity

The long flexor tendon is commonly understood to work as a bowstring. However, all the intrinsic plantar and lateral muscles that insert on the plantar aspect of the proximal phalanx serve to pull the hallux in a plantar and lateral direction, and so contribute to the deforming force.

The next factor, which is not widely appreciated, is tightness of the plantar aponeurosis, which is produced by equinus deformity. This factor applies whether the equinus tendency is caused by isolated gastrocnemius contracture or by global shortening of the calf.

However, there are many cases of plantar aponeurosis tightness that do not result in hallux valgus. It is therefore appropriate to conclude that such tightness increases the risk of hallux valgus when there are other predisposing local factors.

Specific Structural Abnormalities

In acquired hallux valgus, shoes may be considered as a cause. Hallux valgus was extremely rare in Japan until the beginning of the last century, but since Japanese women began to wear high-heeled and pointed shoes, hallux valgus problems have increased significantly. In India, where traditional shoes (thongs) are still used, there are fewer cases of hallux valgus.

Juvenile hallux valgus deformity is present in a high proportion of patients presenting in adulthood. Hardy and Clapham[39] found this in 40%, Piggott in 57%,[42] and Barouk and colleagues[18] in 26%.

There are specific structural abnormalities that can explain the juvenile deformity even without the influence of footwear:

1. Rounded metatarsal head in 50% of cases.[18]
2. On the plantar aspect of the metatarsal head, loss of the sesamoid crest in 70%.[18]
3. Increased DMAA, as noted by Mann and Coughlin,[41] Barouk and colleagues,[18] and Ki Won Young and colleagues.[40]
4. Long first metatarsal. Barouk and colleagues[18] found excess of length in 36% of juvenile cases versus only 20% in acquired deformities.

The high hallux valgus angle (HVA), in association with a low IM angle, as reported by many investigators[18,36,41,42] is not a cause of juvenile hallux valgus, but is specific to this pattern of deformity in its early stages (**Fig. 12**A–D).

Hallux valgus interphalangeus is not more prominent in juvenile cases than in acquired deformity, but Barouk and Maestro[18] observed a dynamic valgus of the distal phalanx when the IPJ is flexed. This dynamic valgus is caused by increased obliquity of the IPJ. In most cases this is combined with pronation of the toe, which increases the overall hallux valgus deformity.

These structural abnormalities are observed in almost all cases of hallux valgus occurring before 12 years of age. Hallux valgus emerging after 15 years of age is less likely to show these structural abnormalities.[18] Hallux valgus in these patients may instead be caused by equinus, particularly isolated gastrocnemius tightness, which is transmitted through the oblique direction of the medial parts of the plantar aponeurosis and weakness of the abductor hallucis.

Even if the structural abnormalities alone explain the juvenile hallux valgus, gastrocnemius tightness still serves to increase the effects of the structural abnormalities. Gastrocnemius equinus leads to tightness of the plantar aponeurosis and together these lead to exacerbation of deforming forces acting on the 1st MTPJ.

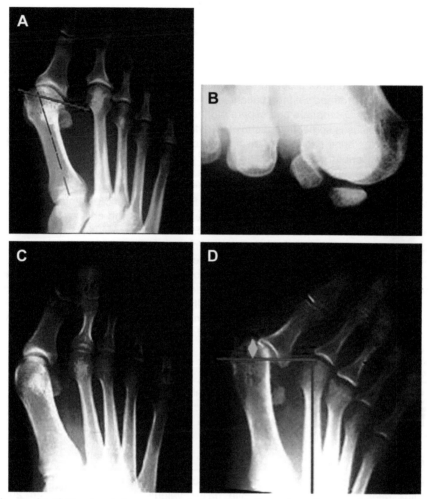

Fig. 12. (*A–D*) Structural abnormalities in juvenile hallux valgus: increased DMAA, loss of sesamoid crest, rounded metatarsal head, long first metatarsal (longer than the second, *green arrow*).

Clinical Consequences

In cases of juvenile hallux valgus there is a need for more research into the influence of gastrocnemius tightness. The next question is whether it is necessary to correct the gastrocnemius tightness and, if nonoperative measures fail, with which operative procedure?

CORRECTION OF HALLUX VALGUS AND GASTROCNEMIUS TIGHTNESS
Gastrocnemius Tightness

Options for correcting gastrocnemius tightness are both nonoperative and operative:
    Stretching the gastrocnemius can have good effect, but there tends to be loss of benefit after stopping these exercises. For many patients the demands in terms of long-term compliance are too great.[43]

Surgical lengthening is becoming increasingly popular as its rationale becomes more widely appreciated, and because of its simplicity and efficacy.

There are 2 main levels for lengthening: distal (midcalf) or proximal.

Distal lengthening was first described in 1950 by Strayer[44,45] in spastic patients then in static tightness. Advantages in the context of forefoot surgery include the ability to perform calf and forefoot procedures simultaneously, because the Strayer technique can easily be performed with the patient supine. Disadvantages are that bilateral procedures are not appropriate and separating the gastrocnemius aponeurosis from the underlying soleus is sometimes technically difficult. Weakness of the triceps, as well as injury to the sural nerve, may also complicate this operation. Endoscopic distal release, as described by Saxena[46] and Rabat,[9] offers solutions to some of these drawbacks and is our preferred distal technique.

The proximal release was first described in spastic patients by Silfverskiold[2] in 1923, and then by Barouk[19] and Barouk and Barouk[47] in static patients. At first the technique released both medial and lateral heads. Barouk and colleagues,[3] Abbassian and colleagues,[1] and De los Santos-Real and Morales-Munoz[35] perform this recession only on the medial head. This technique has been shown to give equally good results compared with a series of patients who had both heads released.[48] Release of the medial head is now preferred because the surgery is easier, quicker, and has minimal complications and no loss of force. The prone or lazy-lateral position is required, and this complicates foot surgery if considered at the same time. However, bilateral surgery (required most of the time) is possible and no postoperative immobilization is required. Our preference is for the proximal-medial gastrocnemius release.

Bunionectomy

In order to address all the structural abnormalities of the juvenile hallux valgus, it is preferable to perform a versatile first metatarsal distal osteotomy. Although either a distal chevron or a scarf osteotomy could be used, we prefer the scarf because of its greater versatility and thus adaptation to wider indications.

Our Series

We studied 182 cases (108 patients) of bunion correction combined with gastrocnemius release (proximal) in juvenile hallux valgus, performed between 2000 and 2005.[23] Bilateral deformity was present in 91% of cases. Follow-up ranged from 1 to 6 years. We performed a proximal gastrocnemius release in all cases (including both the medial and the lateral heads during this time period). It was after this study that Barouk[48] published his comparative study on 30 cases, showing that there is no difference in results when release is by section of the medial head alone.

In 98% of cases we observed correction of the gastrocnemius tightness, and excellent to good results of bunion correction in 97% of cases. We think that this result was caused by the combination of the powerful scarf osteotomy and lengthening of the gastrocnemius.

The weakness of this study is that there was no control group, treated by corrective osteotomy without lengthening of the gastrocnemius. The reason was that it is difficult to leave a patient without gastrocnemius recession when gastrocnemius tightness is observed, because of the exacerbation of the hallux valgus that the gastrocnemius produces. This influences the results, producing undercorrection. We only have cases of bunionectomy without gastrocnemius recession in those patients in whom the gastrocnemius are not tight. We think that gastrocnemius recession is important

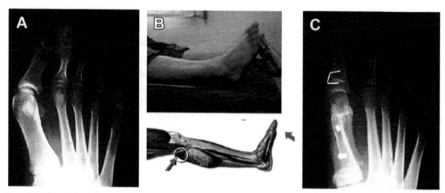

Fig. 13. (*A, B [top]*) Juvenile hallux with gastrocnemius tightness, the usual encountered case. (*B [bottom]*) Gastrocnemius proximal release (*red arrows*). (*C*) Correction with scarf osteotomy.

whenever gastrocnemius tightness is observed because, left untreated, it influences the results (undercorrection, recurrence).

Furthermore, other benefits are frequently seen, with resolution of the associated signs of gastrocnemius tightness (back ache, ankle instability, calf tension or cramps, hindfoot problems). One or more of these symptoms was reported by almost all of these juvenile patients and resolved following treatment.

This study also shows that, in cases with associated metatarsalgia without abnormality on the lesser rays (31%), there is correction of this metatarsalgia in 89% of patients without the need for any surgery on the lateral metatarsals. In this situation gastrocnemius lengthening helps to avoid surgery on the lesser rays, which is particularly important because of the additional morbidity of surgery to the metatarsals.

In a larger series, including both juvenile and acquired bunions (182 cases), in which there was metatarsalgia combined with hallux valgus but this time with notable abnormalities on the lesser rays (37% of cases), we performed gastrocnemius release, and scarf and lesser ray surgery. We observed complete resolution of metatarsalgia in 85% of cases.

We therefore think that the best indication for proximal gastrocnemius recession in bunionectomy is in cases of hallux valgus in which metatarsalgia is associated. The use of the gastrocnemius release allows clinicians to avoid, decrease (or ensure the success of) surgery on the lateral rays (**Fig. 13**A–C).

SUMMARY

Hallux valgus is the most frequent consequence of gastrocnemius tightness in the foot. This condition is particularly evident in juvenile hallux valgus. There are anatomic and biomechanical links between the gastrocnemius muscles and the hallux: Achilles tendon, calcaneum, plantar aponeurosis, plantar plate, and sesamoids. Thus gastrocnemius tightness exerts a deforming force on the hallux, which is well established for hallux limitus (windlass mechanism) but is not widely understood for hallux valgus. It is hoped that the present study addresses this.

Isolated gastrocnemius tightness, through tension in the plantar aponeurosis and the oblique direction of its medial part, results in valgus and plantar deforming forces at the 1st MTPJ. This is defined as the oblique windlass mechanism, and causes, or at least is an exacerbating factor in the pathogenesis of, hallux valgus.

Clinical consequences for clinicians are, first, that it is essential to evaluate the gastrocnemius tightness in any case of juvenile hallux valgus, then to consider correcting this tightness each time it is required. This evaluation not only serves to secure the results of the bunionectomy but also to avoid, diminish, or at least to ensure the success of surgery of the lesser rays in cases of metatarsalgia. In addition, it corrects other signs of gastrocnemius tightness: lumbago, cramps or calf tension, difficulty walking in bare feet or flat shoes, and eventually hindfoot problems (ie, Achilles tendinopathy, plantar fasciitis).

ACKNOWLEDGMENTS

Thanks to P. Barouk MD for his help, and to F. Bonnel and F. Molinier, MD, for their help in their laboratory of anatomy in Montpellier and Toulouse. Thanks to T.S. Roukis, DPM, PhD, FACFAS, for his advice and help with the literature references. A special thanks to M. Solan MD for his help, advices and for studying and spreading gastrocnemius hind foot consequences and the proximal medial release (GPMR).

REFERENCES

1. Abbassian A, Kohls-Gatzoulis J, Solan MC. Proximal medial gastrocnemius release in the treatment of recalcitrant plantar fasciitis. Foot Ankle Int 2012; 33(1):14–9.
2. Silfverskiold N. Reduction of the uncrossed two joints muscles of the leg to one joint muscles in spastic children. Acta Scandinavia 1923;56:315–30.
3. Barouk LS, Colombier P, De los Santos, et al. Brièveté des gastrocnemiens. Symposium AFCP. Maitrise orthopedique Gisep Paris. 2006. N°159:21–28.
4. Barouk P, Barouk S. Diagnostic Clinique de la brièveté des gastrocnemiens. Brièveté des gastrocnémiens. Montpellier (France): Sauramps; 2012. p. 205–13.
5. Carlson RE, Fleming LL, Hutton WC. The biomechanical relationship between the tendoachilles, plantar fascia and metatarso phalangeal dorsi flexion angle. Foot Ankle Int 2000;21(1):18–25.
6. Duthon VB, Lübbeke A, Duc SR, et al. Non insertional Achilles tendinopathy treated with gastrocnemius lengthening. Foot Ankle Int 2011;32(4):375–9.
7. Kiewiet NJ, Holthusen SM, Bohay DR, et al. Gastrocnemius recession for chronic noninsertional Achilles tendinopathy. Foot Ankle Int 2013;34(4):481–5.
8. Maffuli N, Walley G, Sayana MK, et al. Eccentric calf muscle training in Athletic patients with Achilles tendinopathy. Disabil Rehabil 2008;30(20–22):1677–84.
9. Rabat E. Allongement endoscopique du gastrocnemien. Brièveté des Gastrocnémiens. De l'anatomie au traitement. Montpellier (France): Sauramps; 2012. p. 351–73.
10. Gurdezi S, Kohls-Gatzoulis J, Solan MC. Results of proximal medial gastrocnemius release for Achilles tendinopathy. Foot Ankle Int 2013;34(10):1364–9.
11. Snow SW, Bohne WH, DiCarlo E, et al. Anatomy of the Achilles tendon and plantar fascia in relation to the calcaneus in various age groups. Foot Ankle Int 1995; 16(7):418–21.
12. Bolívar YA, Munuera PV, Padillo JP. Relationship between tightness of the posterior muscles of the lower limb and plantar fasciitis. Foot Ankle Int 2013;34(1): 42–8.
13. Erdemir A, Hamel AJ, Fauth AR, et al. Dynamic loading of the plantar aponeurosis in walking. J Bone Joint Surg Am 2004;86-A(3):546–52.
14. Garrett T, Neibert PJ. The effectiveness of a gastrocnemius/soleus stretching program as a therapeutic treatment of plantar fasciitis. J Sport Rehabil 2013;22(4): 22–36.

15. Lee WC, Wong WY, Kung E, et al. Effectiveness of adjustable dorsiflexion night splint in combination with accommodative foot orthosis on plantar fasciitis. J Rehabil Res Dev 2012;49(10):1557–64.
16. Monteagudo M, Maceira E, Garcia-Virto V, et al. Chronic plantar fasciitis: plantar fasciotomy versus gastrocnemius recession. Int Orthop 2013;37(9): 1845–50.
17. Solan MC, Carne A, Davies MS. Brièveté des Gastrocnemiens et Talalgies. Brièveté des gastrocnémiens. Montpellier (France): Sauramps; 2012. p. 241–63.
18. Barouk LS, Diebold P, Goldcher A, et al. Hallux valgus congenital. Symposium. Journées de printemps SFMCP. Med Chir Pied 7(2–3):65–112.
19. Barouk LS. Juvenile hallux valgus. Forefoot reconstruction. Paris: Springer; 2003. p. 175–80.
20. Rogers WA, Joplin RJ. Hallux Valgus, weak foot and the Keller operation. Surg Clin North Am 1947;27:1295–302.
21. Drakos MC, DiGiovanni CW. Importance de la brièveté isolée des gastrocnémiens dans la pathologie du pied. Brièveté des Gastrocnemiens: de l'anatomie au traitement. Montpellier (France): Sauramps; 2012. p. 231–40.
22. DiGiovanni CW, Kuo R, Teiwani M, et al. Isolated gastrocnemius tightness. J Bone Joint Surg Am 2002;84 A(6):962–70.
23. Barouk LS, Barouk P. Hallux valgus et Gastrocnemiens courts: étude de deux series cliniques. Brièveté des gastrocnémiens. Montpellier (France): Sauramps; 2012. p. 265–8.
24. Sarrafian SK. Anatomy of the foot and ankle. 2nd edition. Philadelphia: Lippincott Company; 1993.
25. Arandes R, Viladot A. Biomecanica del Calcaneo. Med Clin 1954;21(1):21–5.
26. Bonnel F. Le triceps sural. Micro anatomie fonctionnelle - Pennation des fascicules musculaire et aponévroses Brièveté des gastrocnémiens. Montpellier (France): Sauramps; 2012. p. 91–118.
27. Golano P, Dalmau AM, Vega J. Anatomie générale et chirurgicale du triceps sural. Brièveté des gastrocnémiens: de l'anatomie au traitement. Montpellier (France): Sauramps; 2012. p. 25–55.
28. Holstein A. Hallux valgus. An acquired pathology of the foot in cerebral palsy. Foot Ankle 1980;1(1):33–8.
29. Pascual Huerta J. Brièveté des gastrocnémiens et son effet sur l'aponévrose plantaire et le comportement sagittal. Brièveté des gastrocnémiens de l'anatomie au traitement. Montpellier (France): Sauramps; 2012. p. 119–40.
30. Maceira E, Orejana A. Hallux limitus fonctionnel et le système suro- Achilleoplantaire Brièveté des gastrocnémiens. De l'anatomie au traitement. Montpellier (France): Sauramps; 2012. p. 147–94.
31. Cazeau C, Stiglitz Y. Analyse des consequences biomecaniques de la brièveté des gastrocnémiens sur l'avant pied Brièveté des gastrocnémiens. Montpellier (France): Sauramps; 2012. p. 79–90.
32. Diebold P. Gastrocnemiens courts et hallux valgus congenital: Dysmorphie globale du membre inférieur. Brièveté des Gastrocnémiens: de l'anatomie au traitement. Montpellier (France): Sauramps; 2012. p. 281–4.
33. Kirby KA, Roukis TS. Precise naming aids dorsiflexion stiffness diagnosis. [Understanding the mechanics of the first ray: hypermobility versus decreased dorsiflexion stiffness]. Biomechanics 2005;12(7):55–63.
34. Kowalski C, Diebold P, Pennecot GF. Le tendon Calcaneen court. Paris: Encyclopedie medico Chirurgicale Elsevier; 1999. p. 27–60.

35. De los Santos-Real R, Morales-Munoz P, Payo J, et al. Gastrocnemius proximal release with minimal incision: a modified technique. Foot Ankle Int 2012;33(9):750–62.

36. Scranton P, Zuckerman J. Bunion surgery in adolescents: results of surgical treatment. J Pediatr Orthop 1984;4(1):39–43.

37. Trott A. Hallux valgus in adolescents. Instructional course lecture. Am Acad Orthop Surgeons 1972;21:262–8.

38. Barouk LS. Les brièvetés musculaires postérieures de l'infirme moteur cérébral. Rev Chir Orthop Reparatrice Appar Mot 1984;70(Suppl 2):163–6.

39. Hardy R, Clapham J. Observations on Hallux Valgus. J Bone Joint Surg Br 1951; 33:376–91.

40. Young KW, Kim JS, Cho JW, et al. Characteristics of male Adolescent Onset Hallux Valgus. Foot Ankle Int 2013;34(8):111–25.

41. Mann R, Coughlin MJ. Juvenile bunions. Surgery of foot and ankle. 6th edition. 1996. vol. 1. p. 297–339.

42. Piggott H. The natural history of hallux valgus in adolescence and early adult life. J Bone Joint Surg Br 1960;42:749–60.

43. Rodineau J. Strategie therapeutique medicale dans la retraction des triceps suraux. Brièveté des gastrocnemiens. Montpellier (France): Sauramps; 2012. p. 287–94.

44. Strayer LM. Recession of the gastrocnemius muscles to relieve spastic contracture of the calf muscles. J Bone Joint Surg Am 1950;32A(3):671–6.

45. Strayer LM. Gastrocnemius recession: five years experience. J Bone Joint Surg Am 1958;40A(5):1019–30.

46. Saxena A. Endoscopic gastrocnemius tenotomy. J Foot Ankle surg 2002;41(1): 45–58.

47. Barouk LS, Barouk P. Hallux valgus congenital. Reconstruction de l'Avant Pied. Paris: Springer; 2006. p. 158–67.

48. Barouk P. Comparaison de deux types de liberation proximale des gastrocnémiens medial et latéral, versus gastrocnémien medial isolé. Med Chir Pied 2006;22:156.

Index

Note: Page numbers of article titles are in **boldface** type.

Foot Ankle Clin N Am 19 (2014) 823–858
http://dx.doi.org/10.1016/S1083-7515(14)00124-7
1083-7515/14/$ – see front matter © 2014 Elsevier Inc. All rights reserved.

United States Postal Service

Statement of Ownership, Management, and Circulation
(All Periodicals Publications Except Requestor Publications)

1. Publication Title	2. Publication Number	3. Filing Date
Foot and Ankle Clinics of North America	0 1 6 - 3 6 8	9/14/14

4. Issue Frequency	5. Number of Issues Published Annually	6. Annual Subscription Price
Mar, Jun, Sep, Dec	4	$315.00

7. Complete Mailing Address of Known Office of Publication (Not printer) (Street, city, county, state, and ZIP+4®)

Elsevier Inc.
360 Park Avenue South
New York, NY 10010-1710

Contact Person: Stephen R. Bushing

Telephone (Include area code): 215-239-3688

8. Complete Mailing Address of Headquarters or General Business Office of Publisher (Not printer)

Elsevier Inc., 360 Park Avenue South, New York, NY 10010-1710

9. Full Names and Complete Mailing Addresses of Publisher, Editor, and Managing Editor (Do not leave blank)

Publisher (Name and complete mailing address)

Linda Belfus, Elsevier Inc., 1600 John F. Kennedy Blvd., Suite 1800, Philadelphia, PA 19103-2899

Editor (Name and complete mailing address)

Jennifer Flynn-Briggs, Elsevier Inc., 1600 John F. Kennedy Blvd., Suite 1800, Philadelphia, PA 19103-2899

Managing Editor (Name and complete mailing address)

Adrianne Brigido, Elsevier Inc., 1600 John F. Kennedy Blvd., Suite 1800, Philadelphia, PA 19103-2899

10. Owner (Do not leave blank. If the publication is owned by a corporation, give the name and address of the corporation immediately followed by the names and addresses of all stockholders owning or holding 1 percent or more of the total amount of stock. If not owned by a corporation, give the names and addresses of the individual owners. If owned by a partnership or other unincorporated firm, give its name and address as well as those of each individual owner. If the publication is published by a nonprofit organization, give its name and address.)

Full Name	Complete Mailing Address
Wholly owned subsidiary of	1600 John F. Kennedy Blvd, Ste. 1800
Reed/Elsevier, US holdings	Philadelphia, PA 19103-2899

11. Known Bondholders, Mortgagees, and Other Security Holders Owning or Holding 1 Percent or More of Total Amount of Bonds, Mortgages, or Other Securities. If none, check box ☐ None

Full Name	Complete Mailing Address
N/A	

12. Tax Status (For completion by nonprofit organizations authorized to mail at nonprofit rates) (Check one)
The purpose, function, and nonprofit status of this organization and the exempt status for federal income tax purposes:
☐ Has Not Changed During Preceding 12 Months
☐ Has Changed During Preceding 12 Months (Publisher must submit explanation of change with this statement)

PS Form 3526, August 2012 (Page 1 of 3 (Instructions Page 3)) PSN 7530-01-000-9931 PRIVACY NOTICE: See our Privacy policy in www.usps.com

---

13. Publication Title			
Foot and Ankle Clinics of North America			

14. Issue Date for Circulation Data Below
September 2014

15. Extent and Nature of Circulation		Average No. Copies Each Issue During Preceding 12 Months	No. Copies of Single Issue Published Nearest to Filing Date
a. Total Number of Copies (Net press run)		839	751
b. Paid Circulation (By Mail and Outside the Mail)	(1) Mailed Outside-County Paid Subscriptions Stated on PS Form 3541. (Include paid distribution above nominal rate, advertiser's proof copies, and exchange copies)	541	505
	(2) Mailed In-County Paid Subscriptions Stated on PS Form 3541 (Include paid distribution above nominal rate, advertiser's proof copies, and exchange copies)		
	(3) Paid Distribution Outside the Mails Including Sales Through Dealers and Carriers, Street Vendors, Counter Sales, and Other Paid Distribution Outside USPS®	121	115
	(4) Paid Distribution by Other Classes Mailed Through the USPS (e.g. First-Class Mail®)		
c. Total Paid Distribution (Sum of 15b (1), (2), (3), and (4))		662	620
d. Free or Nominal Rate Distribution (By Mail and Outside the Mail)	(1) Free or Nominal Rate Outside-County Copies Included on PS Form 3541	57	46
	(2) Free or Nominal Rate In-County Copies Included on PS Form 3541		
	(3) Free or Nominal Rate Copies Mailed at Other Classes Through the USPS (e.g. First-Class Mail)		
	(4) Free or Nominal Rate Distribution Outside the Mail (Carriers or other means)		
e. Total Free or Nominal Rate Distribution (Sum of 15d (1), (2), (3) and (4))		57	46
f. Total Distribution (Sum of 15c and 15e)		719	666
g. Copies not Distributed (See instructions to publishers #4 (page #3))		120	85
h. Total (Sum of 15f and g)		839	751
i. Percent Paid (15c divided by 15f times 100)		92.07%	94.82%

16 Total circulation includes electronic copies. Report circulation on PS Form 3526-X worksheet.

17. Publication of Statement of Ownership.
If the publication is a general publication, publication of this statement is required. Will be printed in the December 2014 issue of this publication.

18. Signature and Title of Editor, Publisher, Business Manager, or Owner

Stephen R. Bushing   Date: September 14, 2014

Stephen R. Bushing – Inventory Distribution Coordinator

I certify that all information furnished on this form is true and complete. I understand that anyone who furnishes false or misleading information on this form or who omits material or information requested on the form may be subject to criminal sanctions (including fines and imprisonment) and/or civil sanctions (including civil penalties).

PS Form 3526, August 2012 (Page 2 of 3)

Moving?

Make sure your subscription moves with you!

To notify us of your new address, find your **Clinics Account Number** (located on your mailing label above your name), and contact customer service at:

Email: **journalscustomerservice-usa@elsevier.com**

800-654-2452 (subscribers in the U.S. & Canada)
314-447-8871 (subscribers outside of the U.S. & Canada)

Fax number: **314-447-8029**

Elsevier Health Sciences Division
Subscription Customer Service
3251 Riverport Lane
Maryland Heights, MO 63043

*To ensure uninterrupted delivery of your subscription, please notify us at least 4 weeks in advance of move.

ELSEVIER

Printed and bound by CPI Group (UK) Ltd, Croydon, CR0 4YY

03/10/2024

01040492-0010